Complete Revision Notes for Medical and Surgical Finals

OF01032

Complete Revision Notes for Medical and Surgical Finals

Second edition

KINESH PATEL BA(Hons) MB BS MRCP
Specialty Registrar, Gastroenterology
St Mark's Hospital
London, UK

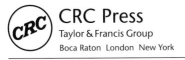

CRC Press
Taylor & Francis Group
Boca Raton London New York

CRC Press is an imprint of the
Taylor & Francis Group, an **informa** business

CRC Press
Taylor & Francis Group
6000 Broken Sound Parkway NW, Suite 300
Boca Raton, FL 33487-2742

© 2011 by Taylor & Francis Group, LLC
CRC Press is an imprint of Taylor & Francis Group, an Informa business

No claim to original U.S. Government works

Printed and bound in India by Replika Press Pvt. Ltd.

Visit the Taylor & Francis Web site at
http://www.taylorandfrancis.com

and the CRC Press Web site at
http://www.crcpress.com

Contents

Contributors

Sophie Atwood MA MBBS MRCPsych PGCME
ST3 Psychiatry Specialty Trainee, Sussex Partnership NHS Foundation Trust, UK

Jane Borley BSc MBBS MRCOG
Clinical Research Fellow, Imperial College London, UK

Simon RJ Bott MD FRCS(Urol)
Consultant Urologist, Frimley Park Hospital, Frimley, UK

Scott Cherry MBChB MRCPsych PGCME
Specialist Registrar, Sussex Partnership NHS Foundation Trust, UK

Sarita Depani MBBS BSc(Hons) MRCPCH
Specialist Registrar in Paediatrics, South Thames Rotation, London, UK

Ben Eddy FRCS(Urol)
Consultant Urologist, Kent and Canterbury Hospital, Canterbury, UK

Gareth G Jones BSc(Hons) MB BS MRCS (Eng)
Specialist Registrar in Trauma and Orthopaedics, Imperial College Healthcare NHS Trust, London, UK

Julian JH Leong MA(Oxon) MBBS MRCS(Eng) PhD DIC
Specialty Registrar, UCLH rotation, London, UK

Alexandra Kent MB ChB MRCP
Research Fellow, John Radcliffe Hospital, Oxford, UK

Kinesh Patel BA (Hons) MB BS MRCP
Specialty Registrar, Gastroenterology, St Mark's Hospital, London, UK

Natasha H Patel BSc(Hons) MB BS MRCP
Consultant in Diabetes and AMU, St George's Hospital, Tooting, London, UK

Nisha Patel BSc (Hons) MB BS MRCP
St Mary's Hospital NHS Trust, London, UK

Kirstin Satherley BSc(Hons) MB BS MRCP
Specialist Registrar in Clinical Oncology, The Royal Marsden Hospital, London, UK

Jagdeep Singh Gandhi BSc MB ChB MRCS FRCOphth
Consultant Ophthalmic Surgeon, Worcester Royal Eye Unit, Worcester, UK

Irfan Syed BSc(Hons) MBBS(Lon) MRCS DO-HNS
Specialist Registrar ENT Surgery, St George's Hospital, Tooting, London, UK

Preface

Finals tend to be a stressful time for medical students, as the requirement to relearn the large volumes of knowledge accumulated over 5 or 6 years is demanding, both physically and emotionally. Often the most difficult part is deciding exactly what level of detail is expected by examiners: the constant fear of not knowing enough inevitably leads students to try to learn too much from complicated texts, and consequently the key points that examiners actually seek are often forgotten.

This book is useful as it uniquely contains the entire undergraduate curriculum examined at finals, from medicine to surgery and ENT to oncology. The salient points needed to pass are featured in an easy to read (and remember!) bulleted format.

As most examinations are now multiple choice question-based, these bullets provide the essential nuggets of information that are often difficult and time-consuming to extract from a conventional textbook. Particular thought has been given to include facts that are repeatedly tested in finals, although explanations have been kept deliberately brief to act more as an aide-mémoire than to provide comprehensive descriptions of diseases.

The content is deliberately broad, but without the unnecessary extensive verbosity that can create real confusion and anxiety in the days running up to exams. The information contained within this book should be sufficient to pass written finals.

I wish you every success in your studies.

Kinesh Patel

Acknowledgements

I would like to thank the contributors to the first edition of the book for their hard work. These include Alexandra Kent and Natasha Patel (Medicine), Simon Phillips (Surgery), Julian Leong (Orthopaedics), Alex Charkin (Ear, Nose and Throat) and Ben Eddy (Urology).

Finally thanks must go to all the staff at Hodder Arnold for their help, support and encouragement to make this book and its companions a success.

The authors of Chapter 11 wish to acknowledge the ICD-10 of the World Health Organization and the NICE guidelines on mental health and behavioural conditions as providing source material for their chapter.

List of icons

A	Aetiology/incidence
Cx	Complications
Ix	Investigations
P	Pathology
Px	Prognosis
Si	Signs
Sy	Symptoms
S	Signs and symptoms
DD	Differential diagnosis
Rx	Treatment

Abbreviations

AAA	abdominal aortic aneurysm
AAFB	acid- and alcohol-fast bacilli
Ab	antibody
ABC	airway, breathing, circulation
ABG	arterial blood gases
ABPI	ankle brachial pressure index
ACA	anticentromere antibody
ACE	angiotensin-converting enzyme
ACS	acute coronary syndrome
ACTH	adrenocorticotrophic hormone
AD	Alzheimer's disease
ADH	antidiuretic hormone
ADHD	attention-deficit hyperactivity disorder
ADLs	activities of daily living
AE	acute endocarditis
AF	atrial fibrillation
AFB	acid-fast bacilli
AFP	α-fetoprotein
Ag	antigen
AGN	acute glomerulonephritis
AIDS	acquired immune deficiency syndrome
AIH	autoimmune hepatitis
AIHA	autoimmune haemolytic anaemia
AITP	autoimmune thrombocytopenic purpura
ALL	acute lymphoblastic leukaemia
ALP	alkaline phosphatase
ALS	amyotrophic lateral sclerosis
ALT	alanine transaminase
AMA	antimitochondrial antibody
AML	acute myelogenous leukaemia
ANA	antinuclear antibodies
ANCA	antineutrophil cytoplasmic antibodies
AP	anteroposterior
APH	antepartum haemorrhage

APKD	adult polycystic kidney disease
APTT	activated partial thromboplastin time
APUD	amine precursor uptake and decarboxylation
ARDS	acute respiratory distress syndrome
ARF	acute renal failure
5-ASA	5-aminosalicylic acid
ASD	atrial septal defect
ASIS	anterior superior iliac spine
ASO	antistreptolysin O
AST	aspartate transaminase
ATLS	advanced trauma life support
ATN	acute tubular necrosis
AV	atrioventricular (node)
AVB	atrioventricular block
AVSD	atrioventricular septal defect
AXR	abdominal X-ray
BaFT	barium follow-through
BAL	broncho-alveolar lavage
BCC	basal cell carcinoma
BCG	Bacille Calmette-Guérin
BE	base excess
BMI	body mass index
BP	blood pressure
BPH	benign prostatic hyperplasia
BSO	bilateral salpingo-oophectomy
BT	breath test
BZD	benzodiazepine
CBD	common bile duct
CBT	cognitive behavioural therapy
CCF	congestive cardiac failure
CCP	cyclic citrullinated peptide
CFA	cryptogenic fibrosing alveolitis
CFM	cerebral function monitor
CFTR	cystic fibrosis transmembrane regulating (gene)
CFU	colony-forming units
CIN	cervical intra-epithelial neoplasia
CJD	Creutzfeldt–Jakob disease
CK	creatine kinase
CMC	carpo-metacarpal
CML	chronic myeloid leukaemia
CMV	cytomegalovirus
CNS	central nervous system
COCP	combined oral contraceptive pill
COMT	catechol O-methyltransferase
COPD	chronic obstructive pulmonary disease
CPAP	continuous positive airway pressure
CPN	common peroneal nerve

CrCl	creatinine clearance
CRF	chronic renal failure
CRL	crown rump length
CRP	*C*-reactive protein
CRT	capillary refill time
CSF	cerebrospinal fluid
CT	computed tomography
CTG	cardiotocograph
CTPA	CT pulmonary angiography
CTR	cardiothoracic ratio
CVA	cerebrovascular accident
CVD	cardiovascular disease
CVP	central venous pressure
CVS	cardiovascular system
CXR	chest X-ray
DCIS	ductal carcinoma *in situ*
DDH	developmental dysplasia of the hip
DEXA	dual-energy X-ray absorptiometry
DI	diabetes insipidus
DIB	difficulty in breathing
DIC	disseminated intravascular coagulation
DIOS	distal intestinal obstruction syndrome
DIP	distal interphalangeal joint
DKA	diabetic ketoacidosis
DLB	Lewy body dementia
DM	diabetes mellitus
DMARD	disease-modifying antirheumatic drugs
DOT	directly observed therapy
DSH	deliberate self-harm
DVT	deep vein thrombosis
EAA	extrinsic allergic alveolitis
EBV	Epstein–Barr virus
ECF	extracellular fluid
ECG	electrocardiogram
ECT	electroconvulsive therapy
EEG	electroencephalogram
EMDR	eye movement desensitization and reprocessing
EMG	electromyogram
ENT	ear, nose and throat
EPS	extrapyramidal symptoms
ERCP	endoscopic retrograde cholangiopancreatography/evacuation of retained products of conception
ESR	erythrocyte sedimentation rate
ESRF	end-stage renal failure
ESWL	extracorporeal shockwave lithotripsy
EUA	examination under anaesthesia
FAP	familial adenomatous polyposis coli syndrome

FB	foreign body
FBC	full blood count
FDP	fibrin degradation products
FEV1	forced expiratory volume in 1 s
FFP	fresh-frozen plasma
FH	family history
FHH	familial hypocalciuric hypercalcaemia
FNA	fine needle aspiration
FSGS	focal segmental glomerulosclerosis
FSH	follicle-stimulating hormone
5-FU	5-fluorouracil
FVC	forced vital capacity
GA	general anaesthetic
GAD	generalized anxiety disorder
GBM	glomerular basement membrane
GBS	Group B *Streptococcus*
GCS	Glasgow Coma Score
G-CSF	granulocyte colony-stimulating factor
GFR	glomerular filtration rate
GGT	gamma glutamyl transferase
GH	growth hormone
GI	gastrointestinal
GM-CSF	granulocyte monocyte colony-stimulating factor
GN	glomerulonephritis
GnRH	gonadotrophin-releasing hormone
GOJ	gastro-oesophageal junction
GORD	gastro-oesophageal reflux disease
GP	general practitioner
G6PD	glucose-6-phosphate dehydrogenase
GTN	glyceryl trinitrate
HAART	highly active antiretroviral treatment
HAV	hepatitis A virus
Hb	haemoglobin
HbA1c	haemoglobin A1c
HBV	hepatitis B virus
HBcAb	hepatitis B core antibody
HBcAg	hepatitis B core antigen
HBeAb	hepatitis B e antibody
HBeAg	hepatitis B e antigen
HBsAb	hepatitis B surface antibody
HBsAg	hepatitis B surface antigen
HCC	hepatocellular carcinoma
hCG	human chorionic gonadotrophin
HCV	hepatitis C virus
HD	Huntingdon's disease
HDV	hepatitis D virus
HEV	hepatitis E virus

HF	heart failure
HHC	hereditary haemochromatosis
5-HIAA	5-hydroxyindoleacetic acid
HiB	*Haemophilus influenzae B*
HIV	human immunodeficiency virus
HLA	human leucocyte antigen
HMSN	hereditary motor and sensory neuropathy
HNPCC	hereditary non-polyposis colon cancer
HOCM	hypertrophic obstructive cardiomyopathy
HONK	hyperosmolar non-ketotic coma
HPA	hypothalamo-pituitary-adrenal (axis))
HPV	human papilloma virus
HR	heart rate
HRCT	high-resolution CT
HRT	hormone replacement therapy
HSP	Henoch–Schönlein purpura
HSV	herpes simplex virus
5-HT	5-hydroxytryptamine
HTLV-1	human T-cell lymphotropic virus type 1
HTN	hypertension
HUS	haemolytic uraemic syndrome
HVS	high vaginal swab
HZV	Herpes zoster virus
IBD	inflammatory bowel disease
IBS	irritable bowel syndrome
ICF	intracellular fluid
ICP	intracranial pressure
ICSI	intracytoplasmic sperm injection
IF	intrinsic factor
IFG	impaired fasting glycaemia
IGF	insulin-like growth factor
IgG	immunoglobulin G
IgM	immunoglobulin M
IGT	impaired glucose tolerance
IHD	ischaemic heart disease
i.m.	intramuscular
INR	international normalized ratio
IOL	induction of labour
IPF	idiopathic pulmonary fibrosis
ITP	idiopathic thrombocytopenic purpura
ITU	intensive therapy unit
IUD	intrauterine death/intrauterine device
IUGR	intrauterine growth restriction
IUGS	intrauterine gestation sac
IUS	intrauterine system
i.v.	intravenous
IVC	inferior vena cava

IVDU	intravenous drug use
IVF	*in-vitro* fertilization
IVU	intravenous urogram
JVP	jugular venous pressure
KUB	kidneys, ureter and bladder
LA	left atrium/local anaesthetic
LDH	lactate dehydrogenase
LDL	low-density lipoprotein
LFT	liver function test
LH	luteinizing hormone
LIF	left iliac fossa
LKM	liver, kidney, microsomal antibody
LLETZ	large loop excision of the transformation zone
LMWH	low molecular weight heparin
LOC	loss of consciousness
LOS	lower oesophageal sphincter
LP	lumbar puncture
LRTI	lower respiratory tract infection
LSE	left sternal edge
LUQ	left upper quadrant
LV	left ventricle/ventricular
MAC	*Mycobacterium avium* complex
MC&S	microscopy, culture and sensitivity
MCUG	micturating cystourethrogram
MCV	mean corpuscular volume
MDR-TB	multi-drug-resistant TB
MDT	multidisciplinary team
MEN	multiple endocrine neoplasia
MI	myocardial infarction
MIBG	metaiodobenzylguanidine
MLF	medial longitudinal fasciculus
MMR	measles, mumps and rubella
MMSE	mini-mental state examination
MR	mitral regurgitation
MRA	magnetic resonance angiography
MRCP	MR cholangiopancreatography
MRI	magnetic resonance imaging
MRSA	methicillin-resistant *Staphylococcus aureus*
MS	multiple sclerosis
MSU	mid-stream urine
MTP	metatarsophalangeal joint
NA	noradrenaline
NaSSA	noradrenaline-serotonin specific antidepressant
NASH	non-alcoholic steatohepatitis
NBM	nil by mouth
NCS	nerve conduction studies
NF1	neurofibromatosis type 1

NGT	nasogastric tube
NHL	non-Hodgkin's lymphoma
NICE	National Institute for Health and Clinical Excellence
NIPPV	non-invasive positive pressure ventilation
NNRTI	non-nucleoside reverse transcriptase inhibitors
NNT	number needed to treat
NPV	negative predictive value
NRTI	nucleoside reverse transcriptase inhibitor
NSAID	non-steroidal anti-inflammatory drug
NSTEMI	non-ST-elevation myocardial infarction
NTD	neural tube defect
OA	osteoarthritis
OCP	oral contraceptive pill
OGD	oesophagogastroduodenoscopy
OGT	oro-gastric tube
OGTT	oral glucose tolerance test
OI	opportunistic infection
ORIF	open reduction and internal fixation
ORT	oral rehydration therapy
OT	occupational therapy
PAPP-A	pregnancy-associated plasma protein-A
PBC	primary biliary cirrhosis
PCO2	partial pressure of carbon dioxide
PCOS	polycystic ovarian syndrome
PCP	Pneumocystis carinii pneumonia
PCR	polymerase chain reaction
PD	Parkinson's disease
PDA	patent ductus arteriosus
PE	pulmonary embolism
PEFR	peak expiratory flow rate
PET	positron emission tomography/pre-eclampsia toxaemia
PGE2	prostaglandin
PH	pulmonary hypertension
PICA	posterior inferior cerebellar artery
PID	pelvic inflammatory disease
PMS	premenstrual syndrome
PO2	partial pressure of oxygen
POC	products of conception
POP	plaster of Paris/progestogen only contraception
PPH	primary pulmonary hypertension/postpartum haemorrhage
PPHN	persistent pulmonary hypertension of the newborn
PPI	proton pump inhibitor
PPV	positive predictive value
PR	per rectum
prn	pro re nata
PRV	polycythaemia rubra vera
PSA	prostate-specific antigen

PSC	primary sclerosing cholangitis
PT	prothrombin time
PTCA	percutaneous transluminal coronary angioplasty
PTH	parathyroid hormone
PTHrP	PTH-related peptide
PUJ	pelvic–ureteric junction
PUVA	psoralen plus ultraviolet A
PV	per vaginam
RA	right atrium/rheumatoid arthritis
RAST	radioallergosorbent test
RBBB	right bundle branch block
RBC	red blood cell
RCC	renal cell carcinoma
RDS	respiratory distress syndrome
Rh	rhesus
RhF	rheumatoid factor
RIF	right iliac fossa
RPOC	retained products of conception
RR	respiration rate
RSV	respiratory syncytial virus
RT	radiotherapy
RUQ	right upper quadrant
RV	right ventricle
SAH	subarachnoid haemorrhage
SALT	speech and language therapy
SBE	subacute bacterial endocarditis
SCC	squamous cell carcinoma
SCID	severe combined immunodeficiency
SCLC	small cell lung carcinoma
SeHCAT	selenium-75-homocholic acid taurine
SFH	symphysis–fundal height
SGA	small for gestational age
SIADH	syndrome of inappropriate antidiuretic hormone
SLE	systemic lupus erythematosus
SMR	standardised mortality ratio
SOB	shortness of breath
SPECT	single photon emission computed tomography
SSRI	selective serotonin reuptake inhibitor
STD	sexually transmitted disease
STEMI	ST-elevation myocardial infarction
STI	sexually transmitted infection
SVC	superior vena cava
T3	tri-iodothyronine
T4	thyroxine
TAH	total abdominal hysterectomy
TB	tuberculosis
TCC	transitional cell carcinoma

TED	thromboembolic deterrent
TFT	thyroid function tests
TIA	transient ischaemic attack
TIBC	total iron binding capacity
TIPS	transjugular intrahepatic portosystemic shunt
TJ	transjugular
TNF-a	tissue necrosis factor-a
TNM	tumour, node, metastasis
TOP	termination of pregnancy
TPHA	Treponema pallidum haemagglutination assay
TPN	total parenteral nutrition
TSH	thyroid-stimulating hormone
TT	thrombin time
tTG	tissue transglutaminase
TURP	trans-urethral resection of the prostate
TVUSS	transvaginal ultrasound scan
UDCA	ursodeoxycholic acid
U&E	urea and electrolytes
URTI	upper respiratory tract infection
USS	ultrasound scan
UTI	urinary tract infection
UVB	ultraviolet B
VATS	video-assisted thoracic surgery
VDRL	venereal diseases research laboratory
VF	ventricular fibrillation
VIP	vasoactive intestinal peptide
V•/Q•	ventilation–perfusion
VRE	vancomycin-resistant enterococcus
VSD	ventricular septal defect
VT	ventricular tachycardia
VTE	venous thromboembolism
VUJ	vesico–ureteric junction
VZV	varicella zoster virus
vWF	von Willebrand factor
WBC	white blood cell
WCC	white cell count
WLE	wide local excision
WPW	Wolff–Parkinson–White syndrome

CHAPTER 1

Medicine

Nisha Patel, Alexandra Kent and Natasha Patel

CARDIOLOGY

CARDIAC INVESTIGATIONS

- **ECG (electrocardiography):** records cardiac electrical activity
- **Echocardiography (echo):** ultrasound imaging of the heart which provides an impression of cardiac chambers, valvular heart disease, the pericardium, great vessels and masses. *Transthoracic echo* is quick and easy to perform, but *trans-oesophageal echo* gives more detailed images, particularly of the posterior structures
- **Doppler echocardiography:** Doppler studies measure the velocity and direction of red blood flow, and are useful for assessing flow across valves, through the great vessels and through cardiac chambers
- **Stress echocardiography:** echo is done at baseline, then immediately after exercise or dobutamine infusion (which increases myocardial oxygen demand); systolic function and regional wall motion abnormalities are recorded to assess for myocardial ischaemia
- **Nuclear imaging:** thallium or technetium-labelled compounds can be used to assess ventricular function and myocardial ischaemia; at rest and during stress; **SPECT (single photon emission computed tomography)** and **PET (positron emission tomography)** are being increasingly used
- **MRI (magnetic resonance imaging)/CT (computed tomography):** used to define anatomy; useful in congenital heart disease, tumours, pericardial disease; **MRA (MR angiography)** can be used to assess the aorta, large vessels and myocardial perfusion, CT calcium
- **Cardiac catheterization:** involves passage of a catheter from a peripheral artery into the heart for pressure measurements or injection of a contrast agent; angiography can assess the left ventricle, coronary arteries and aorta; allows for balloon angioplasty or stent insertion

HEART FAILURE (HF)

(P) Occurs when the heart is unable to pump blood at a rate required by metabolizing tissues

(A) Ischaemic, valvular, hypertensive or congenital heart disease, cardiomyopathy, myocarditis, endocarditis, pulmonary embolism (PE)
Precipitating factors: myocardial infarction, infection, arrhythmia, anaemia, thyrotoxicosis, electrolyte disturbance, PE, pregnancy, vitamin deficiencies such as beriberi.

(S) Left-sided heart failure (HF): dyspnoea, orthopnoea, paroxysmal nocturnal dyspnoea, fatigue, lung crepitations, pleural effusions, cyanosis
Right-sided HF: peripheral oedema, abdominal distension/ascites, tender pulsatile hepatomegaly, ↑ jugular venous pressure (JVP), hepatojugular reflux
Severe HF: reduced pulse pressure, hypotension, cool peripheries, 3rd ± 4th heart sounds, gallop rhythm

(Ix) Full blood count (FBC), urea and electrolytes (U&E), liver function tests (LFT), lipid profile, thyroid function tests (TFT), glucose, cardiac enzymes, ECG, chest X-ray (CXR), echo with colour Doppler studies

(Rx) Treat any risk factor (cholesterol reduction, glycaemic control, weight loss, smoking cessation etc.); remove any precipitant
Diuretics, angiotensin-converting enzyme (ACE) inhibitors or angiotensin receptor blockers, β-blockers, digoxin, glyceryl trinitrate (GTN) infusion

ISCHAEMIC HEART DISEASE

(P) Ischaemia occurs whenever there is an imbalance between oxygen delivery and oxygen demand; the commonest lesion is the atherosclerotic plaque
Ischaemia can also occur when coronary blood flow is limited – rupture of the atherosclerotic plaque, coronary spasm, emboli, aortic stenosis with left ventricular (LV) hypertrophy
It can be precipitated by severe anaemia (due to ↓ oxygen-carrying capacity of the blood) and fluid overload

(A) Obesity, smoking, insulin resistance/Type 2 diabetes mellitus, high-fat diet, hypertension, high cholesterol/low-density lipoprotein (LDL)
Ischaemic heart disease (IHD) is the most common cause of death in the developed world

ACUTE CORONARY SYNDROME (ACS)

This encompasses **angina**, **unstable angina** and **non-ST-elevation myocardial infarction (NSTEMI)**

(S) Central crushing chest pain, ± radiation to neck and left arm, sweating, dyspnoea, pallor, palpitations

(Ix) FBC, U&E, glucose, lipids, cardiac enzymes (troponin, creatinine kinase), CXR, ECG (T wave inversion, ST depression), exercise testing, stress echo/nuclear imaging if patient unable to exercise, ± coronary angiography

(Rx) Acute presentation: oxygen, GTN spray, aspirin, clopidogrel, morphine sulphate, low molecular weight heparin (LMWH), ± GTN infusion, glycoprotein IIb/IIIa inhibitors (e.g. tirofiban)

Long term treatment: nitrates, β-blockers, calcium channel antagonists, aspirin, clopidogrel (for up to 1 year following non-ST elevation myocardial infarction [MI]), nicorandil; coronary revascularization

---

Box 1.1 GRADING OF ANGINA

I   angina on strenuous or prolonged exertion
II   slight limitation of ordinary activity; angina on moderate activity
III   marked limitation of ordinary activity; angina on mild activity
IV   unable to carry out activities without angina; may occur at rest

Source: Campeau L. Grading of angina pectoris [letter]. *Circulation* 1976;54:522–3 (reproduced with kind permission by the Canadian Cardiovascular Society)

ST-ELEVATION MYOCARDIAL INFARCTION (STEMI)

(P) Usually occurs due to atherosclerotic plaque rupture, leading to thrombosis formation, and coronary artery occlusion

(Sy) Similar to that of ACS, but more severe

(Ix) As for ACS; ECG will show ST segment elevation and Q waves evolve
Echo will indicate myocardial damage with abnormal wall motion

(Rx) Acute presentation: oxygen, GTN spray, aspirin, clopidogrel, primary percutaneous transluminal coronary angioplasty (PTCA), fibrinolysis (if PTCA not available)
Long term management: β-blockers, ACE inhibitors, aspirin, statins

(Cx) Heart failure, cardiogenic shock, arrhythmias, pericarditis, ventricular septal rupture, recurrent pain, LV aneurysm

HYPERTENSION

(P) Defined as blood pressure >140/90 mmHg

Box 1.2 CLASSIFICATION OF HYPERTENSION

- *Essential hypertension*: arterial hypertension with no specific cause; >90 per cent of cases
- *Secondary hypertension*: due to conditions including:
  - endocrine disorders
    Cushing's syndrome
    phaeochromocytoma
    acromegaly
    Conn's syndrome
    thyrotoxicosis
  - renal disease
    chronic renal failure
    renal artery stenosis
  - acute porphyria
  - coarctation of the aorta
  - iatrogenic
    ciclosporin
    contraceptives
    steroids

(A) Obesity, salt intake, alcohol, diabetes mellitus, genetic inheritance

(Sy) Headaches, dizziness, blurred vision, epistaxis, angina, syncope, signs of heart failure ± symptoms related to underlying causes

(Si) LV heave, 4th heart sound ± 3rd heart sound, hypertensive retinopathy, carotid/renal bruits

(Ix) FBC, U&E, fasting glucose and lipid profile, haemoglobin A1c (HbA1c), urine for sugar/protein/blood/creatinine clearance, ECG (LV hypertrophy ± strain), CXR
Other investigations would be to rule out secondary causes, e.g. calcium, TFT, cortisol, dexamethasone suppression test (Cushing's), 24-h urine for hydroxyindoleacetic acid (HIAA) (carcinoid)/catecholamines (phaeochromocytoma), aldosterone:renin ratio (Conn's syndrome), renal Doppler flow studies, renal MRA (renal artery stenosis)

(Rx) *Lifestyle*: weight loss, salt restriction, stop smoking, reduce alcohol intake, optimize glycaemic control
Medical: diuretics, ACE inhibitors, angiotensin receptor antagonists, calcium channel blockers, β-blockers

(Cx) Atherosclerosis, heart failure, cerebral infarct, cerebral haemorrhage, renal impairment

MALIGNANT HYPERTENSION

This is a **medical emergency**.

(P) Fibrinoid necrosis of small arteries/arterioles and dilatation of cerebral arteries

(A) ♂ > ♀; usually in 5th decade

(S) Headache, vomiting, visual disturbance, convulsions, papilloedema

(Rx) Intravenous labetalol/GTN, bring blood pressure (BP) down slowly

(Cx) Microangiopathic haemolytic anaemia, renal failure, cerebral haemorrhage, coma, death

ARRHYTHMIAS

ATRIAL FIBRILLATION (AF)

(P) Disorganized atrial activity, resulting in an irregular ventricular response

(A) See Box 1.3.

Box 1.3 CAUSES OF ATRIAL FIBRILLATION	
• Ischaemic heart disease	• Hypercapnia
• Lung disease	• Alcohol
• Hypoxia	• Mitral stenosis
• Hypertension	• Atrial septal defect
• Rheumatic heart disease	• Metabolic abnormalities
• Sepsis	• Thyrotoxicosis

(Sy) Palpitations, dizziness, shortness of breath (SOB) and heart failure

(Si) Irregularly irregular pulse, with or without haemodynamic compromise

(Ix) ECG, investigations into the underlying cause

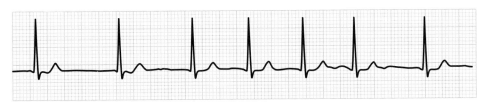

Figure 1.1 Atrial fibrillation: note the absence of P waves and irregularly irregular rhythm

Rx Treatment of underlying cause; rate control (digoxin, β-blockers, diltiazem), anti-arrhythmics (amiodarone, flecainide), anticoagulation (warfarin/heparin), DC cardioversion to return to sinus rhythm

Cx Systemic embolization, rapid ventricular rate leading to hypotension/angina/heart failure

ATRIAL FLUTTER

P Atrial re-entry tachycardia, leading to rapid atrial rate (~300 beats/min); usually occurs with slower ventricular rate due to 2:1 or 3:1 block in the atrioventricular (AV) node

A Acute cardiac or respiratory problems e.g. pericarditis, pneumonia

Sy Palpitations, dizziness and heart failure

Si Tachycardia, with or without haemodynamic compromise

Ix ECG: usually reveals characteristic saw-tooth pattern with AV block

Rx *Rate control*: anti-arrhythmics, anticoagulation
Curative: DC cardioversion, catheter ablation of aberrant pathway

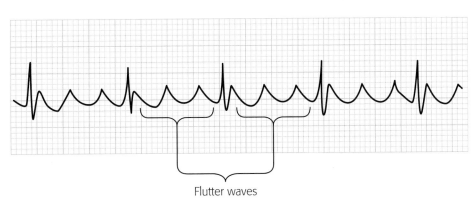

Flutter waves

Figure 1.2 Atrial flutter: note the characteristic 'F' waves

WOLFF–PARKINSON–WHITE SYNDROME (WPW)

P Atrial re-entry tachycardia, with an accessory excitatory pathway linking the atrium to the ventricle (bundle of Kent)

A Idiopathic

Sy Palpitations, dizziness and collapse

Si Tachycardia

Ix ECG: short PR interval, delta wave (slurred upstroke to QRS), wide QRS

Rx DC cardioversion, β-blockers, calcium-channel blockers, catheter ablation

Cx Rarely may progress to ventricular fibrillation (VF)

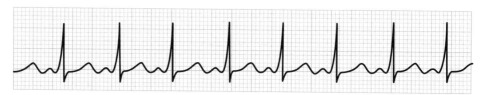

Figure 1.3 Wolff–Parkinson–White syndrome: note the short PR interval and slurred upstroke to the QRS complex

VENTRICULAR TACHYCARDIA (VT)

(P) Sustained VT is VT that lasts for >30 s or causes haemodynamic compromise

(A) Most commonly due to ischaemic heart disease ± MI; cardiomyopathy, metabolic abnormalities, drug toxicity, long QT syndrome

(Sy) Palpitations, chest pain, syncope

(Si) Tachycardia with hypotension, varying 1st heart sound, occasional cannon waves (giant 'a' waves in JVP)

(Ix) ECG (wide complex tachycardia)

(Rx) Anti-arrhythmics (amiodarone, lidocaine), DC cardioversion, implantable cardiac defibrillator to treat recurrence

(Cx) VF

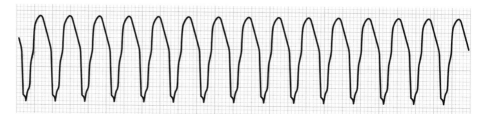

Figure 1.4 Ventricular tachycardia

VENTRICULAR FIBRILLATION

(A) Ischaemic heart disease, post-infarction, torsades de pointes, prolonged QT interval, severe hypoxia; VT can always degenerate into VF

(S) Syncope, cardiac arrest

(Ix) ECG/heart monitor

(Rx) DC cardioversion, anti-arrhythmics, intravenous magnesium, cardiac pacing, implanted cardiac defibrillator

(Cx) Death

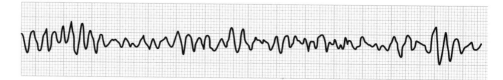

Figure 1.5 Ventricular fibrillation

ATRIOVENTRICULAR BLOCK (AVB)

P Due to damage to the atrial node, AV node or His/Purkinje system

A Myocardial infarction, drugs (digitalis, calcium channel blockers, β-blockers), myocarditis, acute rheumatic fever, sarcoid, infections (e.g. Lyme disease)

Box 1.4 CLASSIFICATION OF AV BLOCK

- *1st degree AVB*: PR interval >0.20 s (five small squares on ECG)
- *2nd degree AVB*: some atrial impulses fail to conduct to the ventricles
   – *Mobitz Type I* (Wenckebach): the PR interval gradually increases in length until there is a 'missed beat'
   – *Mobitz Type II*: occasional dropped QRS complexes are not related to changes in the PR interval
- *3rd degree AVB*: atrial and ventricular impulses are completely dissociated

---

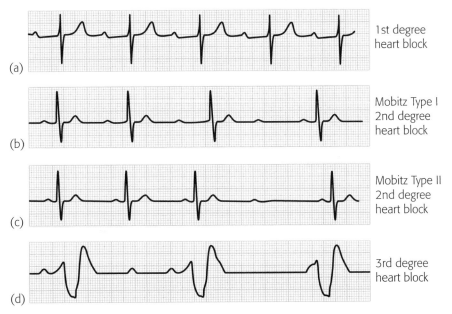

(a)   1st degree heart block

(b)   Mobitz Type I 2nd degree heart block

(c)   Mobitz Type II 2nd degree heart block

(d)   3rd degree heart block

Figure 1.6 (a) 1st degree heart block: prolonged PR interval; (b) Mobitz Type I 2nd degree heart block: progressive PR elongation; (c) Mobitz Type II 2nd degree heart block: fixed PR interval, with occasional P waves not being conducted to the ventricles; (d) 3rd degree AV block, there is no relationship between atrial and ventricular activity. The wide QRS complex is the result of a spontaneous escape rhythm of 35–40 beats/min

S Syncope, dyspnoea, heart failure

Ix ECG, cardiac monitoring

Rx Atropine, isoprenaline (β-agonist); any patients with symptomatic 2nd or 3rd degree heart block should have cardiac pacing

VALVULAR HEART DISEASE

AORTIC STENOSIS

(P) A pressure gradient between the LV and aorta >50mmHg or aortic orifice <1 cm^2 leads to LV outflow obstruction: response is LV dilatation, muscle hypertrophy and ↓ stroke volume; hypertrophy leads to ↑ oxygen demand

(A) Degenerative calcification, rheumatic fever, congenital bicuspid valve

(Sy) Exertional dyspnoea, angina, heart failure, syncope, sudden death

(Si) Narrow pulse pressure, slow rising pulse, heaving apex beat, displaced apex beat, systolic thrill, ejection systolic murmur (heard best over the aortic valve in expiration ± radiation to the carotids), soft S2, paradoxical splitting of S2, 4th heart sound

(Ix) ECG (LV hypertrophy and 'strain'), CXR (LV enlargement, pulmonary congestion), echo, cardiac catheterization

(Rx) *Medical*: treatment aimed at symptoms (diuretics, nitrates, β-blockers)
Surgery: aortic valve replacement

AORTIC REGURGITATION

(P) Regurgitation leads to an increase in LV end-diastolic pressure, which leads to LV dilatation and hypertrophy

(A) Rheumatic fever, endocarditis, hypertension, atherosclerosis, Marfan's syndrome, syphilis, seronegative arthritis, aortic dissection

(Sy) Dyspnoea, arrhythmias, orthopnoea, paroxysmal nocturnal dyspnoea, angina

(Si) Heaving displaced apex beat, diastolic thrill, 3rd heart sound

---

Box 1.5 SIGNS OF AORTIC REGURGITATION

- Wide pulse pressure
- Large volume collapsing 'waterhammer' pulse
- Early diastolic, high-pitched murmur (heard best at lower left sternal edge, patient sitting forward)
- Visible carotid pulsations: Corrigan's sign
- Capillary pulsations in the nail bed: Quincke's sign
- 'Pistol shots' over the femoral arteries: Traube's sign
- Head nodding in time with the pulse: de Musset's sign
- Mid-diastolic murmur heard at the apex: Austin Flint murmur

---

(Ix) ECG (LV hypertrophy and strain, left axis deviation), echo, CXR (LV enlargement), cardiac catheterization

(Rx) *Medical*: treatment aimed at symptoms (diuretics, ACE inhibitors, vasodilators); nifedipine/ACE inhibitors may delay the need for surgery
Surgery: aortic valve replacement

MITRAL STENOSIS

(P) When the mitral valve orifice is <2 cm^2, the left atrium (LA) requires abnormally high pressures to propel blood into the LV and maintain cardiac output; this leads to a high AV pressure gradient; backward transmission of the high LA pressure leads to pulmonary hypertension

A ♀ > ♂; rheumatic heart disease, congenital, endocarditis, systemic lupus erythematosus

Sy Dyspnoea, orthopnoea, paroxysmal nocturnal dyspnoea, palpitations, right-sided heart failure

Si Malar flush, atrial fibrillation, pulmonary oedema, ↑JVP with prominent a waves, tapping apex beat, left parasternal heave, loud 1st heart sound, opening snap, rumbling mid-diastolic murmur (accentuated with exertion, heard with patient on left side), stigmata of systemic embolization, may develop tricuspid regurgitation

Ix ECG (tall P waves in V1 and II; right axis deviation and RV hypertrophy in pulmonary hypertension; AF), echo, CXR (straightening of left border of heart, prominent pulmonary arteries), cardiac catheterization

Rx *Medical*: treatment aimed at symptoms (diuretics, digoxin, β-blockers), warfarin (history of AF or systemic emboli)
Surgery: mitral valvotomy (percutaneous balloon or surgical), mitral valve replacement

MITRAL REGURGITATION (MR)

P Increasing regurgitant jet leads to an increase in LV volume and reduction in cardiac output

A Rheumatic heart disease, ischaemic heart disease, post-infarction, hypertrophic cardiomyopathy, degenerative calcification, infective endocarditis, mitral valve prolapse, LV dilatation, connective tissue disorders

Sy Dyspnoea, fatigue, orthopnoea, right-sided heart failure

Si Jerky pulse, soft 1st heart sound, displaced apex beat, apical thrill, 3rd heart sound, pansystolic murmur, pulmonary oedema

Ix ECG (LA ± RA may be enlarged), CXR (LA may be massively enlarged; ± pulmonary oedema), echo, cardiac catheterization

Rx *Medical*: treatment aimed at symptoms (diuretics, ACE inhibitors, digoxin)
Surgery: mitral valve replacement

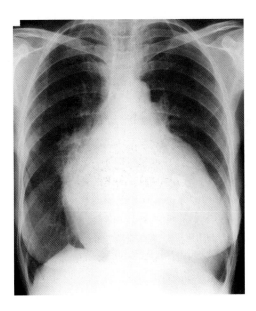

Figure 1.7 Mitral valve disease: enlarged heart with a double contour to the right cardiac border, indicating left atrial enlargement. Prominence of the left cardiac border is from the atrial appendage. Note the calcification in the mitral annulus

MITRAL VALVE PROLAPSE

(P) myxomatous degeneration

(A) ♀ > ♂; idiopathic, rheumatic heart disease, ischaemic heart disease, cardiomyopathy, connective tissue disorders, e.g. Marfan's syndrome, Ehlers–Danlos syndrome

(Sy) May be asymptomatic; palpitations, syncope, chest pain, sudden death (rare)

(Si) Arrhythmias, mid-late systolic click, high pitched late-systolic murmur

(Ix) ECG, echo

(Rx) *Medical*: aimed at symptoms: anti-arrhythmics, antibiotic prophylaxis, β-blockers for chest pain
Surgery: Mitral valve repair/replacement if MR is a problem

(Cx) MR, infective endocarditis

PULMONARY STENOSIS

(P) Outflow obstruction may be valvular, subvalvular or supravalvular; transvalvular gradient grades the severity: <50 mmHg: mild; 50–80 mmHg: moderate; >80 mmHg: severe

(A) Congenital, associated with carcinoid syndrome

(Sy) Asymptomatic; fatigue, dyspnoea, syncope, symptoms associated with heart failure

(Si) a wave in the JVP, soft P2, 4th heart sound, left parasternal heave, thrill and ejection systolic murmur (left upper sternal border), increasing severity leads to a longer murmur,

(Ix) ECG (right axis deviation and RV hypertrophy), CXR (large left atrium), echo

(Rx) Balloon valvuloplasty; valve replacement rarely indicated

TRICUSPID REGURGITATION

(P) Usually functional: due to dilatation of the tricuspid annulus following right ventricular dilatation

(A) Functional (pulmonary hypertension, CCF, cardiomyopathy), rheumatic, tricuspid valve endocarditis, carcinoid, trauma, post-infarction, endomyocardial fibrosis

(Sy) Clinical features are due to venous congestion and reduced cardiac output

(Si) ↑JVP with prominent v waves, pansystolic murmur heard best at left lower sternal edge, pulsatile hepatomegaly, peripheral oedema, ascites, dyspnoea

(Ix) ECG, CXR (enlarged RA and RV), echo

(Rx) Aimed at underlying cause or surgery

CONGENITAL HEART DISEASE

ATRIAL SEPTAL DEFECT

(P) *Ostium primum*: septal defect lies adjacent to AV valve
Ostium secundum: mid-septum; 70 per cent of cases
Sinus venosus: high in septum, near superior vena cava (SVC)

(A) Congenital; ♀ > ♂; Down syndrome associated with ostium primum

(Sy) Usually asymptomatic until adulthood; palpitations (arrhythmias), dyspnoea, cyanosis

Si   Left parasternal heave, wide fixed splitting of 2nd heart sound, mid-systolic murmur at left sternal edge (due to increased flow across the pulmonary valve), cyanosis, clubbing, occasional mid-diastolic murmur

Ix   ECG (ostium primum: left axis deviation, ostium secundum: right axis deviation, right bundle branch block (RBBB); RV or RA hypertrophy), CXR (large hilar arteries, enlarged RV and RA, increased pulmonary vasculature), echo

Rx   Small atrial septal defect (ASD) with minimum left-to-right shunts can be left; surgical closure

Cx   Arrhythmias

VENTRICULAR SEPTAL DEFECT

P   Usually in the membranous portion of the septum

A   Congenital, post-infarction; commonest congenital anomaly; incidence ~0.2 per cent births; associated with Fallot's tetralogy

Sy   Usually develop with reversal of the shunt; dyspnoea, chest pain, syncope, haemoptysis

Si   Cyanosis, clubbing, loud pansystolic murmur

Ix   Echo

Rx   Spontaneous closure occurs in ~50 per cent small ventricular septal defects (VSDs); surgical correction when there is a moderate/large left-to-right shunt

Cx   Congestive cardiac failure (CCF), pulmonary hypertension and reversal of shunt, RV outflow tract obstruction, aortic regurgitation, infective endocarditis

INFECTIVE/INFLAMMATORY CONDITIONS

PERICARDITIS

P   Inflammation of the pericardium

A   Viral, post-MI, uraemia, tuberculosis, rheumatic fever, connective tissue disorders, malignancy

Sy   Substernal sharp chest pain, worse on movement and inspiration; relieved by sitting forward and worse on lying flat

Si   Pericardial friction rub, fever

Ix   ECG (widespread ST elevation, concave in shape, followed by T wave inversion)

Rx   Non-steroidal anti-inflammatory drugs (NSAIDs) for pain; treatment of underlying condition

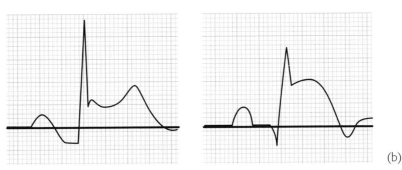

(a)   (b)

Figure 1.8 (a) Pericarditis. Note the concave ST elevation, compared with myocardial infarction (b)

MYOCARDITIS

(A) Infection, drugs, radiation; commonest cause is viruses – *Coxsackie*

(Sy) Variable; may be asymptomatic, chest pain, heart failure, palpitations, death

(Si) Often normal; occasionally 3rd heart sound, pansystolic murmur (MR)

(Ix) ECG (T wave or ST changes), viral screen (stool samples, throat swab, nasopharyngeal washings etc.), cardiac enzymes, echo

(Rx) Usually self-limiting; treatment aimed at symptoms/complications; patients rarely require intensive therapy unit (ITU)/cardiac transplantation

(Cx) Chronic myocarditis, dilated cardiomyopathy, heart failure

INFECTIVE ENDOCARDITIS

(P) Infection of the endothelium; usually involves the valves; vegetations are a mixture of bacteria, fibrin and platelets

(A) Intravenous drug use (IVDU), prosthetic valves, sporadic
Bacteria involved: ~10 per cent no causative organism, *Staphylococcus aureus* (IVDU), *Streptococci*, *Enterococci*, Gram-negative bacteria, *Candida*

(Sy) Separated into acute endocarditis (AE), a rapidly progressive illness, and subacute bacterial endocarditis (SBE), a slowly progressive condition
Fever, anorexia, weight loss, myalgia

(Si) See Box 1.6

Box 1.6 DIAGNOSIS OF ENDOCARDITIS

Duke Criteria: 2 major, 1 major + 3 minor, or 5 minor for diagnosis
- *Major*:
  - blood culture positive for typical organism or persistently positive
  - evidence of endocardial involvement
- *Minor*:
  - fever
  - previous heart condition or IVDU
  - immunological phenomena (due to immune complex deposition): Osler's nodes (raised tender nodules on finger pulps), Roth spots (small retinal haemorrhages), glomerulonephritis, clubbing, petechiae, arthralgia
  - vascular phenomena: mycotic aneurysms, Janeway lesions (painless macules on palm), septic emboli, intracranial haemorrhage, visceral infarct, splinter haemorrhages
  - positive blood culture with atypical bacteria

(Ix) FBC, C-reactive protein (CRP), erythrocyte sedimentation rate (ESR), blood cultures (minimum of 3), rheumatoid factor, immune complex titre, ECG, echo (trans-oesophageal echo is more sensitive)

(Rx) Broad-spectrum intravenous antibiotics until culture results available (check hospital policy, but usually i.v. benzylpenicillin + gentamicin); add flucloxacillin in IVDUs

(Cx) Septic emboli, mycotic aneurysms, meningitis, intracranial haemorrhage, emboli, glomerulonephritis

MISCELLANEOUS

HYPERTROPHIC OBSTRUCTIVE CARDIOMYOPATHY (HOCM)

(P) Left ventricular hypertrophy, especially involving the septum; varying degrees of myocardial fibrosis

(A) ~50 per cent patients have a +ve family history; multiple mutations have been identified; associated with Friedrich's ataxia

(Sy) Many are asymptomatic; dyspnoea, fatigue, palpitations, angina, syncope, sudden death

(Si) *a* wave in the JVP, double apical impulse, ejection systolic murmur at lower left sternal border, pansystolic murmur at the apex, 4th heart sound

(Ix) ECG (LV hypertrophy, Q waves, arrhythmias), CXR (increased cardiothoracic ratio [CTR]), echo (asymmetric septal hypertrophy, systolic anterior motion of the mitral valve, small LV cavity with posterior wall motion, MR)

(Rx) β-blockers/verapamil to improve LV function, amiodarone as anti-arrhythmic, surgery (myotomy/myectomy), ethanol injections into the septum (causes partial infarction of the septum), cardiac pacing; avoidance of any drugs that significantly lower the preload

(Cx) Arrhythmias, ischaemia, sudden death

ATRIAL MYXOMA

(P) Benign tumour; gelatinous polypoid structure attached to the atrial septum; usually left atrium

(A) ♀ > ♂; 3rd–6th decades; most are sporadic; occasionally familial (autosomal dominant)

(Sy) Fever, dyspnoea, weight loss, arthralgia, syncope; can mimic mitral valve disease (stenosis from the tumour prolapsing into the valve, or regurgitation from related valve trauma)

(Si) Loud 1st heart sound, tumour 'plop' (a loud 3rd heart sound), clubbing

(Ix) Echo, FBC (anaemia or polycythaemia), ↑ESR

(Rx) Surgical resection

(Cx) Peripheral or pulmonary emboli

RESPIRATORY

RESPIRATORY INVESTIGATIONS

- **Chest radiography (CXR):** be careful to look at the apices, behind the heart and costophrenic angles
- **Computed tomography (CT):** better at distinguishing between tissue densities and assessing lesions; high-resolution CT shows subtle parenchymal changes useful in the diagnosis of interstitial lung diseases; CT pulmonary angiography (CTPA) can diagnose pulmonary emboli in the segmental and larger pulmonary arteries
- **Ventilation–perfusion scans:** albumin labelled with technetium 99m is administered intravenously to demonstrate blood flow, and radiolabelled xenon gas is inhaled to demonstrate ventilation. This shows mismatches in ventilation and perfusion, and is commonly used to diagnose pulmonary embolism.
- **Positron emission tomography (PET):** used to identify malignant lesions and stage lung cancer. A radiolabelled glucose analogue is injected and is taken up by metabolically active malignant cells.
- **Arterial blood gases:** for interpretation see 'Respiratory failure' section (p. 15)
- **PEFR (peak expiratory flow rate):** useful in asthma
- **Spirometry:** measures inspired and expired gas volume against time:
  - FEV_1 – forced expiratory volume in 1 second
  - FVC – forced vital capacity (total volume exhaled)
    $$\frac{FEV_1}{FVC}:$$
    normal range 0.75–0.80
    <0.75 = obstructive defect
    >0.80 = restrictive defect
- **Sputum:** microscopy, culture, Gram stain, Ziehl-Neelsen stain, cytology and sensitivities.
- **Bronchoscopy:** allowing direct visualization of the bronchial tree. Samples can be taken by biopsy, brushings or broncho-alveolar lavage (BAL).
- **Video-assisted thoracic surgery (VATS):** a rigid endoscope is passed into the pleura to allow visualization and biopsy of pleural or parenchymal disease and pleurodesis.

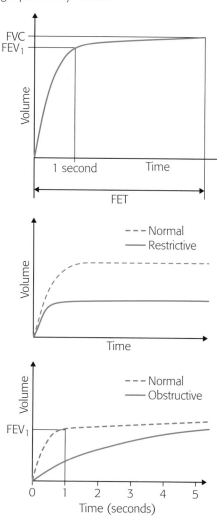

Figure 1.9 Interpretation of spirometry results (adapted with kind permission from Dakin J, Kourteli E and Winter R, *Making Sense of Lung Function Tests A Hands-on Guide*, London: Arnold, 2003)

RESPIRATORY FAILURE

P Respiration requires the integrated function of the nervous system, airways, alveoli, musculature and vasculature. Failure of any of these can lead to respiratory failure:
- Type I respiratory failure: hypoxia with normal partial pressure of carbon dioxide (P_{CO_2})
- Type II respiratory failure: hypoxia and hypercapnia

A See Fig. 1.10

Hypoxaemia has four causes:
- hypoventilation
- ventilation–perfusion ($\dot{V}/\dot{Q}$) mismatch
- shunting
- ↓ in inspired partial pressure of oxygen (P_{O_2})

Rx Management is aimed at the underlying cause:
- initial treatment is to administer high-flow oxygen
- patients may require assisted ventilation; this can be given as non-invasive positive pressure ventilation (NIPPV) – this can eliminate CO_2 (and hence acidosis)
- if this fails they will require mechanical ventilation

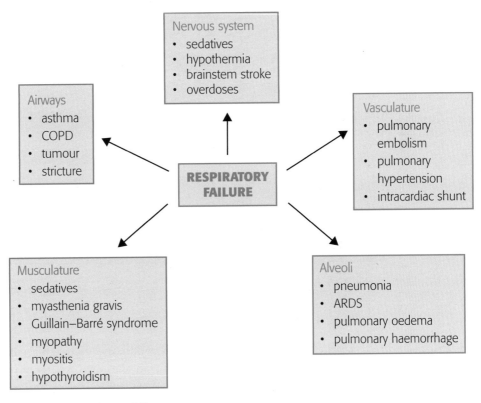

Figure 1.10 Respiratory failure
ARDS: acute respiratory distress syndrome; COPD: chronic obstructive pulmonary disease

AIRWAYS DISEASE

ASTHMA[1]

(P) Chronic reversible inflammation of the airways caused by increased sensitivity to various stimuli; leading to variable airway obstruction

(A) Atopy, family history (especially maternal), parental smoking increases the risk of childhood asthma

Triggers: dust, emotion, exercise, cold weather, NSAID/β-blockers, etc.

(Sy) None when well

Wheeze, cough, dyspnoea, chest tightness, night-time waking

(Si) None when well

Tachypnoea, tachycardia, cyanosis, wheeze

Diurnal variation

(Ix) FBC (includes eosinophil count), U&E, CRP, *PEFR* (peak expiratory flow rate) *and spirometry*: expected >25 per cent variability

CXR: if any atypical symptoms or exacerbations (to rule out pneumothorax/infection, etc.)

(Rx) Avoidance of pollutants/allergens/smoking; weight loss in obesity

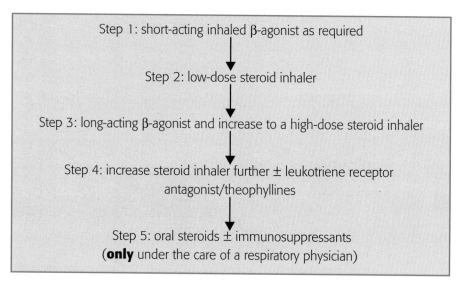

Step 1: short-acting inhaled β-agonist as required

Step 2: low-dose steroid inhaler

Step 3: long-acting β-agonist and increase to a high-dose steroid inhaler

Step 4: increase steroid inhaler further ± leukotriene receptor antagonist/theophyllines

Step 5: oral steroids ± immunosuppressants (**only** under the care of a respiratory physician)

Figure 1.11 Management of chronic asthma

NB:

1   beware the side-effects of long-term steroids: osteoporosis, diabetes mellitus, hypertension, oral candidiasis, easy bruising (see Cushing's syndrome, p. 66)

2   check inhaler technique – need for a spacer device?

Acute asthma

This is a **medical emergency**.

Box 1.7 CLASSIFICATION OF ACUTE ASTHMA

- **Moderate exacerbation**
  - PEFR 50–75% predicted/best
  - Worsening symptoms

- **Severe asthma**
  - PEFR 33–50% predicted/best
  - Unable to complete sentences in one breath
  - Exhaustion/poor respiratory effort
  - Tachycardia (HR >110 beats/min)
  - Tachypnoea (RR >25 breaths/min)

- **Life-threatening asthma**
  - Silent chest
  - Po_2 <8 kPa
  - Normal or rising Pco_2
  - Bradycardia
  - Hypotension
  - Confusion

HR: heart rate
RR: respiration rate

Ix Pulse oximetry, PEFR, arterial blood gases if saturations are <92 per cent
CXR **only** if signs of pneumothorax/consolidation/failure to respond/life-threatening asthma

Rx High-flow oxygen, nebulized beta agonist bronchodilators, nebulized ipratropium bromide, oral steroids
If no improvement: magnesium sulphate infusion ± aminophylline infusion
Call for help early
The patient should be closely monitored with pulse oximetry and PEFR

CHRONIC OBSTRUCTIVE PULMONARY DISEASE (COPD)/EMPHYSEMA

P Chronic inflammatory condition which causes progressive airflow obstruction secondary to parenchymal damage

A Smoking, α1-antitrypsin deficiency

S Breathlessness, cough, sputum production, wheeze
Signs of cor pulmonale (see p. 28)
Very little diurnal variation in symptoms, and less reversibility than asthma (<20 per cent)

Ix CXR, FBC, BMI (body mass index), ECG, theophylline level (if applicable)
Spirometry: FEV_1 <80 per cent predicted, $\frac{FEV_1}{FVC}$ <0.7 (obstructive picture)

Rx *Acute exacerbation*:
- oxygen – beware Type II respiratory failure!
- nebulizers (β_2-agonists/anticholinergics)
- steroids
- aminophylline infusions
- NIPPV

Chronic:
- smoking cessation
- vaccinations
- pulmonary rehabilitation
- surgery

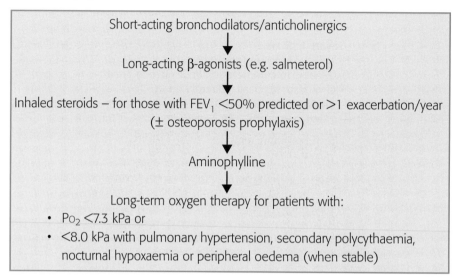

Short-acting bronchodilators/anticholinergics

↓

Long-acting β-agonists (e.g. salmeterol)

↓

Inhaled steroids – for those with FEV_1 <50% predicted or >1 exacerbation/year
(± osteoporosis prophylaxis)

↓

Aminophylline

↓

Long-term oxygen therapy for patients with:
- Po_2 <7.3 kPa or
- <8.0 kPa with pulmonary hypertension, secondary polycythaemia, nocturnal hypoxaemia or peripheral oedema (when stable)

Figure 1.12 Management of COPD/emphysema ('BTS Guidelines on the Management of COPD', *Thorax* 1997;52, Supplement V, adapted with kind permission from BMJ Publishing Group)

α_1-ANTITRYPSIN DEFICIENCY

P Lack of α1-antitrypsin, an enzyme made in the liver, that controls the breakdown of other enzymes in the body

A Autosomal recessive disease; affects all populations

S All symptoms related to emphysema and cirrhosis; onset of these conditions at a younger age, with no other causes

Ix As for emphysema and cirrhosis; serum α1-antitrypsin levels can be measured

Rx As for emphysema and cirrhosis; liver ± lung transplantation

INFECTIONS[2]

COMMUNITY-ACQUIRED PNEUMONIA

P Commonly *Streptococcus pneumoniae*; *Legionella* and *Staphylococcus* are more common in patients admitted to ITU; 'atypical' bacteria include *Chlamydia pneumoniae*, *Mycoplasma pneumoniae*, *Chlamydia psittaci*, *Coxiella burnetii*

A Mortality 4–10 per cent; increased incidence in the elderly, COPD, diabetes, alcoholics, nursing home residents
Epidemics of *Mycoplasma pneumoniae* occur every 4 years in the UK; *Legionella* infection may occur more often in young people and those exposed to poorly maintained air conditioning systems
Staphylococcus is related to the influenza virus

Sy Cough, fever, dyspnoea, tachypnoea, pleuritic pain, myalgia
'Atypical' pneumonias may present with diarrhoea or abdominal pain

Si Crepitations, bronchial breathing, hypoxia/cyanosis

Ix CXR, FBC, U&E, CRP, LFT, sputum culture and Gram stain
In severe community-acquired pneumonia: viral and 'atypical' pathogen serology, pneumococcal and *Legionella* urine antigen detection, blood cultures

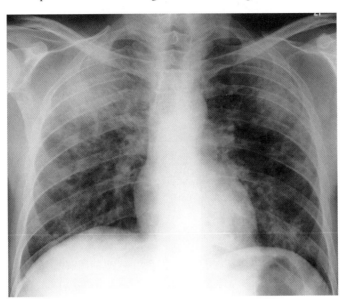

Figure 1.13 Bilateral patchy shadowing throughout both lungfields – bronchopneumonia

---

Box 1.8 CURB-65 SCORE

This is a 6-point score system to assess severity of community acquired pneumonia on presentation to hospital
  One point for each of the following:
- **C**onfusion
- **U**rea >7 mmol/L
- **R**espiratory rate >30/min
- systolic **B**lood pressure <90 mmHg
- diastolic **B**lood pressure <60 mmHg
- age >**65** years

CURB score 0: low risk of death; no need for hospital admission
CURB score 1–2: increased risk of death; should be admitted
CURB score 3 or more: high risk of death; urgent hospital admission

Source: Lim WS, van der Eerden MM, Laing R *et al*. Defining community acquired pneumonia severity on presentation to hospital: an international derivation and validation study. *Thorax* 2003;58:377–82.

Rx *Non-severe*: amoxicillin + erythromycin/clarithromycin (fluoroquinolone if penicillin allergic)
Severe: co-amoxiclav/cefuroxime/3rd generation cephalosporin + erythromycin/clarithromycin
Saline nebulizers may aid expectoration
Intravenous fluids if there are any signs of dehydration/renal impairment

PULMONARY TUBERCULOSIS

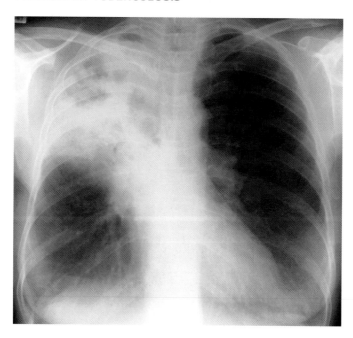

Figure 1.14 Cavitating consolidation in the right upper lobe – active tuberculosis

(P) Due to *Mycobacterium tuberculosis*; transmission through airborne spread
Miliary tuberculosis (TB) is due to haematogenous spread of tubercle bacilli

(A) ~9 million new cases worldwide/year;
↑incidence in the UK through the 1990s due to HIV infection, immigration from countries with high prevalence, social problems/homelessness

(Sy) Can have an acute (often in the young or immunocompromised) or insidious onset
Tachypnoea, cough, haemoptysis, lethargy, weakness, weight loss, anorexia, night sweats, fever

(Si) Often no findings on chest examination; crepitations in upper zones, lymphadenopathy

(Ix) Sputum microscopy and culture for AFB (acid-fast bacilli), CXR, Mantoux
If diagnosis is difficult, consider bronchoscopy and biopsy/brushings/broncho-alveolar lavage (BAL)

(Rx) 6 month regime: 2 months of RIPE:
- Rifampicin,
- Isoniazid,
- Pyrazinamide,
- Ethambutol

followed by rifampicin and isoniazid for 4 months
Multi-drug-resistant TB (MDR-TB): defined as resistance to rifampicin and isoniazid; treatment is complicated and must be done under specialist centres, usually involving five or more drugs to which the bacteria is susceptible for a minimum of 9 months (and often much longer). Directly observed therapy (DOT) may be required in patients who have drug-resistant TB, HIV-infected patients and those that might not comply with treatment.

Cx All anti-TB drugs have serious side-effects:
- pyridoxine is given to prevent peripheral neuropathy from isoniazid
- prior to starting treatment visual acuity should be assessed and renal/liver function monitored throughout
- patients should be warned they are likely to pass red-orange coloured urine while taking rifampicin

All cases of TB should be notified to the local consultant in communicable disease control

Contact tracing should be performed

PLEURAL DISEASE[3]

PLEURAL EFFUSION

A *Transudate* (protein <25 g/L): heart failure, hypoalbuminaemia, cirrhosis, hypothyroidism, peritoneal dialysis, PE, Meigs syndrome

Exudate (protein >35 g/L): carcinoma, pneumonia, TB, rheumatoid arthritis, systemic lupus erythematosus (SLE), lymphoma, mesothelioma, pancreatitis, drugs (amiodarone, nitrofurantoin, methotrexate)

An **empyema** refers to a grossly purulent pleural effusion

Sy Breathlessness

Si Tracheal deviation, decreased expansion, stony dull percussion note, diminished breath sounds

Ix *Imaging*: CXR, bronchoscopy and high-resolution CT (HRCT) scan may be required to determine the underlying cause

Pleural aspirate: for protein, microscopy, Gram stain, culture, cytology, glucose, lactate dehydrogenase (LDH), pH, acid- and alcohol-fast bacilli (AAFB) culture ± amylase/triglycerides

---

Box 1.9 LIGHT'S CRITERIA FOR PLEURAL EFFUSIONS

For pleural protein 25–35 g/L; the fluid is an exudate if:
- pleural fluid protein divided by serum protein > 0.5
- pleural fluid LDH divided by serum LDH > 0.6
- pleural fluid LDH > two-thirds the upper limit of normal serum LDH.

Source: Light RW, Macgregor MI, Luchsinger PC, Ball WC Jr. Pleural effusions: the diagnostic separation of transudates and exudates. *Annals of Internal Medicine* 1972;77:507–13.

---

pH: normal ~7.6; drainage required if pH <7.2 in an infected effusion

Glucose: low in empyema, rheumatoid, lupus, TB, malignancy

Amylase: raised in acute pancreatitis, oesophageal rupture, malignancy

Cytology: positive in ~60 per cent malignancy

Rx Aimed at the underlying cause

If there is any respiratory compromise a pleurocentesis should be performed. If fluid re-accumulates, a chest drain should be considered

PARAPNEUMONIC EFFUSIONS

(A) Pleural fluid will develop in 57 per cent of cases of pneumonia; in rarer cases, there is no obvious precipitant to the effusion

Commonest pathogens include *Streptococcus, Haemophilus influenzae, Escherichia coli, Pseudomonas, Klebsiella*

(S) A combination of the symptoms and signs of pneumonia and pleural effusions

(Ix) As for pneumonia/pleural effusion

Ultrasound imaging can help with diagnosis

Pleural aspiration is *fundamental*

(Rx) Antibiotics

Chest drain is necessary if:
- pleural fluid pH <7.2
- pleural fluid glucose <2.2 mmol/L
- pleural LDH >1000 IU/L
- positive Gram stain/culture
- gross pus is aspirated (this is an empyema)

If the infection fails to resolve, refer to cardiothoracic surgery

SPONTANEOUS PNEUMOTHORAX

(P) Rupture of pleural bleb

(A) Commonest in young men ($\male$:$\female$ 6:1); COPD, asthma, carcinoma, cystic fibrosis, TB, connective tissue disorders

(Sy) Pleuritic pain, breathlessness

(Si) Tachycardia, tachypnoea, deviated trachea, diminished breath sounds, hyper-resonance, decreased vocal resonance

(Ix) CXR, CT scan if differentiating pneumothorax from bullous lung disease

(Rx) High-flow oxygen

Rim of air <2 cm and patient not breathless: discharge with early follow-up (if patient has underlying lung disease, observe for 24 h)

Rim of air >2 cm and breathless: aspirate

If patient is >50 years and has underlying lung disease: insertion of intercostal drain

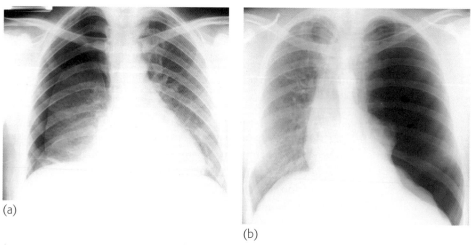

(a)

(b)

Figure 1.15 (a) Right pneumothorax: absence of lung markings beyond the lung edge; (b) left-sided tension pneumothorax. Note the mediastinal shift away from the affected side

If aspiration fails: insertion of intercostal drain
If lung fails to re-expand: refer to respiratory specialist to consider suction ±
pleurodesis (artificial obliteration of the pleural space)

Cx Tension pneumothorax – severe dyspnoea, hypotension, severe tachycardia,
mediastinal shift

PULMONARY FIBROSIS[4]

A See Box 1.10

Box 1.10 CAUSES OF PULMONARY FIBROSIS

- *Occupation* (see below): exposure to pets/birds EAA (extrinsic allergic alveolitis)
- *Previous radiotherapy*
- *Drugs*: amiodarone, methotrexate, nitrofurantoin, penicillamine, bleomycin,
  cyclophosphamide
- *Systemic disorders*: vasculitis (Wegener's granulomatosis, Churg–Strauss
  syndrome, Behçet's syndrome, Goodpasture's syndrome, sarcoidosis)
- *Connective tissue disorders*: SLE, rheumatoid arthritis, Sjögren's syndrome,
  systemic sclerosis, polymyositis
- *Neoplasm*: lymphoma, lymphangitic carcinoma
- *Inherited disorders*: tuberous sclerosis, neurofibromatosis
- *Others*: amyloidosis

Sy Cough, shortness of breath, pleurisy more common in SLE/rheumatoid arthritis
Si Fine end-inspiratory crepitations, finger clubbing, weight loss, fatigue, hypoxaemia,
signs of systemic disease
Ix Bloods: FBC, U&E, LFT, calcium levels, ACE (angiotensin-converting enzyme)
levels
Immunology: anti-GBM (glomerular basement membrane), autoantibodies, ANA
(antinuclear antibodies), ANCA (antineutrophil cytoplasmic antibodies), rheuma-
toid factor, serum precipitins
Imaging: CXR, HRCT
Spirometry: lung function tests: restrictive defect, reduced transfer factor, reduced
lung volume
Endoscopy: bronchoscopy + BAL/biopsy
Rx Treatment for IPF (idiopathic pulmonary fibrosis), EAA, occupational lung disease
and sarcoidosis is mentioned in each individual section
Treatment for fibrosis aimed at systemic/neoplastic conditions is aimed at the
underlying condition

IDIOPATHIC PULMONARY FIBROSIS (IPF)

Previously known as cryptogenic fibrosing alveolitis (CFA)

(A) Prevalence 6–15 per 100 000; incidence increases with age

(Si) Bilateral fine end-inspiratory crepitations in 90 per cent of patients; finger clubbing in 50–70 per cent

(Rx) Steroids and azathioprine; if azathioprine fails/is not tolerated cyclophosphamide

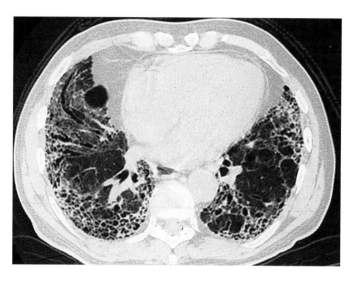

Figure 1.16 CT scan showing extensive interstitial thickening with small cystic spaces in a patient with idiopathic pulmonary fibrosis

EXTRINSIC ALLERGIC ALVEOLITIS (EAA)

(P) Hypersensitivity reaction to various antigens

(A) Less likely to be smokers than the general population
Farmer's lung (*Thermoactinomyces* in mouldy hay) and bird fancier's lung (avian protein on feathers) are most common; other antigens include isocyanates (chemical workers), *Aspergillus* spp. (tobacco workers)

(S) Symptoms usually regress when the causative agent is removed

(Ix) Serum precipitins to potential allergens, e.g. *Micropolyspora faeni*, *Thermoactinomyces vulgaris*: eosinophilia is not a feature
CXR often shows apical sparing

(Rx) Removal from exposure to the antigen; steroids speed up recovery

OCCUPATIONAL LUNG DISEASE

(A) Asbestos, silica, cobalt, coal worker's pneumoconiosis, siderosis (iron), copper sulphate, aluminium, beryllium, cotton dust, grain dust

(S) Variable, some dusts are more toxic/fibrogenic

(Rx) Protective apparatus to prevent inhalation

ASBESTOSIS

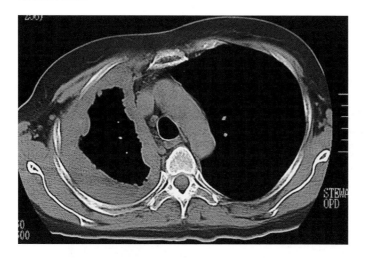

Figure 1.17
Mesothelioma: CT showing extensive right-sided pleural thickening

P Diffuse interstitial fibrosis
Usually manifests >10 years post-exposure
Pleural plaques indicate exposure to asbestos, not pulmonary involvement
A >80 per cent mesotheliomas are associated with asbestos exposure
Increased risk of lung cancer (squamous cell and adenocarcinoma)
Smoking increases the risk further, therefore patients should be advised to stop
Ix CXR may show fibrosis ± pleural plaques
Rx Palliation is the mainstay of treatment for mesothelioma
Px 50 per cent mesotheliomas metastasize, but most are locally invasive
Very poor prognosis

PULMONARY SARCOIDOSIS

P Chronic multisystem disorder; accumulation of non-caseating granulomas and
T lymphocytes
A Unknown cause; 75 per cent are aged 20–40 years, however it can affect all sexes,
ages, races and places of origin
S This depends on the organs involved
Pulmonary sarcoidosis can present subacutely or insidiously
Fever, malaise, weight loss, dyspnoea, cough
Combination of erythema nodosum and bilateral hilar lymphadenopathy is
pathognomonic

Ix   CXR shows abnormalities in 90 per cent

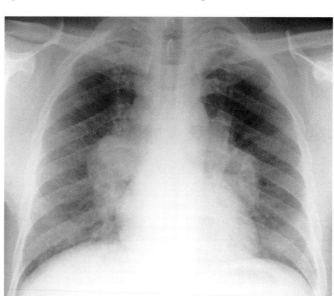

Figure 1.18 Bilateral hilar lymphadenopathy in sarcoidosis

Table 1.1 Chest X-ray grading in sarcoidosis

Grade	Abnormality
0	No abnormality
1	Lymphadenopathy alone
2	Lymphadenopathy and infiltrates
3	Infiltrates alone
4	Fibrosis

$\uparrow Ca^{2+}$, echocardiogram, $\uparrow$ serum ACE levels are poorly specific, but can be used to monitor disease activity

Rx   Majority of patients do not need treatment

For persistent symptoms, steroids can be given and reduced slowly over months

For resistant disease consider methotrexate or chloroquine

SUPPURATIVE LUNG CONDITIONS

BRONCHIECTASIS

P   Chronic inflammation and infection of the bronchial walls, leading to permanent dilatation of the airways

A   Cystic fibrosis, pertussis, measles, TB, mechanical obstruction, Kartagener's syndrome (situs inversus and ciliary dysfunction), immunoglobulin deficiency

Sy   Copious purulent sputum, recurrent chest infections

Si   Clubbing, coarse inspiratory and expiratory crackles

Ix   CXR, sputum culture, HRCT chest, immunoglobulins

Rx   Postural drainage, antibiotics (commonest pathogens: *Staphylococcus aureus*, *Haemophilus influenzae*, *Pseudomonas aeruginosa*), bronchodilators, surgery

Cx   Massive haemoptysis, cerebral abscess

CYSTIC FIBROSIS

P Autosomal recessive; abnormal chloride channels in the luminal surface lead to increased re-absorption of sodium and water leading to increased viscosity of airway secretions

Sy Recurrent childhood chest infections, failure to thrive, meconium ileus, steatorrhoea, bronchiectasis, male infertility, diabetes mellitus, gallstones

Si Clubbing, purulent sputum, central cyanosis, bilateral coarse crackles

Ix Sweat testing, genetic testing, immunoreactive trypsin assay

Rx Antibiotics, postural drainage, pancreatic supplements, low-fat diet, bronchodilators, heart–lung transplantation

MISCELLANEOUS

PULMONARY EMBOLISM

A Immobility, trauma, recent surgery, pregnancy, malignancy, pro-thrombotic disorders, air travel, oral oestrogens

Sy Dyspnoea, tachypnoea, pleuritic pain, haemoptysis, cough

Si Tachycardia, hypotension, ↑ JVP, clinical deep vein thrombosis (DVT)

Ix *Bloods*: arterial blood gases, D-dimer (beware false positives),
ECG: S1Q3T3 pattern only seen in 10 per cent of PE
Imaging: CXR, V̇/Q̇ scan, CTPA, Doppler ultrasound scan (USS) leg, echo (only useful in massive central PE)

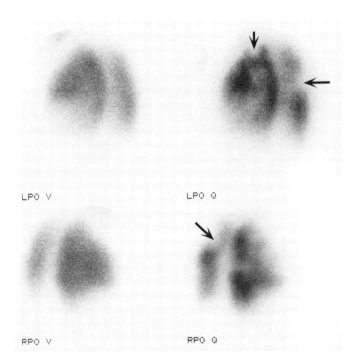

LPO V

LPO Q

RPO V

RPO Q

Figure 1.19 Isotope ventilation and perfusion scan: normal ventilation scan (V̇) but the perfusion (Q̇) scan shows multiple defects in pulmonary embolus

Rx Oxygen, analgesia
Anticoagulation: usually with LMWH until PE confirmed, and then with warfarin
Thrombolysis: only in massive PE with haemodynamic compromise
Surgery: embolectomy, inferior vena cava (IVC) filters (to prevent recurrence)

PULMONARY HYPERTENSION/COR PULMONALE

P Pulmonary hypertension (PH) refers to ↑ pulmonary artery pressure – it can be primary or secondary
Cor pulmonale refers to right ventricular enlargement secondary to pulmonary disease
Primary pulmonary hypertension (PPH): extremely rare
Secondary pulmonary hypertension: lung disease leads to increased pulmonary vascular resistance; to preserve cardiac output the right ventricle has to increase its output

Sy Dyspnoea, fatigue, weakness, angina (RV [right ventricle] ischaemia), syncope

Si ↑ JVP, peripheral oedema, loud P2, right-sided 4th heart sound, RV heave, tricuspid regurgitation, pulsatile hepatomegaly

Ix Investigations to diagnose secondary causes of PH: CXR, ventilation-perfusion scan, HRCT, pulmonary function tests, lung biopsy, FBC (polycythaemia)
Investigations confirming PH: ECG (right axis deviation/RV hypertrophy), echocardiogram (RV and RA enlargement), cardiac catheterization (not usually necessary)

Rx Treat the underlying cause; cor pulmonale is treated as for right heart failure (diuretics/oxygen)

BRONCHIAL CARCINOMA

P Squamous cell 48 per cent, small cell (SCLC) 24 per cent, adenocarcinoma 13 per cent, large cell 10 per cent, other 5 per cent

A Smoking (85 per cent), asbestos, nickel, air pollution
Commonest cancer of the Western world (and rapidly rising incidence in the developing world)

Sy Cough, dyspnoea, haemoptysis, hoarse voice (laryngeal nerve invasion), weight loss

Si Horner's syndrome (Pancoast's tumour), superior vena caval obstruction, lymphadenopathy, clubbing, hypertrophic pulmonary osteoarthropathy

Box 1.11 FEATURES OF HORNER'S SYNDROME
• Miosis (constricted pupil)
• Ptosis
• Anhidrosis (loss of sweating over half of face)
• Apparent enophthalmos

Ix CXR, bronchoscopy + biopsy/brushings, sputum cytology, CT of the thorax/abdomen, lung function tests

Rx *Surgery*: only possible if FEV$_1$ >1.5 L for lobectomy/>2 L for pneumonectomy
Radiotherapy (RT): radical RT for inoperable non-SCLC patients
Chemotherapy: first-line treatment for SCLC

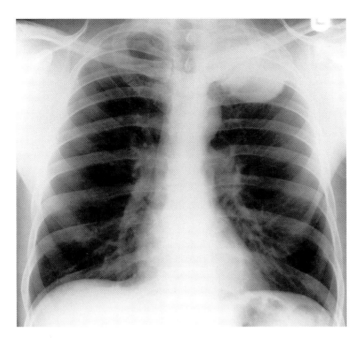

Figure 1.20 Pancoast's tumour at the left apex

REFERENCES

1   The British Thoracic Society/Scottish Intercollegiate Guidelines Network British Guideline on the Management of Asthma. *Thorax* 2003;58(Suppl I).
2   British Thoracic Society Guidelines for the Management of Community Acquired Pneumonia in Adults. *Thorax* 2001;56(Suppl IV) and 2004 update.
3   British Thoracic Society Guidelines for the Management of Pleural Disease. *Thorax* 2003;58 (Suppl II).
4   British Thoracic Society and Standards of Care Committee. The diagnosis assessment and treatment of diffuse parenchymal lung disease in adults. *Thorax* 1999;54:1–28.

GASTROENTEROLOGY

GASTROINTESTINAL INVESTIGATIONS

- **Iron, folate, calcium:** absorbed in proximal small intestine
- **B_{12}:** absorbed in the terminal ileum
- **Endoscopy:**
    allows direct visualization of gastrointestinal (GI) tract and therapeutic procedures, OGD (oesophagogastroduodenoscopy)/jejunoscopy/sigmoidoscopy/colonoscopy therapies include variceal banding, injection of bleeding points with sclerosants, dilatation of strictures, stent placement, video capsule endoscopy
- **Contrast studies:** (including barium and Gastrografin studies) allow visualization of GI mucosa
- **Urinary D-xylose test:** tests carbohydrate absorption; D-xylose is absorbed in proximal small intestine and excreted in the urine, therefore low excretion reflects poor absorption
- **Breath tests (BT):** commonly lactose–hydrogen BT (for lactose intolerance) or glucose–hydrogen BT (for bacterial overgrowth)

- **SeHCAT scan:** (selenium-75-homocholic acid taurine) nuclear medicine scan which assesses bile salt malabsorption; radiolabelled bile salts ingested, then scanned at 3 h and 7 days; if <15 per cent present at 7 days this suggests bile acid malabsorption
- **3-day faecal fat collection:** patient is given a high-fat diet during this test and every stool sample collected for 3 days; normal faecal fat is <18 mmol/day; increased in fat malabsorption or bile salt malabsorption
- **Faecal elastase:** reduced in chronic pancreatitis or pancreatic insufficiency
- **Pancreolauryl test:** test of pancreatic exocrine function

MALABSORPTION

(P) Can be malabsorption of fat, carbohydrate, protein, vitamins or a combination of all

(A) See Box 1.12

Box 1.12 CAUSES OF MALABSORPTION
- Coeliac disease - Protein-losing enteropathy - Whipple's disease - Bacterial overgrowth - Short bowel syndrome - Tropical sprue - Crohn's disease - Lactose intolerance - Chronic pancreatitis

History will give clues to potential diagnoses, e.g. recent travel, recent bowel resection, dairy product intolerance, chronic pancreatitis, etc.

(Sy) Diarrhoea, steatorrhoea, weight loss

(Si) Anaemia, oedema, hypovitaminosis

(Ix) FBC, U&E, LFT, albumin, calcium, folate, iron, B_{12}, vitamin D, coagulation, coeliac serology, thyroid function[1]

Further investigations depend on history and results of blood tests indicating possible region of bowel involved:

- *Imaging*: OGD + small bowel biopsy, barium follow-through (BaFT), sigmoidoscopy/colonoscopy, barium enema, SeHCAT scan
- *Functional testing*: 24-h faecal fat, faecal elastase, urinary D-xylose test, 24-h urinary protein (if albumin low), gut hormones

(Rx) aimed at underlying cause:

- *Whipple's disease/bacterial overgrowth/tropical sprue*: antibiotics
- *coeliac disease*: gluten-free diet
- *lactose intolerance*: avoidance of dairy products
- *short bowel syndrome*: anti-diarrhoeals, low-fat, high-fibre diet; nutritional replacement
- *chronic pancreatitis*: enzyme supplements

COELIAC DISEASE

P Gluten sensitivity leading to small intestinal enteropathy

A Affects all ages; peak in 3rd decade

Sy Lethargy, weakness, diarrhoea, reduced fertility, weight loss

Si Anaemia

Ix *Diagnostic tests*: OGD + intestinal biopsy showing subtotal villous atrophy, coeliac antibodies (including antibodies to gliadin, endomysium and tissue transglutaminase [tTG]). OGD and video capsule endoscopy may show scalloping of the duodenal mucosa
Tests for malabsorption: FBC, iron, folate, B_{12}, albumin and calcium

Rx Gluten exclusion lifelong

Cx Small intestinal lymphoma/adenocarcinoma, osteopenia, dermatitis herpetiformis, hyposplenism

IRRITABLE BOWEL SYNDROME

P GI symptoms in the absence of structural pathology; abnormal autonomic reactivity, visceral hypersensitivity

A Post-infective, stress, adverse life events, psychological problems: anxiety, depression

Sy Abdominal discomfort, relief with defaecation, alternating bowel habit, bloating

Ix In a patient <45 years with a long history of typical symptoms, further investigations, beyond routine blood tests, should not be required
In a patient >45 years, with a short history or atypical symptoms, investigations should be done to exclude other pathologies – FBC, TFT, coeliac antibodies, inflammatory markers, sigmoidoscopy, diarrhoea/malabsorption screen

Rx *Supportive*: explanation and reassurance, lifestyle advice
Medical: drug treatment is aimed at particular symptoms: antispasmodics (e.g. mebeverine), antidepressants, treatment for diarrhoea (loperamide, codeine), treatment for constipation, peppermint oil
Dietary: symptom diary to assess dietary factors, exclusion diets
Psychological: cognitive–behavioural therapy

INFLAMMATORY BOWEL DISEASE

CROHN'S DISEASE

P Affects any part of the GI tract from mouth to anus; segmental; transmural process; ulceration, cobblestone appearance, pseudopolyps, non-caseating granulomas, fissures, fistulae

A Genetic predisposition, smoking

Sy Depends on site affected; abdominal pain, diarrhoea, weight loss, per rectum (PR) mucus/pus, arthritis

Si Fever, malaise, anaemia, palpable inflammatory mass, fistulae, erythema nodosum, pyoderma gangrenosum

Ix Stool microscopy/culture, ↑CRP, ↑ESR, ↓Hb, ↓albumin, sigmoidoscopy/colonoscopy with biopsies, white cell scan, BaFT; tests for malabsorption: vitamin B_{12}, folate, vitamin D, calcium

(Rx) 5-aminosalicylic acid (5-ASA) (e.g. mesalazine), steroids, antibiotics, azathioprine/6-mercaptopurine, methotrexate, infliximab (anti TNF-α [tissue necrosis factor-α]), enteral therapies (elemental diet, TPN [total parenteral nutrition]), surgery

(Cx) Stricturing, bowel obstruction, perforation, cholelithiasis, fatty liver

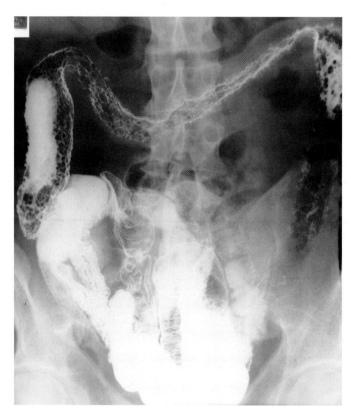

Figure

1.21 Cobblestone mucosa of the colon in Crohn's disease

ULCERATIVE COLITIS

(P) Involves the rectum and extends proximally; inflammation confined to mucosa and submucosa; distorted crypt architecture, cryptitis, crypt abscesses, inflammatory cell infiltrate, vascular congestion

(A) Genetic predisposition, non-smokers

(Sy) Diarrhoea, rectal bleeding and mucus, abdominal pain

(Si) Weight loss, fever, erythema nodosum, pyoderma gangrenosum

(Ix) ↑CRP, ↑ESR, ↑platelets, ↓albumin, ↓Hb (haemoglobin); stool microscopy/ culture, abdominal X-ray (AXR) (need to rule out toxic dilatation), sigmoidoscopy with biopsies, pANCA +ve (~70 per cent)

(Rx) 5-ASA, steroids, azathioprine/6-mercaptopurine, ciclosporin, surgery

(Cx) Haemorrhage, toxic megacolon, colorectal carcinoma, fatty liver, primary sclerosing cholangitis

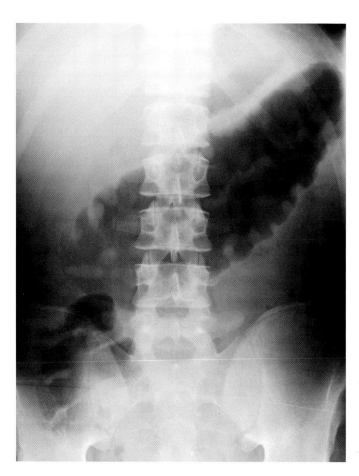

Figure 1.22 Toxic megacolon: dilatation of the transverse colon with loss of the normal haustral pattern and extensive mucosal irregularity

Table 1.2 Differences between Crohn's disease and ulcerative colitis

	Crohn's disease	Ulcerative colitis
Distribution	Can affect any part of GI tract – from mouth to anus	Affects large bowel only
Endoscopy findings	Rectum frequently spared Some areas of healthy bowel between diseased segments (skip lesions) Bowel wall is thickened and has 'cobblestone' appearance due to deep ulceration	Rectum always affected Continuous inflammation Bowel wall is thin and featureless in severe disease
Histology	Granuloma is characteristic finding Transmural inflammation (extends all the way through the bowel wall)	Inflammation usually confined to mucosa

Radiology	Strictures, fissures and fistulae are common	Less common in ulcerative colitis
	Asymmetrical inflammation	Symmetrical inflammation
Smoking	Strongly associated with smoking	Associated with non-smokers or ex-smokers
	Predicts a worse course of disease Increases risk of surgery and further surgery	Appears to protect against disease

INFECTIOUS DIARRHOEA

(P) Organisms causing diarrhoea produce their effect by invasion and destruction of mucosal cells, and toxin production

(A) Travel, contact, age (<5 years and >70 years have increased mortality), food, recent antibiotic use (*Clostridium difficile*)

(S) Fever, diarrhoea (may be bloody), nausea, dehydration, abdominal pain
Bloody diarrhoea is more common with *Campylobacter*, *Shigella*

(Ix) FBC, U&E, CRP, stool microscopy, culture and sensitivity (MC&S), blood cultures if septic

(Rx) Majority of cases are self-terminating and require rehydration and electrolyte correction; antibiotics are considered in immunocompromised patients, the very young or the very septic; always liaise with microbiologists

(Cx) Renal failure, septic shock; *E. coli* is associated with the haemolytic–uraemic syndrome

DYSPEPSIA[2]

(P) 'Dyspepsia' encompasses a group of symptoms, including heartburn, nausea, epigastric/retrosternal pain, bloating, anorexia and early satiety. Several disorders can cause dyspepsia, including peptic ulcers, oesophagitis, gastritis, gastric cancer and gallstones.

(S) *Alarm symptoms/signs*: unintentional weight loss, unexplained iron deficiency, dysphagia, GI bleeding, persistent continuous vomiting, epigastric mass, previous gastric surgery, previous gastric ulcer

GASTRO-OESOPHAGEAL REFLUX DISEASE (GORD)

(P) Decreased lower oesophageal sphincter tone; sustained or transient

(A) Usually no obvious cause; secondary causes include smoking, pregnancy, scleroderma, drugs, trauma, alcohol, obesity
Helicobacter pylori is **not** associated with GORD

(Sy) Heartburn, regurgitation

(Ix) OGD, 24-h pH monitoring in difficult cases

(Rx) *Conservative*: weight loss, avoidance of smoking and alcohol
Medical: simple antacids, H_2 blockers (e.g. ranitidine), proton pump inhibitor (PPI) (e.g. omeprazole)
Surgery: Nissen fundoplication (see p. 109)

(Cx) Reflux oesophagitis, peptic stricture, Barrett's oesophagus

BARRETT'S OESOPHAGUS

(P) Squamous → columnar metaplasia in lower oesophagus, premalignant
(A) Secondary to chronic GORD
(S) As GORD
(Ix) Serial OGDs to detect progression of dysplasia
(Rx) Surgical removal, endoscopic ablation
(Cx) Adenocarcinoma

PEPTIC ULCER DISEASE

(P) Break in mucosal surface >5 mm
(A) *Helicobacter pylori* is associated with 95 per cent duodenal ulcers and 70 per cent gastric ulcers; NSAIDs, smoking, alcohol
(S) As above
(Ix) Anyone >55 years with new-onset dyspepsia, or anyone with alarm symptoms should undergo an OGD and testing for H. pylori; if <55 years with no alarm symptoms, then the patient can simply undergo a urea breath test, FBC
(Rx) Antacids, H_2-receptor blockers, eradication of *H. pylori*, PPI, sucralfate, avoidance of smoking, NSAIDs and alcohol
All patients with gastric ulcers should have repeat OGD to ensure healing
(Cx) GI bleed, perforation, gastric outlet obstruction

REFERENCES

1   Thomas PD, Forbes A, Green J *et al*. Guidelines for the investigation of chronic diarrhoea, 2nd edition. *Gut* 2003;52(Suppl V):v1–v15.
2   National Institute for Clinical Excellence. *NICE clinical guideline 17: Dyspepsia: management of dyspepsia in adults in primary care*. London: National Institute for Clinical Excellence, 2004.

HEPATOLOGY

HEPATOLOGY INVESTIGATIONS

Blood tests
- **Hepatocellular integrity:**
  - alanine transaminase (ALT)/aspartate transaminase (AST)
  - lactate dehydrogenase (LDH): markedly raised in liver metastases and obstructive jaundice
  - gamma glutamyl transferase (GGT): raised in hepatocellular, hepatobiliary and alcoholic liver disease
  - iron/ferritin: raised in haemochromatosis, liver necrosis, alcoholic liver disease, acute viral hepatitis
- **Disorders of excretion:**
  - bilirubin: jaundice occurs at levels >40 mmol/L:

     Hyperbilirubinaemia:
     Indirect bilirubin is produced as a water-insoluble, albumin-bound form which is conjugated in the liver to form direct bilirubin, a water-soluble form.

Jaundice can be divided into three forms:

1 pre-hepatic: due to haemolysis – LDH:AST ratio >12, no bilirubinuria
2 intrahepatic: hepatocellular damage – LDH:AST ratio <12, bilirubinuria
3 post-hepatic: due to cholestasis, bilirubinuria

- alkaline phosphatase (ALP): raised in cholestasis (NB also found in bone, kidney, intestine and lung – isoenzymes can differentiate the source)
- total copper: raised in cholestasis; decreased in Wilson's disease
- cholesterol: marked increase in cholestasis
- **Synthetic function:**
  - coagulation: clotting factors I, II, V, VII, XI–XIII are synthesized in the liver; monitored using prothrombin time (PT)/international normalized ratio (INR)
  - albumin
  - A preliminary 'liver screen' includes: viral hepatitis (hepatitis A, B and C) serology, cytomegalovirus (CMV), Epstein–Barr virus (EBV), autoantibodies, immunoglobulin levels, ferritin, copper, caeruloplasmin, α_1-antitrypsin, α-fetoprotein, Ca 19-9, amylase and ultrasonography

Imaging

- **USS:** can comment on echogenicity, nodularity, lesions and the biliary system; Doppler can assess venous flow
- **CT:** gives further details of hepatic parenchyma; contrast media is used in triple phase CT (looking at the arterial, parenchymal and venous phase) to help differentiate between liver parenchyma and pathological structures
- **MRI:** allows cross- and longitudinal sections; further differentiation between tissues than USS and CT; MR angiography and MRCP (cholangiopancreatography) available
- **Angiography:** delineates vascular supply to liver
- **Nuclear medicine**

Liver biopsy

- Can be done directly at the bedside, under ultrasound guidance or via the transjugular (TJ) route. TJ biopsies are less readily available and usually reserved for high-risk patients, in whom bleeding is more likely

CIRRHOSIS

P Necrosis of hepatic parenchyma with connective tissue proliferation and nodular regeneration

A Multiple causes, discussed below; commonest cause is chronic alcohol abuse

Ix Investigations are aimed at finding the cause
LFT, FBC, U&E
Albumin and coagulation to assess synthetic function
Liver biopsy will show degree of activity and fibrosis and help diagnose a cause

S Related to the underlying cause: lethargy, splenomegaly, jaundice, leuconychia, telangiectasia, spider naevi, gynaecomastia, xanthelasma/xanthoma, Dupuytren's contracture, clubbing, dilated chest/abdominal wall veins, scratch marks, fetor hepaticus, palmar erythema, weight and height for the calculated body mass index, Kayser-Fleischer rings, tatoos, intravenous track marks

Rx Aimed at the underlying cause and preventing complications; supportive treatment includes laxatives (prevent encephalopathy), vitamin K (correct clotting), nutritional support, terlipressin and human albumin solution (to correct hepatorenal syndrome), antibiotics ± liver transplant

The Child–Pugh scoring shown in Table 1.3 is used to predict the prognosis of cirrhotic patients.

Table 1.3 Child–Pugh scoring system for cirrhotic patients

Indices	1 point	2 points	3 points
Albumin (g/L)	>35	30–35	<30
Bilirubin (μmol/L)	<34	34–51	>51
INR	<1.7	1.7–2.3	>2.3
Ascites	No	Mild–moderate	Severe
Encephalopathy	No	Stages I and II	Stages III and IV

Total score: 5–6, Child–Pugh A; 7–9, Child–Pugh B; 10–15 Child–Pugh C

Box 1.13 COMPLICATIONS OF CIRRHOSIS

MALNUTRITION

1 Catabolism
2 Reduced glycogenolysis and increased gluconeogenesis
3 Hypoglycaemia/impaired glucose tolerance

HEPATIC ENCEPHALOPATHY

(A) Infection, constipation, drugs/toxins, GI bleed, electrolyte disturbance
(S) Affects conscious level, behaviour and intellectual function
(Ix) Psychometric testing, EEG (electroencephalography), ammonia
(Rx) Removal of causative factors, antibiotics, laxatives, branched-chain amino acids

ASCITES/OEDEMA

(P) Portal hypertension, hypoalbuminaemia and increased capillary permeability leads to fluid seepage, with stimulation of the renin–angiotensin system
(S) Abdominal distension, breathlessness with gross ascites, pleural effusions and peripheral oedema
(Ix) Ascitic aspirate: protein, cell count, microscopy/culture, cytology
(Cx) Spontaneous bacterial peritonitis (white cell count [WCC] >250/mm³), respiratory compromise, hernia, compression of renal vein/IVC (inferior vena cava), hepatorenal syndrome, encephalopathy, electrolyte disturbance
(Rx) Fluid restriction, salt restriction, diuretics, paracentesis, TIPS (transjugular intrahepatic portosystemic shunt, see Information Box, p. 39)

VITAMIN DEFICIENCY

Typically B vitamins (especially thiamine)

COAGULOPATHY

IMPAIRED IMMUNE SYSTEM

VARICES

(P) Portal hypertension leads to the formation of collateral circulations; occur when portal pressure exceeds 12 mmHg
(Rx) *Acute variceal bleed*: ABC, fluid resuscitation, endoscopic treatment (sclerosant, band ligation), balloon tamponade (Sengstaken–Blakemore tube), terlipressin, antibiotics
Prevention: β-blockers (propranolol), endoscopic screening, TIPS, liver transplantation

---

HEPATORENAL SYNDROME

Renal failure in the presence of severe liver disease, where all other causes have been excluded

HEPATOCELLULAR CARCINOMA (HCC)

Cirrhosis is found in 65–90 per cent of patients with HCC

ALCOHOLISM

P Steatosis, fibrosis, cirrhosis

A Degree of liver damage dependent on genetic susceptibility and coexisting liver disease; women progress to cirrhosis faster

S CAGE questionnaire:
- do you feel you should Cut down your alcohol consumption?
- do you feel Annoyed when people criticize your drinking?
- do you feel Guilty?
- do you ever drink first thing in the morning – an Eye-opener?

Otherwise, the symptoms/signs depend on the degree of liver damage

Ix As for cirrhosis: LFT ($\uparrow$ GGT), $\downarrow$ albumin, coagulation, FBC: $\uparrow$ MCV (mean corpuscular volume), $\downarrow$ platelets, U&E, $\uparrow$ IgA, $\uparrow$ cholesterol; USS; liver biopsy will give the exact degree of damage, but is not required for diagnosis

Rx Abstinence, nutrition, vitamin replacement, laxatives, liver transplantation

ACUTE ALCOHOLIC HEPATITIS

S Fever, nausea, RUQ (right upper quadrant) pain, jaundice, ascites, oedema, encephalopathy

Rx All the above measures ± steroids/pentoxifylline

Px Mortality rate ~10 per cent

HEPATIC FAILURE

There are three types of acute liver failure:

1. *hyperacute or fulminant liver failure* – encephalopathy develops within 1 week
2. *acute liver failure* – encephalopathy develops within 2–4 weeks
3. *subacute liver failure* – encephalopathy develops within 4–8 weeks.

P Acute necrotizing hepatitis leading to cell destruction

A Viral hepatitis, infections (viral, bacterial, parasitic), drugs, toxins, alcohol, ischaemic, complications associated with pregnancy, malignancy

Sy Lethargy, weakness, nausea, anorexia, sleep disturbance

Si Jaundice, fever, fetor hepaticus, encephalopathy, cerebral oedema leading to bradycardia, hypertension, tachypnoea

Ix Liver screen to look for an underlying cause; poor prognostic indicators include: $\uparrow$ bilirubin, severe hyponatraemia, rising lactate, acidosis, rapid drop in transaminases, renal failure

Cx Renal failure, coagulopathy, respiratory failure, sepsis, circulatory failure, hypoglycaemia, pancreatitis

Rx Supportive treatment in an intensive care setting; liver transplantation

BUDD–CHIARI SYNDROME

P   Hepatic venous outflow obstruction; this leads to increased hepatic sinusoidal pressure and portal hypertension

A   Hypercoagulable states; myeloproliferative disorders are the most common cause

S   Depends on speed of onset; abdominal pain, hepatomegaly, ascites; varices and splenomegaly can be seen in the chronic form; nausea and jaundice in the acute form

Ix $\uparrow\uparrow$ ALT/AST, $\uparrow$ ALP/bilirubin, $\downarrow$ albumin, USS with Doppler studies of the hepatic vein, CT/MRI

Rx Anticoagulation

Ascites is controlled with sodium restriction and diuretics $\pm$ paracentesis

Thrombolysis, angioplasty, TIPS, liver transplant

INFORMATION BOX: TIPS

A **T**ransjugular **I**ntrahepatic **P**ortosystemic **S**hunt is a procedure performed by a radiologist whereby a connection is made between the portal vein and the hepatic vein via a catheter introduced into the jugular vein. This aims to reduce the portal hypertension causing some of the symptoms of liver disease, but can precipitate encephalopathy. *Patency of stent can be checked using Doppler USS. Stenosis ✓ revise.*

VIRAL HEPATITIS

HEPATITIS A VIRUS (HAV)

P   RNA virus; transmitted by faecal-oral route. Does not cause cirrhosis

A   Poor hygiene correlates with increased risk

Sy Nausea, anorexia, vomiting, diarrhoea, weakness, fever, malaise, arthralgia, dark urine

Si Jaundice, hepatomegaly, splenomegaly, lymphadenopathy

Ix LFT: raised transaminases and bilirubin, HAV IgM (immunoglobulin M)

Rx Supportive

HEPATITIS B VIRUS (HBV)

P   DNA virus

A   Parenteral, sexual, vertical transmission

Sy Similar to hepatitis A, but often more severe; often found on antenatal testing

Si Jaundice, pruritus, tender hepatomegaly, lymphadenopathy, splenomegaly

Ix See Box 1.14

Box 1.14 SEROLOGY IN HEPATITIS B INFECTION

- *HBsAg*: first serological marker; usually becomes undetectable at 6 months
- *HBsAb*: detectable once HBsAg clears; remains indefinitely
- *HBcAg*: not detected routinely
- *HBcAb*: detectable 1–2 weeks after HBsAg (IgM initially, then IgG)
- *HBeAg*: occurs shortly after HBsAg; correlates with viral replication

- *HBeAb*: correlates with lower viral replication and infectivity
- *HBV DNA by PCR* (polymerase chain reaction): quantifies viral replication

HBsAg, hepatitis B surface antigen; HBsAb, hepatitis B surface antibody; HBcAg, hepatitis B core antigen; HBcAb, hepatitis B core antibody; HBeAg, hepatitis B e antigen, HBeAb, hepatitis B e antibody

Rx   alcohol avoidance, antivirals e.g. lamivudine, pegylated interferon, adefovir, tenofovir, entecavir, telbivudine, interferon α

Cx   >90 per cent patients will clear the virus
Carrier state: HBsAg persists for >6 months with no signs of acute hepatitis
10–20 per cent of carriers will develop cirrhosis
↑ risk of hepatocellular carcinoma

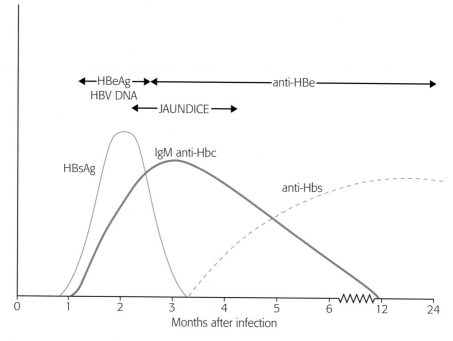

Figure 1.23 Changes in hepatitis B enzymes after acute infection

HEPATITIS C VIRUS (HCV)

P   RNA virus; six genotypes
A   Spread parenterally or sporadically
Sy   Prodromal symptoms usually mild or absent; fatigue may be pronounced
Si   Jaundice, hepatomegaly
Ix   HCV antibody, HCV RNA by PCR
Rx   Antiviral therapy: usually peginterferon α and ribavirin, although many new treatments in development
Cx   >80 per cent develop chronic HCV infection
~30 per cent develop cirrhosis
↑ risk of hepatocellular carcinoma

HEPATITIS D VIRUS (HDV)

P RNA virus, dependent on presence of HBV for infectivity
A Corresponds to HBV infection
S As for HBV
Ix HDAg, HDV RNA by PCR
Anti-HDV and RNA are markers of replication; persistent HDV antibody is consistent with chronic HDV
Rx Treatment is usually supportive; limited response to antivirals
Prevention is only by immunity to HBV; HBV carriers should avoid HDV endemic areas
Cx As for HBV

HEPATITIS E VIRUS (HEV)

P RNA virus, faecal–oral transmission
S Very similar to hepatitis A
Ix HEV antibody, HEV RNA
Rx Supportive, prevention by improvements in sanitation
Cx Fulminant hepatic failure: 20 per cent incidence in pregnant women

AUTOIMMUNE DISEASE

AUTOIMMUNE HEPATITIS (AIH)

P Periportal piecemeal necrosis/bridging necrosis; fibrosis
A More common in young women
Sy Fatigue, abdominal discomfort, decreased appetite, myalgia
Si Hepatomegaly, icterus, signs of chronic liver disease/cirrhosis
Ix Raised transaminases, $\uparrow$ ESR, ANA +ve, smooth muscle antibody +ve, anti-LKM (liver, kidney, microsomal antibodies) +ve, $\uparrow$ IgG, liver biopsy
Rx Steroids, azathioprine, ursodeoxycholic acid (UDCA), liver transplantation

PRIMARY BILIARY CIRRHOSIS (PBC)

P Chronic inflammation and destruction of the small and medium bile ducts
A 80–90 per cent women; age 30–60 years

S Fatigue, pruritus, arthralgia, xanthelasma, hepatomegaly, splenomegaly, jaundice, signs of chronic liver disease, osteoporosis
Ix cholestatic LFTs; $\uparrow$ IgM, antimitochondrial antibody (AMA) +ve (in ~95 per cent), ANA +ve (in ~40 per cent), liver biopsy
Rx *Pruritus*: colestyramine, UDCA, antihistamines
Osteoporosis and hypercholesterolaemia: bisphosphonates, statins
Immunosuppression: prednisolone, azathioprine
Liver transplantation

PRIMARY SCLEROSING CHOLANGITIS (PSC)

(P) Progressive fibrosis and obliteration of the biliary ducts

(A) 70 per cent men; 3rd–5th decade; associated with inflammatory bowel disease (mainly ulcerative colitis)

(S) Can be asymptomatic; fatigue, weight loss, fever, pruritus, RUQ discomfort, hepatomegaly; may have relapsing cholangitis

(Ix) Cholestatic LFTs; pANCA +ve, ANA +ve, ↑IgM, MRCP/ERCP (endoscopic retrograde cholangiopancreatography), liver biopsy

(Rx) *Medical*: UDCA, prednisolone and methotrexate
Endoscopy: therapeutic ERCP: sphincterotomy/stent insertion
Surgery: liver transplantation

METABOLIC DISORDERS

NON-ALCOHOLIC STEATOHEPATITIS (NASH)

(P) When liver fat content >12 per cent = fatty liver; this can lead to inflammation and fibrosis

(A) ♀ > ♂
Viral hepatitis and autoimmune conditions **must** be excluded
Multiple other causes – commonest are obesity, diabetes and hyperlipidaemia

(S) Often asymptomatic and found after routine blood tests reveal abnormal LFTs, hepatomegaly, fatigue

(Ix) LFT-raised transaminases, liver screen to rule out other causes of liver disease, lipid screen, HbA_{1c}, USS, liver biopsy is diagnostic

(Rx) No specific treatments; aim at removing any causative factors; alcohol abstinence

HEREDITARY HAEMOCHROMATOSIS (HHC)

(P) Autosomal recessive mutations in the *HFE* gene leading to abnormal absorption of iron

(A) ♂:♀ ratio = 5–10:1

(Si) Iron overload in multiple sites throughout the body, leading to a wide variety of signs: hepatomegaly, stigmata of chronic liver disease, ascites, splenomegaly, fatigue, arthralgia, pigmentation

(Sy) Symptoms of cardiomyopathy, diabetes mellitus, hypothyroidism, hypogonadism, hypoparathyroidism, joint pain

(Ix) ↑ferritin, iron and transferrin saturation; HFE genotyping and family genotyping; raised transaminases, ↑IgG, USS/CT/MRI, liver biopsy

(Rx) Venesection, desferrioxamine, low iron diet, alcohol abstinence, liver transplantation, screening for HCC

(Cx) HCC, liver failure

WILSON'S DISEASE

(P) Autosomal recessive; abnormal hepatobiliary copper excretion

(S) Related to the degree and sites of copper deposition

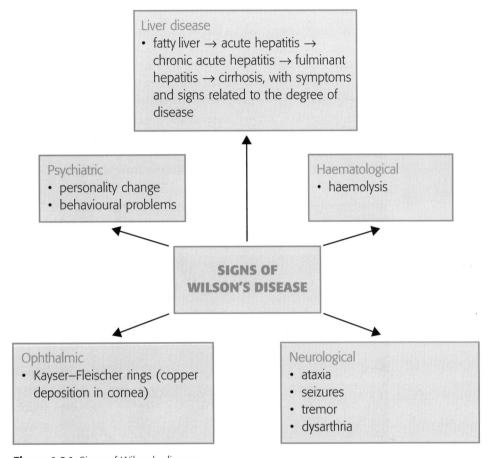

Figure 1.24 Signs of Wilson's disease

Ix   ↑ serum free copper and urinary copper, ↓ caeruloplasmin, USS, liver biopsy, penicillamine test
To assess other organ involvement: slit lamp eye examination, MRI, ECG, echo, EEG, EMG (electromyogram)

Rx   D-penicillamine (chelates copper), low copper diet, liver transplantation

INFECTIONS

LIVER ABSCESS

P   Bacterial, helminthic, fungal or protozoal
Spread via blood, post-traumatic, directly or via the biliary tree

S   Fever, RUQ pain/tenderness, right-sided pleural effusion, septicaemia, rupture

Ix   FBC, LFT, CRP, ESR, CXR, USS ± CT, angiography is required to assess arterial anatomy pre-operatively, USS/CT-guided aspiration

Rx   Intravenous antibiotics, aspiration, percutaneous drainage, surgery

HYDATID DISEASE

(P) Majority due to *Echinococcus cysticus*, a tapeworm; commonly found in areas of cattle breeding; spread via faecal–oral route

Larvae travel to the portal system via the intestine and form fluid-filled cysts (hydatids) in the liver; these can grow up to 1 cm/year

(Sy) RUQ pain once the cyst is large enough

(Si) Hepatomegaly due to hydatid growth

(Ix) Eosinophilia, LFT, serology, USS

(Rx) ~10 per cent spontaneously regress; surgical removal, mebendazole/albendazole

(Cx) Rupture of the hydatid will cause an anaphylactic reaction

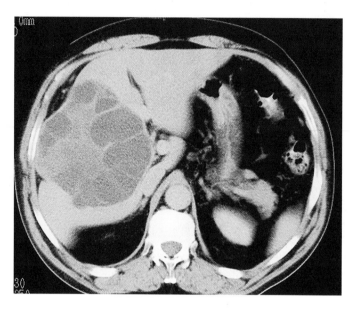

Figure 1.25 Hydatid cyst: a well-delineated multiloculated cystic mass, with orderly internal septations (daughter cysts), in the right lobe of the liver

HEPATIC TUMOURS

HEPATIC ADENOMA

(P) Vary in size and number, usually solitary and found in the right lobe

(A) Found in women in their reproductive years; often associated with oral contraceptives

(S) Usually asymptomatic and found by chance; if large, they may be associated with abdominal discomfort; haemorrhage: severe pain

(Ix) LFTs normal; USS, CT, MRI, liver biopsy

(Rx) Embolization, surgery

HEPATOCELLULAR CARCINOMA (HCC)

(A) Affects all age groups; slight increased incidence in men (ratio 2–3:1)

Liver disease: cirrhosis, HBV, HCV, HDV, haemochromatosis, α_1-antitrypsin deficiency, autoimmune hepatitis, PBC

Alcohol, smoking; drugs, genetics

(Sy)   Weight loss, anorexia, abdominal pain
(Si)   Cachexia, hepatomegaly, fever, lymphadenopathy
        Metastases may also add to the symptoms and signs: lungs, bone, lymph nodes
(Ix)   Raised transaminases, ↑ alpha-fetoprotein, CRP and ESR may be raised; there may
        be cholestasis if the tumour affects the intrahepatic bile ducts; USS (microbubble
        contrast), CT, MRI; liver biopsy (only if diagnosis is in question, as the procedure
        may cause tumour spread)
(Rx)   Resection, liver transplant, chemoembolization, ethanol injection, laser ablation

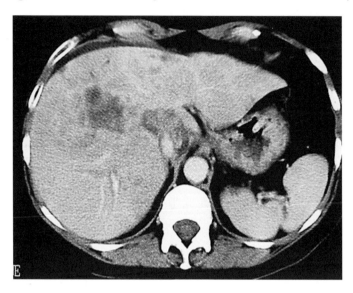

Figure
1.26 Hepatocellular
carcinoma: localized
poorly marginated mixed
density area in the right
lobe of the liver

NEUROLOGY

NEUROLOGY INVESTIGATIONS

- **CT:** study of choice in acute trauma and haemorrhage; usually given with contrast to help enhance tumours, infections and infarcts
- **MRI:** T_1-weighted images enhance acute haemorrhage; T_2-weighted images enhance oedema, infarction, demyelination and chronic haemorrhage
- **Angiography** can also be performed with or without contrast
- **EEG:** electrodes are placed on the scalp and electrical activity of the brain is recorded; particularly important in evaluating epilepsy
- **Evoked potentials:** electrical potentials are measured while nerves are repetitively stimulated; the commonest use is in visual evoked potentials to diagnose multiple sclerosis
- **Nerve conduction studies:** nerves are stimulated and the electrical activity is measured from different points; conduction velocity can be recorded
- **EMG:** electromyography records electrical potentials from needle electrodes in muscle at rest and during contraction; this can differentiate between neuropathic and myopathic disorders
- **Lumbar puncture:** cerebrospinal fluid (CSF) is taken via a needle inserted into the spinal column between L3/4 or L4/5
- **Tensilon test:** a short-acting anticholinesterase (edrophonium) is given intravenously to see if there is any improvement in those with suspected myasthenia gravis

ISCHAEMIA

CEREBROVASCULAR DISEASE/ISCHAEMIC STROKE

(P) Acute occlusion of an intracranial vessel leading to hypoxia and infarction; if blood flow is restored prior to significant cell death there may be transient symptoms: transient ischaemic attack (TIA)

(A) Diabetes mellitus, hypertension, smoking, hypercholesterolaemia, family history, age, atrial fibrillation, valvular lesions, cardiac congenital defects, hypercoagulable states, vasculitis

(S) Symptoms are variable and dependent on the area and arteries involved; Box 1.15 gives an idea of symptoms related to territories.

Box 1.15 SYMPTOMS OF CEREBROVASCULAR DISEASE ACCORDING TO TERRITORIES

Anterior cerebral artery occlusion
- Contralateral hemiplegia
- Gait apraxia
- Abulia (severe apathy)
- Urinary incontinence
- Lower limb sensory loss

Middle cerebral artery occlusion
- Contralateral hemiplegia
- Homonymous hemianopia
- Contralateral sensory loss
- Dysarthria, dysphasia
  Non-dominant symptoms include:
  - Aphasia
  - Neglect
  - Constructional apraxia

Posterior cerebral artery occlusion
- Homonymous hemianopia ± macular sparing
- Contralateral hemiplegia
- Ataxia/hemiballismus
- Visual agnosia
- Cortical blindness

Posterior inferior cerebellar artery (PICA) occlusion
- Syncope
- Vertigo
- Hemiplegia
- Dysarthria
- Ipsilateral face numbness
- Contralateral limb numbness

Basilar artery occlusion
- Dizziness
- Vertigo
- Diplopia
- Dysarthria
- Facial numbness
- Ipsilateral hemiparesis

Ix FBC, U&E, lipids, ESR, CRP, fasting glucose CT, MRI with diffusion-weighted imaging (DWI), MR angiography, carotid dopplers, echo, ECG, 24-hour tape

Rx *Medical*: aspirin, clopidogrel, dipyridamole, anticoagulation
Thrombolysis is not yet in widespread use
Collateral blood flow is blood pressure dependent, therefore BP should not be lowered unless there are signs of malignant hypertension
Surgery: carotid endarterectomy

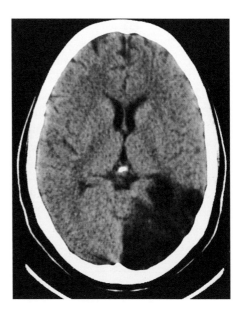

Figure 1.27 Large left posterior cerebral artery infarct

CEREBELLAR SYNDROME

A Vascular lesion, alcohol, demyelination, tumours, paraneoplastic phenomenon, hypothyroidism, phenytoin toxicity, metabolic disorders (e.g. Wilson's disease)

Sy Poor balance, dysphasia

Si 'DANISH', see Box 1.16

Box 1.16 FEATURES OF CEREBELLAR SYNDROMES
Dysdiadochokinesis **A**taxia **N**ystagmus **I**ntention tremor, past pointing **S**canning speech, dysarthria **H**ypotonia, hyporeflexia

Ix MRI

Rx Treatment aimed at underlying disorder

INFECTION

MENINGITIS

P Infection of the meninges; commonest pathogen is *Streptococcus pneumoniae*; other bacterial pathogens include *Neisseria meningitidis*, *Haemophilus influenzae*, *Listeria monocytogenes* and *Mycobacterium tuberculosis*
Can also be caused by viruses and fungal infection

A Higher risk in immunosuppressed individuals

(Sy)   Headache, photophobia, nausea, vomiting, neck pain

(Si)   Fever, neck stiffness, confusion, drowsiness, petechiae, Kernig's sign (hamstring spasm when attempting to straighten leg)

(Ix)   FBC, U&E, LFT, coagulation, blood cultures, CXR, lumbar puncture (LP). NB do not perform LP if patient has a petechial rash, without the results of clotting profile (need to exclude DIC [disseminated intravascular coagulation]); if there are any neurological signs or conscious level is reduced, perform a CT head prior to LP (? brain abscess)

CSF samples can also be sent for PCR to identify meningococcus, AFB and viruses

Table 1.4 Lumbar puncture results

	Neutrophils (×10^6/L)	Lymphocytes (×10^6/L)	Protein (g/L)	Glucose (ratio CSF/ serum)
Normal	0	<5	<0.4	>0.6
Bacterial	↑↑↑	↑	>1.0	<0.4
Viral	↑	↑↑↑	0.4–1.0	Usually normal
Tuberculosis	↑	↑↑↑	>1.0	<0.4

(Rx)   Start empirical antibiotics immediately; most hospitals advocate third generation cephalosporins (e.g. cefotaxime), plus ampicillin if *Listeria* is suspected

Specific treatment for TB can usually be held off until CSF results are available

Chemoprophylaxis is often offered to close contacts of meningococcal meningitis (e.g. rifampicin)

Close liaison with microbiologist is essential

(Cx)   Seizures, hydrocephalus, cerebral venous/sagittal sinus thrombosis, neurological sequelae, DIC, multi-organ failure, death

ENCEPHALITIS

(P)   Infection of the brain parenchyma

(A)   Can be primary or secondary to viral infections from other areas of the body; 10 per cent caused by herpes simplex virus, which is dealt with here

(S)   Prodromal viral symptoms; headaches, fever, meningism, confusion, delirium, seizures, neurological deficits

(Ix)   FBC, U&E, clotting, septic screen

Specific tests: MRI, EEG, LP with CSF results as for viral meningitis, CSF HSV PCR

(Rx)   Aciclovir; supportive and symptomatic treatment (e.g. for seizures) with close liaison with microbiologist and ITU

(Cx)   Fatal if untreated and causes death in 7–10 days; neurological sequelae e.g. seizures, amnesia, motor deficits, etc.

DEMYELINATION

MULTIPLE SCLEROSIS (MS)

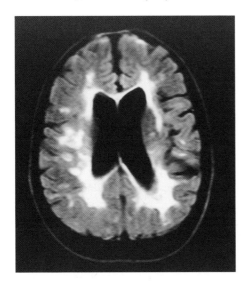

Figure 1.28 Multiple areas of increased signal in the periventricular deep white matter are demyelination plaques in multiple sclerosis

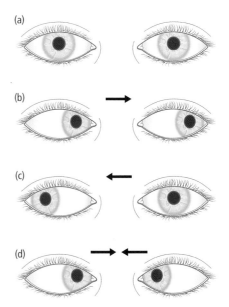

Figure 1.29 Left internuclear ophthalmoplegia. The lesion affects the left medial longitudinal fasciculus (MLF) and prevents adduction of the ipsilateral eye during conjugate gaze (c); convergence is usually normal (d)

P   Chronic disease of the central nervous system (CNS), characterized by white plaques (areas of demyelination and perivascular inflammation) disseminated in time and occurring anywhere within the CNS

A   Affects people within their reproductive years; ? immune dysfunction ? viral association
Incidence ↑ with distance from the equator

S   Symptoms depend on the position of plaques; usually follows a relapsing–remitting course but can be primary progressive, secondary progressive or progressive relapsing. Commoner presentations include internuclear ophthalmoplegia (see Fig. 1.29), optic neuritis, cerebellar syndrome, weakness, sensory disturbance, Lhermitte's sign (electric sensation down spine on neck flexion)

Ix   Lumbar puncture/CSF (↑ protein, ↑ immunoglobulin levels, oligoclonal bands), visual evoked potentials, sensory evoked potentials, MRI (demyelinating lesions)

Rx   High-dose steroids for exacerbations; interferon-β; treatments for muscle spasm (e.g. baclofen), tremor (e.g. clonazepam), pain (e.g. gabapentin), urinary incontinence (e.g. anticholinergics), antidepressants

Px   Increased risk of suicide; mean prognosis 25–35 years

GUILLAIN–BARRÉ SYNDROME

(P) Autoimmune response causing demyelination

(A) Usually follows a respiratory or GI infection; associated with infections, malignancies, drugs, pregnancy, vaccinations

(Sy) Progressive ascending weakness, sensory loss, paraesthesia, pain, dysphasia, dysarthria

(Si) Dysreflexia, hypotonia, papilloedema, bulbar palsy, labile vital signs due to autonomic involvement
Cranial nerves are involved in 45–70 per cent

(Ix) Pregnancy test, LFT ($\uparrow$), lumbar puncture ($\uparrow$ CSF protein; normal cell counts), nerve conduction studies (may take 2–3 weeks to develop abnormalities), antibody screen, ECG, MRI, spirometry

(Rx) Intravenous immunoglobulin, plasmapheresis; close monitoring for cardiac arrhythmias and respiratory failure, and close liaison with ITU; DVT (deep vein thrombosis) prophylaxis

(Cx) Mortality 5–10 per cent; autonomic lability, pneumonia, respiratory failure, cardiac arrhythmias, neurological sequelae

AUTOIMMUNE DISORDERS

MYASTHENIA GRAVIS

(P) Autoimmune condition with antibodies directed against the acetylcholine receptors on the post-synaptic muscle membrane

(A) Thymus is abnormal in ~75 per cent: 65 per cent have hyperplastic thymus, ~10 per cent have thymic tumours; prevalence 1 in 7500; ♀:♂ 3:2

(S) Weakness and fatiguability; often affects cranial muscles early leading to ptosis, diplopia, dysarthria, dysphagia; limb weakness is often proximal
If respiratory function is affected this is a myasthenic crisis

(Ix) Acetylcholine receptor antibodies, CXR/CT (to look at the thymus), anticholinesterase/edrophonium test (Tensilon test), nerve conduction studies, thyroid function, spirometry

(Rx) Medical: anticholinesterases e.g. pyridostigmine
Surgery: thymectomy: improvement in ~85 per cent of patients
Immunosuppression: steroids, azathioprine, ciclosporin, mycophenolate mofetil, cyclophosphamide (rarely)
Emergency treatment: intravenous immunoglobulins, plasmapheresis

PERIPHERAL NEUROPATHY

(A) Sensory neuropathy: diabetes, alcohol, rheumatoid arthritis, drugs, malignancy, B$_{12}$ deficiency, chronic renal failure
Motor neuropathy: Guillain–Barré syndrome, lead toxicity, porphyria, Charcot–Marie–Tooth disease

(S) Commonly there is a sensory loss in a stocking distribution; usually a full history and examination will give clues as to the underlying cause

(Ix) Urine dipstick, blood sugar, FBC, B$_{12}$ levels, history of alcohol consumption

(Rx) Aimed at underlying cause

CHARCOT–MARIE–TOOTH DISEASE/HEREDITARY MOTOR AND SENSORY NEUROPATHY (HMSN)

(P) Several types of hereditary motor and sensory neuropathies, classified according to the genetic mutations

Neuronal degeneration; caused by mutations to genes coding the proteins involved in the structure or function of nerve axons or myelin sheaths

(A) Inherited disorder; mostly autosomal dominant, but there are X-linked varieties

(Sy) Gradual onset; some asymptomatic patients are picked up on screening

Loss of balance, foot deformities (high arches/hammer toes), weakness

(Si) Weakness, atrophy, hyporeflexia/areflexia, sensory loss, nerve enlargement

(Ix) NCS (nerve conduction studies), EMG, nerve biopsy, genetic testing

Differential diagnosis: need to exclude other causes of neuropathy, including infectious, immunological, endocrinological causes, and vitamin and nutritional deficiencies

(Rx) Physiotherapy, occupational therapy, orthopaedic devices to maintain mobility, analgesia

(Px) Normal life expectancy

NERVE DISORDERS

FACIAL NERVE PALSY

(A) Bell's palsy, acoustic neuromas, multiple sclerosis, infarcts, tumours, Lyme disease, sarcoidosis

Ramsay Hunt syndrome: facial palsy due to herpes zoster affecting the geniculate ganglion

(S) Facial weakness

Upper motor neurone palsy: the frontalis and orbicularis oculi function are preserved, i.e. the patient can raise their eyebrows

Lower motor neurone palsy: this function is lost

Ramsay Hunt syndrome: vesicular eruptions of herpes zoster

Acoustic neuromas: involvement of the 8th cranial nerve

Sarcoidosis: parotid gland enlargement/tenderness

(Ix) Bell's palsy/Ramsay Hunt syndrome (lower motor neurone palsy) do not require further investigation; other conditions listed are described in their own relevant sections

(Rx) *Medical*: steroids for Bell's palsy, aciclovir if any evidence of herpes zoster

Supportive: taping down eyelids overnight to prevent corneal drying

TRIGEMINAL NEURALGIA

(P) Pathophysiology unknown ? vascular compression leading to demyelination

(A) Usually idiopathic; can occur secondary to brain tumours, MS, cranial neuropathies or cerebral aneurysms, but this is rare without other neurological features

(Sy) Sudden, severe, unilateral electric shock-like or stabbing pain typically felt on one side of the jaw or cheek; affects right side > left side

Triggers include talking, chewing, smiling, brushing teeth, touching the face, or swallowing

Attacks recur at varying intervals (up to hundreds per day) and last for days, weeks, or months at a time, and then remit for months or years

Attacks rarely occur during sleep

(Si) Neurological examination is normal

(Ix) No specific investigation required as diagnosis is clinical; if any neurological deficits are present trigeminal neuralgia is unlikely and brain imaging should be performed

(Rx) Anticonvulsants (carbamazepine, gabapentin); neurosurgical treatment may be required if medical treatment fails

PUPILLARY ABNORMALITIES

HORNER'S SYNDROME/PTOSIS

(P) Interrupted sympathetic innervation to the eye, at any level from a central lesion to the post-ganglionic fibres

(A) *Central lesions*: basal meningitis, demyelinating disease, cerebrovascular accident (CVA), basal skull tumours, pituitary tumour, intrapontine haemorrhage, neck trauma, syringomyelia

Preganglionic lesions: Pancoast's tumour, cervical rib, aneurysm/dissection of aorta, trauma/surgical injury, lesions of the middle ear, neuroblastoma

Post-ganglionic lesions: Herpes zoster, migraine, internal carotid dissection

Drugs: e.g. chlorpromazine, levodopa, prochlorperazine, oral contraceptive pill (OCP), reserpine

(S) Miosis, ptosis, anhidrosis

(Ix) Diagnosis is clinical; further investigations depend on the location of the lesion, but usually include CT/MRI

(Rx) Aimed at underlying cause

HOLMES–ADIE SYNDROME

(P) Normal variant; rarely a result of a lesion in the efferent parasympathetic pathway

(A) Commoner in young women

(S) Holmes–Adie pupil is a large irregular pupil; pupillary constriction to light (direct and consensual) is slow and incomplete, and the pupil remains constricted for an abnormally long time; usually unilateral

When associated with absent deep tendon jerks, termed Holmes–Adie syndrome

(Ix) Diagnosis is clinical

(Rx) No treatment required

ARGYLL ROBERTSON PUPIL

(A) Neurosyphilis, diabetes mellitus, multiple sclerosis, syringobulbia

(S) Miosis, irregular pupil, absent light reflex, intact accommodation reflex

(Ix) Syphilis serology, urine dipstick (blood/ketones), blood sugar ± CT/MRI brain

(Rx) Based on underlying cause

DEGENERATIVE DISORDERS

ALZHEIMER'S DISEASE (AD)

(P) Cerebral atrophy; neurofibrillary tangles and senile plaques

(A) Most common cause of dementia

Affects >40 per cent of over 80 year olds; <10 per cent are familial

(Sy) Progressive memory loss

(Si) Cognitive impairment; as disease progresses it can affect behaviour, extrapyramidal and cerebellar systems

(Ix) Required to exclude other causes of confusion/memory impairment; this includes FBC, B_{12}, U&E, LFT, TFT, syphilis serology, cortisol, glucose, CT brain; EEG and LP occasionally required to rule out other conditions e.g. Creutzfeldt–Jakob disease (CJD), neurosyphilis, normal pressure hydrocephalus

(Rx) Symptomatic therapy: anxiolytics, antidepressants, antipsychotics; cholinesterase inhibitors (e.g. donepezil), N-methyl-D-aspartate antagonists (e.g. memantine)

FRIEDREICH'S ATAXIA

(P) Degeneration of neurones in the spinal column, due to a gene mutation, causing reduction in the protein 'frataxin'; it affects the posterior columns, corticospinal columns, and ventral and lateral spinocerebellar tracts; also affects myocardial and spinal muscle fibres

(A) Autosomal recessive

(S) Onset usually <20 years; foot deformities (hammer toes, clubfoot), ataxia (sensory ± cerebellar), weakness, distal wasting, loss of lower limb tendon reflexes, extensor plantar reflex, gradual sensory loss, nystagmus, dysarthria, dysphagia

(Ix) Genetic testing, MRI (cervical spinal cord atrophy, with no signs of cerebellar atrophy), sensory nerve action potentials (absent in >90 per cent), visual evoked potential (reduced amplitude and delayed), ECHO, ECG

(Rx) No effective cure or treatment

(Cx) Prognosis 15–20 years; other complications: optic atrophy, deafness, diabetes mellitus, cardiomyopathy, heart block, myocardial fibrosis, scoliosis

PARKINSON'S DISEASE (PD)

(P) Degeneration of the dopaminergic neurones of the substantia nigra

(A) Increased incidence in males, rural living, exposure to well water, positive family history

Important to check drug history to ensure the patient does not have drug-induced parkinsonism (commonly from neuroleptics)

(S) Resting tremor, rigidity, bradykinesia

Other symptoms: masked facies, stooped posture, micrographia, hypophonia, shuffling gait, instability, anosmia, depression, aching pain, sleep disorders, cognitive impairment

(Ix) PD is normally diagnosed clinically

In young (<40 years) patients Wilson's disease (see Hepatology section, p. 42) and mass lesions should be ruled out

(Rx)   *Medical*: dopamine agonists (cabergoline), levodopa/carbidopa, monoamine oxidase B inhibitor (selegiline), catechol *O*-methyltransferase (COMT) inhibitors (entacapone), anticholinergics, amantadine
Surgery: pallidotomy/thalamotomy (radio-frequency ablation), deep brain stimulation (implanted electrodes)

HUNTINGDON'S DISEASE (HD)

(P)   Autosomal dominant; gene on chromosome 4 encodes a protein called *huntingtin*, which accumulates in the brain cells causing damage

(A)   Affects males and females equally; usually presents >35 years

(Sy)   Involuntary movements, erratic/argumentative behaviour, depression

(Si)   Chorea, rigidity, dystonia, loss of saccadic eye movements, behavioural problems, dementia, weight loss

(Ix)   Family history is the most important diagnostic tool; DNA analysis to identify the *HD* gene; CT/MRI

(Rx)   Nil specific; antidepressants ± tranquillizers to control chorea

(Px)   Progressive illness, with death within 15–20 years of diagnosis

MUSCLE DISEASE

MOTOR NEURONE DISEASE (AMYOTROPHIC LATERAL SCLEROSIS)

(P)   Degeneration of upper and lower motor neurones, of unknown cause

(A)   5–10 per cent of cases follow an autosomal dominant pattern; the rest are sporadic ♂ > ♀; 40–60 years

(S)   See Box 1.17

Box 1.17 COMMON PRESENTATIONS OF MOTOR NEURONE DISEASE

- *Spinal muscular atrophy*: limb weakness due to involvement of spinal cord anterior horn cells
- *Primary lateral sclerosis*: spastic limb weakness due to upper motor neurone involvement of the spinal cord
- *Progressive bulbar palsy*: involvement of bulbar motor neurons; it is a progressive disease
- *Amyotrophic lateral sclerosis* (ALS): a mixture of all the above

---

Cardiac and smooth muscle are not involved; ocular muscles very rarely
Autonomic dysfunction occurs late; emotional lability (associated with pseudo-bulbar palsy)

(Ix)   No specific test; diagnosed clinically when other causes of motor neurone damage have been excluded; EMG confirms fasciculations and fibrillations

(Rx)   Antispasmodics (e.g. baclofen), glutamate antagonists (e.g. riluzole); emotional and symptomatic support

(Cx)   Fatal within 3–5 years; death commonly from cardiac arrhythmias or respiratory failure

MYOTONIC DYSTROPHY (DYSTROPHIA MYOTONICA)

(P) Autosomal dominant condition

(S) Atrophy of temporalis, masseter and facial and neck muscles; dysarthria and dysphagia (secondary to pharyngeal, palatal and tongue involvement), myotonia, frontal balding, mitral valve prolapse, heart block, congestive heart failure, cataracts, intellectual impairment, insulin resistance, hypersomnia

(Ix) Diagnosis usually clinical with family history
Creatine kinase (CK), muscle biopsy (showing atrophy), EMG (myotonia)

(Rx) Rarely requires treatment; phenytoin very occasionally used

METABOLIC DISORDERS

SUBACUTE COMBINED DEGENERATION OF THE SPINAL CORD

(P) B_{12} deficiency leading to degeneration of the posterior column and corticospinal tracts of the spinal cord

(A) Pernicious anaemia, dietary deficiency, malabsorption

(Sy) Constant and progressive; paraesthesiae, weakness, sensory deficits

(Si) Sensorimotor neuropathy, lower limb spasticity, ataxia, extensor plantar response, loss of ankle jerk, optic atrophy/neuritis, variable mood changes

(Ix) FBC, B_{12} levels, intrinsic factor antibody

(Rx) B_{12} replacement

(Cx) Prognosis in terms of neurological sequelae is reduced by speed of treatment

MISCELLANEOUS

EPILEPSY

(P) Abnormal neuronal activity leads to seizures

(A) Idiopathic, genetic defects, metabolic abnormalities (e.g. alcohol withdrawal, low blood glucose), post-trauma, hypoxic damage, brain tumour, cerebrovascular disease, Alzheimer's disease

---

Box 1.18 CLASSIFICATION OF EPILEPSY

- *Partial seizures*: abnormal electrical discharge originates from discrete regions of the brain; they can be simple (patient fully conscious) or complex (decreased awareness)
- *Generalized seizures*: abnormal electrical discharge involves the entire brain
- *Absence seizures*: 'petit mal'; sudden brief lapses of consciousness without loss of postural control
- *Tonic–clonic seizures*: 'grand mal'; involve jerking movements
- *Atonic seizures*: sudden loss of postural muscle tone; lasts 1–2 s
- *Myoclonic seizures*: sudden contractions of the limbs, usually followed by unconsciousness

---

(Ix) FBC, U&E, calcium, glucose, magnesium, LFT, urine/serum toxins, EEG, CT/MRI brain, EEG

(Rx) Anti-epileptics

(Cx) Status epilepticus

SYRINGOMYELIA/SYRINGOBULBIA

(P) Formation of a fluid-filled cavity (or syrinx) within the spinal column; when this involves the brainstem it is termed 'syringobulbia'

(A) Meningeal carcinomatosis, Arnold–Chiari malformation, intramedullary tumours, spinal cord injury, haemorrhage, meningitis, idiopathic

♂ > ♀

(S) Usually slowly progressive
- Dissociated sensory loss: loss of pain and temperature, while light touch, vibration, and position senses are preserved; it may affect the upper limbs in a 'shawl' distribution
- Muscle atrophy due to extension into the anterior horns of the spinal cord; this begins in the hands and progresses proximally
- Pain
- Lower limb upper motor neurone signs: spasticity, weakness, hyperreflexia
- Autonomic dysfunction

Syringobulbia: characterized by nystagmus, dysphagia, tongue atrophy, palatal weakness and sensory loss in the distribution of the trigeminal nerve

Other manifestations: Charcot joints

(Ix) MRI; CSF pressure/protein may be raised

(Rx) Surgery, physiotherapy

NEUROFIBROMATOSIS

(P) Genetic disorders that affect growth of nerve cells and lead to the formation of tumours on nerves; separated into Type I and Type II

(A) Autosomal dominant, although many new presentations are due to genetic mutations

(S) See Box 1.19

Box 1.19 DIAGNOSIS OF NEUROFIBROMATOSIS

Neurofibromatosis 1
Two or more of the following:
Five or more light *café au lait* macules (diameter > 5 mm in prepubertal patients or >15 mm across in postpubertal individuals)
Two or more neurofibromas or one plexiform neurofibroma
First-degree relative with neurofibromatosis 1
Two or more Lisch nodules (iris hamartomas)
Freckling in the armpit or groin areas
Optic glioma
Severe scoliosis
Other bony enlargement or deformity

Neurofibromatosis 2
Bilateral tumours of the VIIIth cranial nerve

or

First-degree relative with neurofibromatosis 2 *plus* unilateral VIIIth cranial nerve tumour

or

Two neurofibroma, glioma, schwannoma, meningioma, or juvenile cataracts

(Ix) Family history, genetic testing, MRI, slit lamp testing for Lisch nodules
(Rx) Supportive e.g. excision of tumours causing hearing loss or bony deformities
(Cx) Increased risk of malignancy

MIGRAINE

(P) Exact pathogenesis unknown; ? vasoconstriction, ? neurotransmitters, ? vasoactive substances
(A) ♀ > ♂ (ratio 2–3:1)
(Sy) Headache: throbbing, usually unilateral initially, becoming diffuse over 1–2 h, lasting up to 24 h; nausea/vomiting, photophobia, some have a preceding aura
(Si) Patients normally have a normal neurological examination; occasional sensory or motor deficits; visual deficits, e.g. scotoma, field defects
(Ix) Migraines can be diagnosed clinically, but if a patient presents to the emergency department for the first time (especially with neurological deficits) other causes must be excluded
(Rx) *Prophylaxis*: anti-epileptics, β-blockers, amitriptyline, selective serotonin reuptake inhibitor (SSRI) antidepressants, serotonin antagonists (e.g. methysergide)
Acute attacks: analgesics (paracetamol, NSAIDs, opioids), anti-emetics, 5-HT$_1$ agonists (e.g. sumatriptan), ergot alkaloids (e.g. ergotamine)

NEPHROLOGY

RENAL INVESTIGATIONS

- **Colour:** see Table 1.5

Table 1.5 Variations in urine colour

Colour	Cause
Clear light yellow	Normal
Lighter	Dilute
Darker	Concentrated
Red	Haematuria
White	Pyuria/phosphate crystals
Green	Amitriptyline/propofol
Black	Malignancy/haemolysis

- **Urine dipstick:** can detect albumin but not pathological proteins (i.e. Bence–Jones proteins or microalbuminuria)

- **Urine microscopy – casts:**
  - hyaline (not pathological, can be caused by diuretics)
  - red cell casts (glomerulonephritis, vasculitis)
  - white cell casts (tubulo-interstitial disease, acute pyelonephritis and some glomerulonephritis), epithelial cells (acute tubular necrosis [ATN], acute glomerulonephritis [AGN])
- **Urine microscopy – crystals:**
  - uric acid (+ ARF [acute renal failure] = tumour lysis syndrome)
  - calcium phosphate
  - oxalate
  - cystine (cystinuria)
- **Renal biopsy:**
  - *indication*: unexplained CRF (chronic renal failure) with normal/large kidneys, unexplained progressive renal impairment, nephrotic syndrome, renal impairment + proteinuria + haematuria ± systemic disorders, intrinsic ARF
  - *complications*: bleeding, localized bruising and pain, haematuria, sepsis, perforation of other organs
- **Glomerular filtration rate (GFR):** GFR is the volume of fluid filtered from the renal glomerular capillaries into Bowman's capsule per unit time. Clinically, this is often measured to determine renal function by the approximation:

$$\frac{\text{urine creatinine concentration} \times \text{urine volume (24 h)}}{\text{plasma creatinine concentration}}$$

  - normal GFR: male: 97–137 mL/min.; female: 88–128 mL/min
- **24-h protein:** normal <150 mg/day

GLOMERULONEPHRITIS (GN)

(A) Either primary or secondary (i.e. part of a systemic illness – Wegener's, SLE, diabetes, vasculitis)

(P) Inflammation of the glomeruli affecting both kidneys simultaneously
Histological classification:
- minimal change
- focal and segmental proliferative
- focal and segmental glomerulosclerosis
- mesangial proliferative GN (± IgA)
- crescentic GN
- membranous GN
- mesangiocapillary GN

(S) Features of either nephritic, nephrotic syndrome or non-specific, i.e. weight loss, nausea and vomiting, anorexia, hiccups, pruritus, oliguria, nocturia (see Table 1.6)

Table 1.6 Presentations of renal disease

GN type	Renal failure	Nephrotic syndrome	Nephritic syndrome
Post-infection	++	−	+
Vasculitis	++	+	+
Crescentic mesangiocapillary	++	+	++
Membranous FSGS	+	++	++
Minimal change	+	++	+
Chronic infection	−	+	++

FSGS: focal segmental glomerulosclerosis

Ix Bloods: renal profile, blood film (haemolysis → haemolytic uraemic syndrome), arterial blood gases (ABG) (metabolic acidosis), C3 + C4 (low),
Auto-antibodies:
- ANA (SLE)
- cANCA (Wegener's granulomatosis)
- pANCA (polyarteritis nodosa)
- anti-GBM (Goodpasture's syndrome)
- antistreptolysin O (ASO) titres (post-streptococcal GN)

Urine: 24-h urine collection, protein and creatinine clearance, urine dipstick, urine MC&S
Radiology: USS renal tract
Histology: renal biopsy

Rx Treatment depends on underlying cause (i.e. steroids, immunosuppressants)
Symptomatic; tight control of BP, diuretics; may need to consider dialysis/renal transplant

Cx CRF, end-stage renal failure

ACUTE NEPHRITIC SYNDROME

P Group of disorders that cause inflammation of the glomeruli

A Associated with post-group A β-haemolytic streptococcal sore throat (occurs about 2–3/52 later)
Other causes are haemolytic uraemic syndrome, IgA nephropathy, SLE

Sy Asymptomatic, occasionally oliguria, oedema, haematuria, arthralgia, myalgia, nausea, vomiting

Si Hypertension, oedema

Ix *Urine*: haematuria, mild proteinuria, urine microscopy for renal tubular cells, casts, red blood cells (RBCs), white blood cells (WBCs)
Bloods: FBC (↓ Hb, ↑ WBC), U&E, blood cultures
Immunology: ANA, ANCA, anti-GBM, C3, C4
Imaging: Renal USS, renal biopsy

Rx Bed rest, salt restriction, careful fluid monitoring, tight BP control, may need to consider steroids

Cx ARF, CRF, end-stage renal failure (ESRF)

Px Good: adults 60 per cent resolve, children 80–90 per cent

NEPHROTIC SYNDROME

P Classic triad of:
- proteinuria
- hypoalbuminaemia
- oedema (some add hyperlipidaemia)   & prothrombotic ·

A Long-standing diabetes mellitus (DM), GN (minimal change, membranous, focal segmental), amyloid (primary myeloma), autoimmune (SLE), drugs (gold, penicillamine)

Sy Weight gain, loss of appetite, nausea, vomiting, frothy urine, thrombosis

Si Mild hypertension, oedema (dependent sites plus face and hands)

Ix *Bloods*: renal profile, ↑ cholesterol, glucose, protein electrophoresis (myeloma), auto-antibodies (SLE, systemic vasculitis), albumin, clotting, hypogammaglobulinaemia

Urine: 24-h urine creatinine and protein, Bence–Jones protein

Imaging: renal USS/renal biopsy

Cx Hypercoagulability, hypercholesterolaemia, infection

Rx Diuretics, ACE inhibitors, anticoagulation, lipid-controlling agents

HAEMOLYTIC URAEMIC SYNDROME (HUS)

P Combination of haemolysis with red cell fragmentation, thrombocytopenia and acute renal failure

A Often post-infections, classically after pathogenic *E. coli O157*

Si As for acute renal failure

Ix Blood film, FBC, renal profile

Rx *Supportive*: fluids, blood/plasma transfusions

Dialysis

Cx Hypertension, chronic renal failure

ADULT POLYCYSTIC KIDNEY DISEASE (APKD)

P Numerous fluid-filled cysts in the kidneys

A Genetic disorder (autosomal dominant)

8–10 per cent of all ESRF

Presents in early adult life

Sy Dysuria, haematuria, loin pain (renal abscess), polyuria, nocturia, oliguria

Si ↑BP, feature of renal disease, neurological signs secondary to subarachnoid haemorrhage (due to associated cerebral artery berry aneurysm)

Ix Anaemia, clotting, CT, USS

Rx *Patient education*: prognosis, genetic counselling

Medical: treat hypertension and infection

Surgery: transplantation

Cx Liver and pancreatic cysts, cerebral artery berry aneurysms, abnormal heart valves

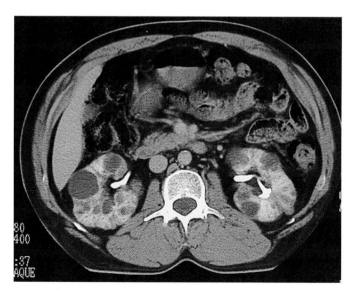

Figure 1.30 Adult polycystic kidney disease with well-defined low-density lesions in both kidneys

RENAL ARTERY STENOSIS

P Narrowing of the artery supplying the kidney

A Atherosclerosis, fibromuscular dysplasia, scar formation

Box 1.20 RISK FACTORS FOR RENAL ARTERY STENOSIS

- Carotid artery disease
- Coronary artery disease
- Smoking
- Peripheral vascular disease
- Diabetes
- Obesity

Sy Difficult to control BP, renal failure with ACE inhibitors

Si ↑BP, renal bruit, flash pulmonary oedema

Ix *Imaging*: renal USS, MRA, renal Doppler USS, angiogram

Rx Control ↑BP, renal balloon angioplasty and stenting

Cx Malignant hypertension, CRF, pulmonary oedema

GOODPASTURE'S SYNDROME

P Autoimmune: antibodies directed against Type IV collagen found in the glomerular and pulmonary alveolar basement membrane

A Commonly young males age 5–40 years (♂:♀ 6:1)

Rx Haematuria, proteinuria, renal failure, pulmonary haemorrhage, haemoptysis

Ix As for any cause of renal failure or pulmonary haemorrhage
Diagnostic markers are anti-GBM antibodies (present in >90 per cent)
Renal biopsy

Rx Plasmapheresis, steroids, immunosuppressants (cyclophosphamide/azathioprine), renal transplantation

URINARY TRACT INFECTION

See 'Urology', p. 194

RENAL FAILURE

ACUTE RENAL FAILURE (ARF)

P Rapid potentially reversible decline in GFR over days to weeks

S *General*: malaise, lethargy, myopathy
Genitourinary: oliguria, polyuria, nocturia
Dermatological: pruritus, rashes, purpura
Cardiovascular: ↑BP, palpitations, pericarditis, oedema
GI: nausea, vomiting, hiccough
Respiratory: pulmonary oedema, Kussmaul's respiration
CNS: peripheral neuropathy, encephalopathy, fits

Ix *Bloods*: FBC, U&E, blood film, blood cultures, ABG
Urine: MC&S
Imaging: CXR, renal USS

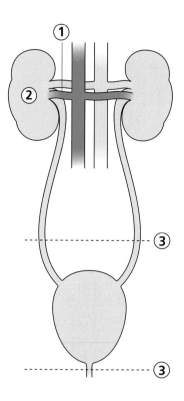

Figure 1.31 Causes of acute renal failure:

1 **Pre-renal:**
   hypovolaemia
   multiple organ failure
   rhabdomyolysis

2 **Renal:**
   acute GN
   acute allergic
     interstitial nephritis
   vasculitis
   acute tubular necrosis

3 **Post-renal:**
   prostatic hypertrophy
   blocked catheter
   extra-ureteric tumour
   retroperitoneal fibrosis

Rx Treat underlying cause

Fluid monitoring (central venous pressure (CVP) line, accurate fluid input and output)

Indications for dialysis:
- pulmonary oedema
- $K^+ > 6.5$ mmol/L (refractory)
- pH < 7.2
- pericarditis
- encephalopathy

Box 1.21 TREATMENT OF HYPERKALAEMIA

- Calcium gluconate (decreases effect of potassium on heart)
- Dextrose and insulin infusion (transfers potassium intracellularly)
- Salbutamol nebulizer (transfers potassium intracellularly)
- Calcium resonium (removes potassium from body)

CHRONIC RENAL FAILURE (CRF)

P Abnormal GFR for >3/12

A GN, interstitial nephritis, reflux nephropathy, polycystic kidneys, DM, renovascular diseases, ↑BP, obstructive uropathy

Sy Malaise, lethargy, nausea, vomiting, headache, hiccups, pruritus, SOB (shortness of breath, secondary to anaemia/pulmonary oedema)

Ix *Bloods*: chronic normochromic anaemia, hypocalcaemia + hyperphosphataemia (can develop hypercalcaemia due to tertiary hyperparathyroidism), metabolic acidosis, hyperkalaemia, low erythropoietin, low ferritin, ↓ activity of von Willebrand factor
Urine: MC&S, creatinine clearance (CrCl)
Imaging: renal USS

Rx Treat underlying cause, low-protein diet, BP control (reduces speed of deterioration), correct calcium, anaemia, acidosis, water retention. Dialysis once CrCl < 20 mL/min

ENDOCRINOLOGY

DIABETES MELLITUS

P Chronic elevation of blood glucose

Ix Oral glucose tolerance test (OGTT): 75 g glucose to a fasting patient, measure baseline fasting glucose and then 2 h post glucose load (see Table 1.7)

Table 1.7 Diagnosis of diabetes and pre-diabetic conditions

	Normal	IFG	IGT	Diabetes
Fasting	≤6.0	6.1–6.9	< 7.0	≥7.0
2 h post-glucose load	< 7.8	< 7.8	7.8–11.0	≥11.1

IFG: impaired fasting glycaemia; IGT: impaired glucose tolerance

Cx *Macrovascular*: CVA, MI, peripheral vascular disease
Microvascular: retinopathy, nephropathy, neuropathy

TYPE 1 DIABETES

P Autoimmune destruction of the β cells in the islets of Langerhans in the pancreas leading to absolute insulin deficiency

A Twin studies: monozygotic concordance rate 45 per cent
Strong association with either HLA-DR3 or DR4 or both
Peak age of onset approximately 12 years

Sy Polyuria, polydipsia, weight loss ± ketoacidosis
Develops over days – months

Si Other features of autoimmune diseases

Ix *Blood*: U&E, FBC, glucose, antibodies
Immunology: anti-islet cell Ab (antibody), anti-GAD Ab
Urine: ketones, ABG

Rx *Supportive*: patient education
Glycaemic control: commence insulin, aim HbA_{1c} < 7 per cent, dietary advice
Complications surveillance: annual review (fundoscopy, feet examination → neurological and vascular), check insulin sites, BP monitoring, monitor renal function, thyroid function

DIABETIC KETOACIDOSIS

(A) Precipitants include infections, MI, omitting insulin

(Sy) As above and nausea, vomiting, abdominal pain, tachypnoea (Kussmaul respiration secondary to metabolic acidosis)

(Ix) *Blood*: glucose, VBG (metabolic acidosis, large anion gap), ketones, bicarbonate
Urine: ketones ++++
Septic screen: CXR, urine, blood, stool cultures

(Rx) Weight-based fixed intravenous insulin infusion, aggressive fluid replacement, monitor K^+ and replace, treat underlying cause

(Cx) Cerebral oedema, hypoglycaemia, hypokalaemia, hyperkalaemia, pulmonary oedema

TYPE 2 DIABETES

(P) Combination of insulin resistance and inadequate production (β cell destruction) / impaired secretion of insulin (β cell dysfunction)

(A) Obesity, chronic pancreatitis, Cushing's syndrome
Twin studies: monozygotic concordance rate 90 per cent
Peak age of onset approx 50 years

(Sy) Often with complications of diabetes (e.g. peripheral vascular disease, CVA, MI), hyperosmolar non-ketotic coma (HONK), recurrent infection, pruritus

(Si) Increased BMI, retinopathy, peripheral neuropathy

(Ix) U&E, FBC, glucose, serum osmolality

(Rx) *Supportive*: patient education, dietary advice
Glycaemic control: initially treat with diet, if unsatisfactory glycaemic control consider oral hypoglycaemics, aim for HbA_{1c} <7 per cent. Some patients may require insulin therapy
Complications surveillance: annual review (fundoscopy, feet examination → neurological and vascular), check insulin sites, BP monitoring, monitor renal function, urine protein dipstick, thyroid function

Table 1.8 Oral agents used in Type 2 diabetes

Class	Example	Mechanism
Biguanides	Metformin	Improve sensitivity to insulin
Sulphonylureas	Gliclazide, glimepiride	Stimulate pancreatic insulin release
Thiazolidinediones	Rosiglitazone	Improve sensitivity to insulin
α-Glucosidase inhibitors	Acarbose	Prevent intestinal sugar absorption

HYPEROSMOLAR NON-KETOTIC COMA (HONK)

(A) Precipitant: infection, increased sugary intake, MI

(Sy) Polydipsia, polyuria, decreased consciousness, thrombosis

(Ix) ↑Na+, glucose (often >50 mmol/L), ↑↑ osmolality

(Rx) CVP monitoring, fluid replacement, insulin, anticoagulation

(Px) Mortality 20–40 per cent

DIABETIC EYE DISEASE

See 'Ophthalmology', p. 199

HYPOGLYCAEMIA

(A) *SAIL:*
  – Sulphonylureas
  – Alcohol/Addison's
  – Insulinomas/Insulin/Infection (malaria, meningococcal)
  – Liver failure

(Sy) Cold sweat, tremor, irritability, confusion, loss of consciousness, collapse

(Si) Sweating, tachycardia, tremor, ↓ GCS (Glasgow Coma Score), fits

(Ix) Plasma glucose < 2.5 mmol/L
  If non-diabetic: insulin + C-peptide + pro-insulin (during hypoglycaemic episode), LFT, ethanol levels, cortisol (short Synacthen test)

(Rx) Oral glucose (e.g. Lucozade), i.m. (intramuscular) glucagon (avoid in alcoholics), i.v. glucose

PITUITARY DISEASE

The pituitary consists of two main parts: anterior and posterior (see Table 1.9)

Table 1.9 Hormones of the pituitary gland

	Origin	Hormones
Anterior pituitary	Derived from Rathke's pouch	ACTH, TSH, LH, FSH, GH, prolactin
Posterior pituitary	Neural origin, nerve fibres originating in supraoptic and paraventricular nuclei in the hypothalamus	ADH, oxytocin

ACTH, adrenocorticotrophic hormone; TSH, thyroid-stimulating hormone; LH, luteinizing hormone; FSH, follicle-stimulating hormone; GH, growth hormone; ADH, antidiuretic hormone

HYPERPROLACTINAEMIA

(P) Elevated prolactin levels

(A) *Physiological*: pregnancy, breast feeding
  Drugs: methyldopa, metoclopramide, haloperidol, oestrogen
  Neoplasia: prolactinoma
  Polycystic ovarian syndrome

(Sy) ♀: amenorrhoea, infertility, galactorrhoea (milk production)
  ♂: loss of libido, impotence, infertility, galactorrhoea
  Pressure effects, i.e. bitemporal hemianopia, hypopituitarism, cranial nerve palsies

(Ix) Full pituitary hormone profile, MRI pituitary, perimetry (visual field measurement)

(Rx) *Microprolactinoma* (<10 mm diameter): bromocriptine, cabergoline (dopamine agonists)
  Macroprolactinoma (>10 mm diameter): trial of bromocriptine/cabergoline, if affecting visual fields then trans-sphenoidal surgery

(Cx) Untreated ↑ risk of osteoporosis

CUSHING'S SYNDROME

(P) Excess cortisol secretion

(A) See Box 1.22

Box 1.22 CAUSES OF CUSHING'S SYNDROME

- *Exogenous*: iatrogenic, steroids, pseudo Cushing's, excess alcohol, depression
- *ACTH dependent*: pituitary overproduction of ACTH stimulating adrenal gland to produce cortisol, Cushing's disease, ectopic ACTH secretion, small-cell lung cancer, carcinoid
- *ACTH independent*: autonomous cortisol secretion, adrenal adenoma/carcinoma/hyperplasia

---

(Sy) ↑ weight gain, poor wound healing, recurrent infections, depression, menstrual disturbances, low libido, hirsutism, headache, osteoporosis

(Si) Plethoric moon face, buffalo hump, angry purple abdominal striae, centripetal obesity, proximal myopathy, hirsutism, thin skin, easy bruising, hypertension, acne

(Ix) *24-h urinary collection*: free cortisol
Random blood cortisol: loss of circadian rhythm
Low-dose dexamethasone suppression test: confirm whether ACTH can be suppressed
High-dose dexamethasone suppression test: differentiate between pituitary and ectopic ACTH secretion
Once Cushing's syndrome is confirmed locate source

(Rx) Cushing's disease:
Surgery: trans-sphenoidal surgery
Cushing's syndrome:
Medical: metyrapone, ketoconazole
Surgery: adrenalectomy

(Cx) *Post-adrenalectomy*: Nelson's syndrome (↑ pigmentation, ↑ pituitary size), adrenal insufficiency
Post-transphenoidal surgery: hypopituitarism

(Px) If untreated poor

ACROMEGALY/GIGANTISM

(P) ↑ GH secretion

(Sy) Sweating, increase in size of hands and feet, headache, oligo/amenorrhoea, infertility

(Si) Macroglossia (enlarged tongue), prominent supra-orbital ridges, prognathism (prominent lower jaw), increased interdental spacing, doughy spade-like hands, carpal tunnel syndrome, bitemporal hemianopia, goitre, heart failure, greasy skin, coarse facial lines, hypertension

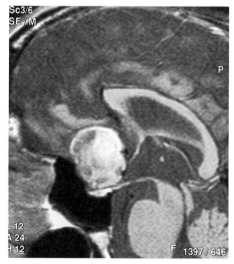

Figure 1.32 Sagittal MRI section shows a large pituitary tumour of mixed signal

(Ix) Failure of suppression of GH in OGTT, insulin-like growth factor-1 (IGF-1), full pituitary hormone profile, MRI pituitary, visual fields, fasting glucose

(Rx) *Medical*: cabergoline, octreotide (somatostatin analogue)
Surgery: transphenoidal surgery ± radiotherapy

(Cx) Diabetes mellitus, heart failure, osteoporosis, obstructive sleep apnoea, ↑ risk of colonic polyps and colonic carcinoma (hence patients require colonoscopy every 3 years), hypopituitarism

(Px) If untreated mortality is high

THYROID DISEASE

THYROTOXICOSIS

(P) Excess thyroxine production

(A) Viral thyroiditis, hyperthyroidism (toxic adenoma, toxic nodule in a MNG, Graves' disease), drugs (amiodarone, lithium), struma ovarii (rare ovarian cancer)
Most commonly affects young females

(Sy) Weight loss, increased appetite, diarrhoea, palpitations, tremor, agitation, psychosis, heat intolerance, increased sweating, SOB, oligomenorrhoea

(Si) Tachycardia, warm, sweaty, fine tremor, lid lag, lid retraction, palmar erythema, hair loss, myopathy, goitre
Specific for Graves': thyroid acropachy (like clubbing), pre-tibial myxoedema
Eye signs: peri-orbital oedema, exophthalmos, proptosis, ophthalmoplegia

(Ix) ↑ thyroxine (T_4), ↑ tri-iodothyronine (T_3), ↓ thyroid-stimulating hormone (TSH), TSH receptor antibody (specific for Graves'), ^{99m}Tc uptake scan, ESR

(Rx) *Medical*: antithyroid drugs e.g. carbimazole often first-line treatment, β-blockers (e.g. propranolol) for symptom relief
Radiation ablation: radio-iodine only for patients over 45 years
Surgery: partial thyroidectomy (see p. 148 for details)
Viral thyroiditis: analgesia, steroids

(Cx) Heart failure, osteoporosis. Small incidence of agranulocytosis with carbimazole (measure FBC regularly)

HYPOTHYROIDISM

(P) Deficiency of T_4

(A) See Box 1.23

Box 1.23 CAUSES OF HYPOTHYROIDISM

- *Autoimmune*: Hashimoto's thyroiditis
- *Dietary*: iodine deficiency
- *Congenital*
- *Panhypopituitarism*
- *Iatrogenic*: post-surgery/radio-iodine
- *Drugs*: amiodarone, lithium

(Sy) Fatigue, lethargy, cold intolerance, constipation, weight gain, carpal tunnel syndrome, menorrhagia, oligo/amenorrhoea, low mood, dry skin, hair loss

(Si) Peri-orbital puffiness, loss of lateral third of eyebrows, cerebellar signs, slow reflexes

(Ix) TFTs ($\uparrow$ TSH, $\downarrow$ T4)

(Rx) Replacement with levothyroxine

(Cx) If untreated can result in myxoedema coma

PARATHYROID GLAND DISORDERS

Classically, the parathyroids are four glands lying behind the thyroid (number and position vary). They secrete parathyroid hormone (PTH) which $\uparrow Ca^{2+}$ and $\downarrow PO_4^{3-}$

HYPERCALCAEMIA

(A) Most commonly bone metastasis (lung, breast) and hyperparathyroidism
Myeloma, sarcoidosis, thyrotoxicosis, FHH (familial hypocalciuric hypercalcaemia)

(Sy) 'Bones, stones, moans and groans' (see Box 1.24); polydipsia, polyuria

(Ix) *Bloods*: Ca^{2+}, albumin, ALP, PTH, PTH-related peptide (PTHrP), vitamin D, ACE, TFTs, tumour markers, urinary Ca^{2+}
ECG: shortened QT interval
Imaging: bone scan, sestamibi scan, CXR, mammogram (if suspicious of breast cancer)

(Rx) Aggressive fluid rehydration, then loop diuretics
Treat underlying cause:
 – *hyperparathyroidism*: surgery (if Ca^{2+} >3 mmol/L + symptomatic or renal stones), bisphosphonates (e.g. alendronate)
 – *bone metastases*: bisphosphonates
 – *sarcoidosis*: steroids

PRIMARY HYPERPARATHYROIDISM

(P) 85 per cent due to solitary parathyroid adenoma, 15 per cent due to hyperplasia, <1 per cent carcinoma

(A) Associated with multiple endocrine neoplasia (MEN) syndromes I and II

(Sy) 50 per cent asymptomatic. For the other 50 per cent, remember the aide mémoire in Box 1.24

Box 1.24 FEATURES OF HYPERCALCAEMIA
• Painful bones (± fractures)
• Renal stones
• Abdominal groans (abdominal pain)
• Psychic moans (depression)

(Ix) Bloods $\uparrow$ PTH in the setting of $\uparrow Ca^{2+}$
Raised 24-h urinary calcium
Sestamibi nuclear medicine scan used to identify position of adenomas

(Rx) High fluid intake (prevent renal stone formation)
Surgical resection indicated if symptoms are significant

(Cx) Risk of transient hypocalcaemia post-operatively

SECONDARY HYPERPARATHYROIDISM

P   Raised PTH in response to low calcium (e.g. renal failure, vitamin D deficiency)

TERTIARY HYPERPARATHYROIDISM

P   Prolonged secondary hyperparathyroidism results in autonomous excessive production of PTH and resultant hypercalcaemia

HYPOCALCAEMIA

A   Hypoalbuminaemia, hypomagnesaemia, hyperphosphataemia, medication effects, surgical effects, PTH deficiency or resistance, and vitamin D deficiency or resistance, acute pancreatitis

Sy   Muscle ache, pins and needles, tetany, bony pain

Si   Chvostek's sign, Trousseau's sign, arrhythmias

Ix Ca^{2+}, PO_4, ALP, vitamin D, PTH, Mg^{2+}, U&E

Rx   Calcium replacement

INFORMATION BOX: SIGNS OF HYPOCALCAEMIA

- *Chvostek's sign*: tap over the facial nerve about 2 cm anterior to the tragus of the ear (twitching first at the angle of the mouth, then by the nose, the eye, and the facial muscles)
- *Trousseau's sign*: inflation of a blood pressure cuff above the systolic pressure causes local ulnar and median nerve ischaemia, resulting in carpal spasm

---

PRIMARY HYPOPARATHYROIDISM

A   Most commonly iatrogenic: inadvertent removal during thyroidectomy or post-radiation

Sy   Tetany, depression, paraesthesiae

Si   Chvostek's sign, Trousseau's sign

Ix   *Bloods*: $\downarrow Ca^{2+}$ and $\uparrow PO_4^{3-}$

Rx   Calcium and vitamin D supplementation

PSEUDOHYPOPARATHYROIDISM

P   Cells resistant to PTH

Si   Pixie face, short metacarpals and metatarsals

PSEUDOPSEUDOHYPOPARATHYROIDISM

P   Same morphological features as pseudohypoparathyroidism, but normal biochemical profile

ADRENAL GLAND DISORDERS

PHAEOCHROMOCYTOMA

P   Tumour of the adrenal medulla secreting noradrenaline and adrenaline
90 per cent benign, unilateral
10 per cent malignant, multiple

(A)   Can be part of MEN IIA/B

(Sy)   Episodic flushing, palpitations, sweating, headache

(Si)   Hypertension, pallor

(Ix)   24-h urinary catecholamines ×3

   If positive: MRI adrenal, ^{131}I-MIBG nuclear medicine scan, exclude MEN II

(Rx)   *Medical*: phenoxybenzamine, needs adequate a blockade prior to β blockade

   Surgery: laparoscopic adrenalectomy

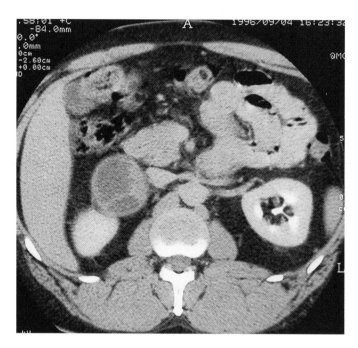

Figure 1.33
Phaeochromocytoma: a well-circumscribed mass in the right adrenal gland

CONN'S SYNDROME

(P)   60 per cent unilateral adrenocortical adenoma producing excess aldosterone
   40 per cent bilateral adrenal hyperplasia

(Si)   ↑BP

(Ix)   *Blood*: hypokalaemia, hypernatraemia, metabolic alkalosis, aldosterone/renin ratio
   Radiology: iodine ^{131}I iodocholesterol scanning, CT/MRI

(Rx)   *Medical*: spironolactone (aldosterone antagonist)
   Surgery: resection

ADDISON'S DISEASE

(P)   Destruction of the adrenal cortices, resulting in steroid and mineralocorticoid deficiency

(A)   Autoimmune (90 per cent), TB, metastasis

(Sy)   Weight loss, abdominal pain, lethargy, malaise, nausea, vomiting, diarrhoea

(Si)   Hyperpigmentation, postural hypotension, vitiligo

(Ix)   Hyponatraemia, short Synacthen, exclude other autoimmune conditions

(Rx)   Hydrocortisone (to replace steroid), fludrocortisone (to replace mineralocorticoid)

CONGENITAL ADRENAL HYPERPLASIA

P Autosomal recessive condition resulting in partial to complete deficiency of an enzyme necessary for the synthesis of aldosterone or cortisol production in the adrenal gland

Si *21-hydroxylase deficiency*: most common, can present with either salt-losing crisis or female virilization
11β-hydroxylase deficiency: presents with female virilization, hypertension
17α-hydroxylase deficiency: presents with male undervirilization, hypokalaemia, hypertension

Rx Long-term replacement with glucocorticoid or aldosterone or both

DISORDERS OF WATER REGULATION

DIABETES INSIPIDUS (DI)

P Inability of the kidneys to conserve water, which leads to frequent urination and pronounced thirst

Table 1.10 The causes of diabetes insipidus

	Pathology	Causes
Cranial	Failure of posterior pituitary to produce vasopressin	Idiopathic Brain tumours Surgery Head trauma Meningitis
Nephrogenic	Failure of kidneys to respond to vasopressin	Hypercalcaemia Hypokalaemia Demeclocycline, lithium Chronic renal disease

Sy Polyuria, polydipsia

Ix Urine/plasma osmolality
Water deprivation test (in cranial DI urine osmolality will ↑ when given desmopressin, no response in nephrogenic DI)

Rx *Cranial*: desmopressin (ADH analogue)
Nephrogenic: treat underlying cause, thiazide diuretics (paradoxical effect)

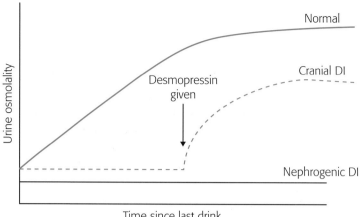

Figure 1.34 Water deprivation test

SYNDROME OF INAPPROPRIATE ANTIDIURETIC HORMONE (SIADH)

P ADH (vasopressin) causes water retention by increasing the permeability of the nephrons

ADH is produced by the hypothalamus and released from the posterior pituitary gland

---

Box 1.25 CAUSES OF THE SYNDROME OF INAPPROPRIATE ADH

- *CNS disorders*: meningitis, encephalitis, tumour, CVA, subarachnoid haemorrhage (SAH)
- *Pulmonary*: TB, empyema, asthma, COPD
- *Malignancy*: lung, pancreas, lymphoma
- *Drugs*: antidepressants, carbamazepine, cyclophosphamide, diuretics, neuroleptics, barbiturates

---

Sy Acute anorexia, nausea and vomiting

Na^+ *110–115 mmol/L*: headache, irritability, disorientation and weakness

Na^+ *<110 mmol/L*: delirium, psychosis, ataxia, tremor

Si Euvolaemic, papilloedema, severe myoclonus

Ix ↓ Na^+, ↓ serum osmolality, inappropriately dilute urine (250–1400 mosmol/kg), TFTs, 09:00 cortisol/short Synacthen, CT head

Rx Fluid restriction, correct Na^+ at a rate < 12 mEq/L/day

Cx If Na^+ increased too rapidly: central pontine myelinolysis (usually fatal)

RHEUMATOLOGY

RHEUMATOID ARTHRITIS (RA)

(P) Systemic autoimmune disorder affecting the synovial joints with extra-articular manifestations

(A) Prevalence is 1–3 per cent, ♀ > ♂, peak age of onset 40 years

(Sy) Joint pain exacerbated by movement, morning stiffness, joint swelling
Extra-articular manifestations (see below)
Systemic: fever (mild), anorexia, malaise, weight loss, lethargy

(Si) Joints: swollen, warm, tender joints,
Joint deformities (swan neck, boutonnière), subluxation
Lymphadenopathy, splenomegaly
Rheumatoid nodules
Muscle weakness, evidence of amyloidosis and vasculitis

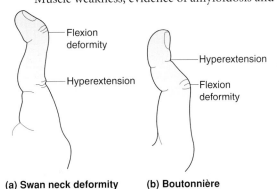

(a) Swan neck deformity   **(b) Boutonnière**

Figure 1.35 Joint deformities in rheumatoid arthritis (figure 1.35(a) adapted with kind permission from Model D, *Making Sense of Clinical Examination of the Adult Patient*, London: Hodder Arnold, 2006)

Box 1.26 DIAGNOSTIC CRITERIA FOR RHEUMATOID ARTHRITIS

(need 4 out of 7 – 'RF RISES')
- **R**heumatoid factor
- **F**inger/hand joint involvement
- **R**heumatoid nodules
- **I**nvolvement of 3 or more joints
- **S**tiffness – early morning
- **E**rosions/decalcification on x-rays
- **S**ymmetrical arthritis

(Ix) *Bloods*: ESR + CRP (degree of synovial inflammation), anaemia of chronic disease, low albumin (correlates directly with disease severity), neutropenia (in Felty's syndrome)
Immunology: rheumatoid factor (RhF), anti-CCP (cyclic citrullinated peptide) Ab (may be a better predictor of progression to erosive joint disease than titres of RhF),
X-rays: soft tissue swelling, joint space narrowing, peri-articular osteoporosis, bony erosions, deformities, atlanto-axial subluxation
Synovial fluid: ↑WBC, ↑protein

Ⓡ Goals: pain relief, protection of remaining articular structure, maintenance of function
Patient education: encourage rest alternating with exercise
Physiotherapy and occupational therapy
Medical: analgesics, NSAIDs, glucocorticoids, DMARDs (disease-modifying antirheumatic drugs)

Table 1.11 Disease-modifying antirheumatic drugs

Non-biological	Biological
Methotrexate	Soluble interleukin-1 (IL-1) receptor therapy (anakinra)
Hydroxychloroquine	Tumour necrosis factor inhibitors (e.g. etanercept, infliximab)
Sulfasalazine	Cytotoxic agents (azathioprine, cyclophosphamide and ciclosporin A)
Leflunomide	
Penicillamine	
Gold	

Ⓒ *Respiratory*: pulmonary nodules, fibrosing alveolitis, pleural effusion, Caplan's syndrome (rheumatoid arthritis in coal miners with pneumoconiosis) and bronchiolitis obliterans
CVS (cardiovascular system): endocarditis, pericarditis, myocarditis, nodules
CNS: entrapment neuropathies, peripheral neuropathy
Eyes: episcleritis, scleritis, kerato-conjunctivitis, scleromalacia
Others: Felty's syndrome (RhF +ve, splenomegaly and neutropenia)

Ⓟ Variable. Poor prognostic factors include systemic involvement, insidious onset, rheumatoid nodules, RhF > 1:512, persistent activity for >12 months and early bone erosions

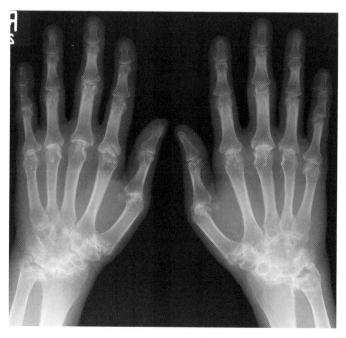

Figure 1.36 Rheumatoid arthritis: erosions at the metacarpophalangeal joints; note peri-articular soft tissue swelling and the severe changes at both wrists

REITER'S SYNDROME

P   Triad of:
- seronegative oligoarticular asymmetrical arthritis
- urethritis and/or cervicitis
- conjunctivitis

A   Male predisposition, age 16–25 years, associated with human leucocyte antigen (HLA) B27
Triggered by *Chlamydia, Salmonella, Shigella, Yersinia* and *Campylobacter*

Sy   Malaise, fever, arthritis, urethritis, conjunctivitis

Si   Joint swelling and pain, dactylitis (sausage finger/toe), circinate balanitis, keratoderma blennorrhagica (papules on palms, soles and glans penis)

Ix   No specific tests. ↑CRP and ESR, −ve RhF and synovial fluid, urinalysis, culture – urine, stool, synovial fluid, high urethral/vaginal swab and serology for *Chlamydia*

Rx   Bed rest, intra-articular steroids, NSAIDs, for recurrent or chronic symptoms consider DMARDs

Px   33 per cent have recurrent/sustained disease
15–22 per cent permanent disability

SEPTIC ARTHRITIS

P   Can occur due to either haematological spread, direct spread from an adjacent source, or through direct introduction of the organism via trauma/instrumentation

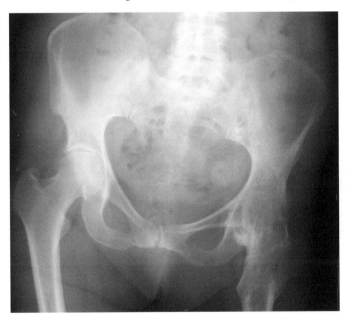

Figure 1.37 Complete ankylosis of the hip joint following a septic arthritis

A   Bacterial causes include *Staphylococcus aureus, Streptococcus pyogenes* and *Neisseria gonorrhoea* (young adults), *Salmonella* (sickle cell)

S   Fever, warm, red, swollen, painful joint, may also be an erythematous rash

Ix   *Bloods*: ↑WBC, uric acid (exclude gout), antibodies (exclude RA), cultures
Synovial fluid: cloudy, ↑leucocytes, culture
Urine: MC&S
Microbiology: urethral, cervical and anorectal swabs

X-rays: soft tissue swelling, joint distension, later juxta-articular osteoporosis, periosteal elevation, joint space narrowing, bony erosions and possible osteomyelitis

(Rx) Physiotherapy, analgesia, antibiotics, aspiration and drainage

(Cx) Joint destruction

SYSTEMIC LUPUS ERYTHEMATOSUS (SLE)

(P) Multisystemic disease in which antibodies and immune complexes may cause cellular and tissue damage

(A) Most common in African–Caribbean women aged 25–35 years
Concordance in twins, plus familial tendency

Box 1.27 DIAGNOSTIC CRITERIA FOR SLE

(need 4 out of 11 – 'ORDER HIS ANA')
- **O**ral ulcers
- **R**ash (malar)
- **D**iscoid rash
- **E**xaggerated photosensitivity
- **R**enal disease
- **H**aematological abnormality
- **I**mmunological abnormality
- **S**erositis
- **A**rthralgia
- **N**eurological disease
- **A**NA

(Sy) Malaise, fever, arthralgia

(Si) Malar 'butterfly' rash, discoid lupus, mucosal ulcers, vasculitic rash, symmetrical arthritis, Raynaud's, Sjögren's, episcleritis, retinal infarcts, optic neuritis

(Ix) *Bloods*: Coombs' +ve haemolytic anaemia, neutropenia, lymphocytopenia, thrombocytopenia, $\uparrow$ ESR, $\rightarrow$ CRP, renal profile,
Antibodies: ANA, anti-dsDNA, anti-smRNA, antiphospholipid Ab, anti-Ro/La, $\downarrow$ C3 + C4

(Rx) *Minor symptoms*: NSAIDs, anti-malarials, low-dose steroids
Major symptoms: Steroids and immunosuppressants

(Cx) *Renal*: 50 per cent can develop lupus nephritis
CNS: psychosis, stroke, fits
CVS: pericarditis, myocarditis, Libman–Sacks endocarditis (autoimmune)
Respiratory system: pleural effusion, pneumonitis, ARDS

ANTIPHOSPHOLIPID SYNDROME

(A) Can be primary or associated with other autoimmune conditions, e.g. SLE

(Sy) Recurrent venous/arterial thrombosis (i.e. CVA, Budd–Chiari syndrome, DVT)
Recurrent spontaneous miscarriages

(Si) Livedo reticularis, purpura, splinter haemorrhages, valvular heart disease

(Ix) $\uparrow$ activated partial thromboplastin time (APTT), thrombocytopenia, haemolytic anaemia, anticardiolipin Ab, lupus anticoagulant

(Rx) Aspirin 75 mg daily; if the patient develops a thromboembolic event, warfarin anticoagulation

SYSTEMIC SCLEROSIS

(A) Associated with malignancy

(P) Multisystemic connective tissue disease causing inflammation, fibrosis and vascular damage to the skin and internal organs

Syndromes:
- limited cutaneous systemic sclerosis (skin involvement distally, systemic involvement occurs late and is rare, anticentromere antibody (ACA) +ve 70 per cent)
- diffuse cutaneous systemic sclerosis (early systemic involvement, Scl-70 (topoisomerase) antibody +ve 30 per cent)

(Sy) Pruritus, Raynaud's, dysphagia, nausea, vomiting, abdominal pain, diarrhoea, faecal incontinence, SOB, non-productive cough, palpitations, weakness, arthralgia, dry eyes

(Si) *Major features*: centrally located skin sclerosis – arms, face ± neck.
Minor features: sclerodactyly (tight skin over fingers), erosions, atrophy of the fingertips, and bilateral lung fibrosis

(Ix) *Bloods*: $\uparrow$ MCV, $\rightarrow$ ESR, $\uparrow$ urea + creatinine (if there is renal involvement), $\uparrow$ CK (mild), $\uparrow$ Ig, ANA (90 per cent)
Imaging: CXR/CT of the chest (linear/nodular interstitial fibrosis)

(Rx) Patient education + counselling
Physiotherapy + occupational therapy (OT)
Drugs:
- *Raynaud's*: Ca^{2+} channel antagonists (nifedipine), prostaglandin infusions
- *GI symptoms*: antacids, H_2 blockers, laxatives
- *myositis*: corticosteroids
- *renal crisis*: ACE inhibitors
- *cardiac*: anti-arrhythmics
- *early stage diffuse form*: immunosuppressants
- *late stage*: antifibrotics, e.g. penicillamine

PSORIATIC ARTHRITIS

(P) Chronic seronegative inflammatory arthritis associated with psoriasis

(A) 10 per cent of patients with psoriasis develop arthritis, mean age of onset 40–50 years
Associated with HLA-B27

(Sy) Asymmetric large joint oligoarthritis, axial arthritis, asymmetrical sacroiliitis, peripheral small joint arthritis, distal interphalangeal joint (DIP) arthritis and arthritis mutilans; stiffness

(Si) Enthesitis, dactylitis, psoriasis,
Nail changes: onycholysis, transverse ridging, nail pitting

(Ix) *Bloods*: $\uparrow$ ESR, RhF –ve, ANA –ve
Synovial fluid: –ve
Imaging: X-rays: para-marginal erosions, fluffy periosteal bone formation, bony ankylosis, asymmetric sacroiliitis

(Rx) Physiotherapy, occupational therapy, NSAIDs, DMARDs

ANKYLOSING SPONDYLITIS

(P) Chronic seronegative disease of unknown aetiology, resulting in inflammation of multiple articular and para-articular structures – bony ankylosis

(A) Associated with HLA-B27 (up to 95 per cent of patients)
Onset occurs in late teens/early adulthood, ♂ > ♀

(Sy) Lower back pain and early morning stiffness, enthesitis, anterior uveitis, pain in hips, buttocks and shoulders

(Si) Tenderness over the sacroiliac joint, ↓ anterior flexion of the lumbar spine, thoracic spinal fusion, ↓ lateral spine flexion, ↓ chest expansion, aortic regurgitation, apical lung fibrosis

(Ix) *Bloods*: chronic anaemia, RhF −ve, ↑ ESR
Imaging: X-ray – sacroiliitis, juxta-articular sclerosis, syndesmophyte formation, marginal erosion, fusion of adjacent vertebrae (bamboo spine), disk calcification, pseudarthrosis; MRI

(Rx) Physiotherapy, occupational therapy, NSAIDs, DMARDs

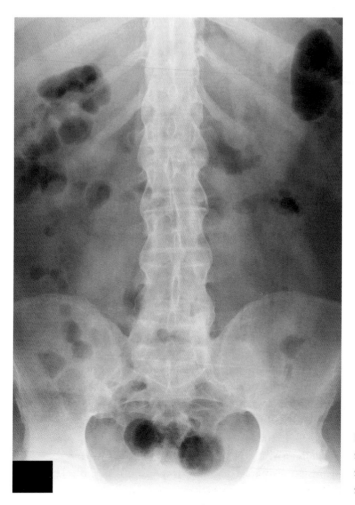

Figure 1.38 Ankylosing spondylitis: 'bamboo spine' with fusion of the sacroiliac joints

MYOSITIS: POLYMYOSITIS/DERMATOMYOSITIS

(P) Inflammatory disease of skeletal muscle of unknown aetiology
Dermatomyositis = polymyositis (muscle involvement only) + skin involvement

(A) Primary or secondary associated with autoimmune rheumatic disease or malignancy

(Sy) Progressive proximal muscle weakness, myalgia, dysphagia, SOB

(Si) Dermatomyositis: periorbital oedema, heliotrope rash, Gottron's papules (erythematous scaly lesions affecting the dorsum of the hands), periungual telangiectasias

(Ix) ↑CK, ANA, Anti-Jo1 Ab, exclude malignancy, EMG, muscle biopsy

(Rx) Medical: high-dose glucocorticoids, azathioprine/methotrexate, immunoglobulin
Physiotherapy

SJÖGREN'S SYNDROME

(P) Autoimmune disease that causes progressive destruction of exocrine glands and polyarthritis

(A) Primary or associated with other autoimmune rheumatic diseases
♀ > ♂

(Sy) Oral soreness, eye dryness, mild relapsing non-erosive polyarthritis

(Si) Angular stomatitis, eye redness, xeroderma

(Ix) ESR, RhF, ANA, anti-Ro, anti-La, lip biopsy

(Rx) *Supportive*: artificial tears, mouthwash

(Cx) Acute/chronic pancreatitis, nephrogenic DI, renal tubular acidosis, interstitial nephritis, glomerulonephritis, neuropathy (peripheral sensory, sensorimotor, cranial)

POLYARTERITIS NODOSA

(P) Necrotizing vasculitis of small and medium-sized vessels

(A) Associated with HBV, hepatitis C, CMV, HIV

(Sy) Weight loss, fever, malaise, myalgia, polyarthritis, rapid renal failure

(Si) ↑BP, acute abdomen, mononeuritis multiplex, fever, livedo reticularis,

(Ix) *Bloods*: FBC (neutrophilia), U&E ↑ESR, ↑ALP, ANCA, viral serology, blood cultures
Urine: microscopy, creatinine clearance
Imaging: CXR, arteriography (multiple small aneurysms)

(Rx) Corticosteroids, cytotoxic drugs

(Px) Worse prognosis with heavy proteinuria, renal insufficiency (creatinine >140 mmol/L), cardiomyopathy, GI manifestations, CNS involvement

POLYMYALGIA RHEUMATICA

(A) Older patients, ♀:♂ 2:1

(Sy) Bilateral proximal muscle stiffness and ache, systemic features (weight loss, fever, malaise)

(Si) Normal muscle power

(Ix) FBC (normocytic normochromic anaemia), ↑ESR

(Rx) Low-dose corticosteroids, often for months/years

WEGENER'S GRANULOMATOSIS

(P) Systemic vascular disease characterized by necrotizing granulomas in the respiratory tract and focal necrotizing glomerulonephritis

(Sy) Cough, pleurisy, SOB, haemoptysis, general malaise, haematuria, arthralgia, purulent/bloody nasal discharge

(Si) Purpura, oral ulceration, pleural effusion, conjunctivitis

(Ix) *Bloods*: FBC (leucocytosis, thrombocytosis), cANCA
Blood film: schistocytes, Burr cells
Urine: proteinuria, haematuria, red cell casts
Imaging: CXR – migrating rounded opacities ± cavitation, pleural effusions, infiltrates; CT scan
Biopsy: affected organs show granulomatous changes

(Rx) Immunosuppressants, corticosteroids

TEMPORAL ARTERITIS

(P) Systemic inflammatory vasculitis of unknown aetiology that affects medium- and large-sized arteries

(A) Mostly in those aged over 50 years; ♀ > ♂

(Sy) Headache, malaise, transient visual disturbance, blindness, fever, lethargy, jaw claudication

(Si) Tender, non-pulsatile temporal arteries, proximal muscle tenderness

(Ix) ↑ESR, temporal artery biopsy

(Rx) High-dose glucocorticoids – do not wait for biopsy

(Cx) Blindness, aortitis, aortic dissection/aneurysm

TAKAYASU'S ARTERITIS

(P) Chronic, progressive, inflammatory, occlusive disease of the aorta and its branches (i.e. large blood vessels)

(A) Young females, 15–35 years

(Sy) Systemic illness + tenderness over palpable arteries, bruits, loss of pulses, claudication pain

(Rx) Steroids ± immunosuppressants; angioplasty/surgical repair for stenosed vessels

(Cx) Renovascular hypertension

BEHÇET'S DISEASE

(P) Chronic autoimmune vasculitis causing characteristic skin, eye and mucosal lesions

(A) ♂ > ♀, common in Turkey, Iran

(S) *Major criteria*: recurrent aphthous stomatitis, sterile pustules at site of skin trauma (pathergy test), uveitis, genital ulceration
Minor criteria: inflammatory large joint arthritis, intestinal ulceration, meningoencephalitis, epididymitis, thrombophlebitis

(Rx) Steroids/ciclosporin A

GOUT

(P) Uric acid arthropathy

(A) ♂ > ♀

↑ dietary purine intake, alcohol, ↑ cell turnover (i.e. malignancy), low-dose aspirin, diuretics, inherited enzyme deficiencies

(Sy) *Acute*: monoarthritis, severe pain lasting 7–10 days, most commonly first metatarsophalangeal joint (podagra)

Chronic: gouty tophi on pinnae, hands ± polyarthritis

(Ix) Uric acid levels, synovial fluid microscopy for crystals (negatively birefringent)

Imaging: X-ray: cortical erosions, sclerotic margins

(Rx) Dietary changes, decrease alcohol intake, NSAIDs, colchicine, allopurinol (to prevent recurrence, but avoid in acute attack)

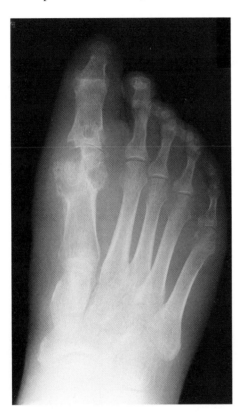

Figure 1.39 Gout of the big toe with soft tissue swelling and sharp well-defined erosions

PSEUDOGOUT

(P) Calcium pyrophosphate arthropathy

(A) Primary or secondary to hyperparathyroidism, haemochromatosis, diabetes, Wilson's disease, hypothyroidism

(Ix) *Imaging*: X-ray shows chondrocalcinosis

Joint aspiration: positively birefringent crystals

(Rx) NSAIDs, colchicine

PAGET'S DISEASE

(P) Chronic disorder of bone remodelling leading to disorganized structure of woven and lamellar bone

(A) ♂ > ♀, >70 years

(Sy) Pain at affected site, most commonly pelvis, lumbar spine, femur; hearing loss due to VIIIth nerve compression

(Si) Sabre tibia, ↑ warmth over affected area, ↑ head size ± frontal bossing, conductive/sensory hearing loss, basilar invagination

(Ix) *Bloods*: ↑ ALP, → Ca^{2+},
Imaging: X-ray: expansion + deformity of affected long bones with mixed osteolytic + sclerotic areas

(Rx) Bisphosphonates (e.g. alendronate) for active disease, calcitonin for severe pain/extensive lytic disease

(Cx) Osteosarcoma, fractures, high-output cardiac failure, hypercalcaemia, secondary immobility

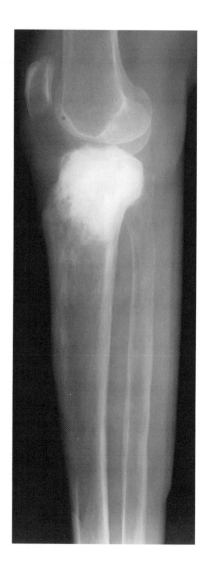

Figure 1.40 Paget's disease: tibial bowing, cortical thickening and abnormal modelling

OSTEOPOROSIS

P ↓ quantity of bone/unit volume, resulting in decreased skeletal strength

A ♀ > ♂, occurs in up to 30 per cent of post-menopausal women

Idiopathic or secondary to endocrine disorders (e.g. Cushing's syndrome, thyrotoxicosis, osteomalacia), corticosteroids, chronic renal failure, multiple myeloma, alcoholism, hereditary

Sy Fractures

Ix DEXA (dual-energy X-ray absorptiometry), bone density scan

Rx Exclude secondary causes, prevention with exercise, ↑ dietary intake, stop smoking, Ca^{2+} supplements (e.g. Calcichew), bisphosphonates, strontium ranelate, selective oestrogen receptor modulators (e.g. raloxifene), parathyroid hormone (e.g. teriparetide)

OSTEOMALACIA

P Heterogeneous disorders characterized by defective bone mineralization of newly synthesized bone

A Most common in children/elderly

Causes: dietary, malabsorption, chronic pancreatitis, CRF (unable to hydroxylate vitamin D), Fanconi syndrome, phenytoin

Si Bony deformities, bone pain + tenderness, proximal myopathy

Ix *Bloods*: ↓ Ca^{2+}, ↓ PO_4, ↑ ALP, ↑ PTH, ↓ 25-OH vitamin D

Imaging: X-ray: Looser's zones (radiolucent areas occurring at right angles to the cortex)

Rx Vitamin D replacement

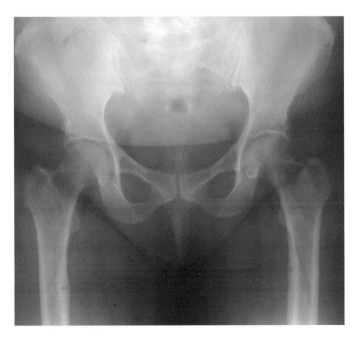

Figure 1.41
Osteomalacia: Looser's zones in the medial aspects of both femora

HAEMATOLOGY

ANAEMIA

- **P** ↓ Hb, classified according to either aetiology or red cell morphology
- **Sy** Lethargy, SOB, palpitations, chest pains, headaches
- **Si** Pallor, systolic flow murmur, specific signs to the underlying condition

MICROCYTIC ANAEMIA (↓ MEAN CORPUSCULAR VOLUME [MCV])

IRON DEFICIENCY ANAEMIA

- **P** Daily requirements, females 1.5 mg/day, pregnancy 7.5 mg/day, males 1 mg/day
  Iron is absorbed from the small intestine, transported in the blood via transferrin and stored attached to ferritin
- **A** Chronic blood loss (GI, menstruation), malabsorption, GI malignancy (in the elderly, assume iron deficiency anaemia is due to colon cancer until proven otherwise)
- **Si** Koilonychia, sore tongue, angular stomatitis, Plummer–Vinson syndrome (dysphagia secondary to oesophageal web), painless gastritis
- **Ix** FBC, ↓ ferritin, ↓ serum iron, ↑ TIBC, ↓ transferrin saturation, OGD, colonoscopy/barium enema
- **Rx** Diagnose and treat underlying cause
  Ferrous sulphate until Hb and MCV normal
  Blood transfusion only if patient is symptomatic or a cardiac patient (keep Hb >10 g/dL)

β THALASSAEMIA

- **A** Most common autosomal recessive inherited haematological disorder
  Commonest in Mediterranean, Middle East, Asia
- **P** ↓ β-globin production, leading to chronic anaemia
- **Si** *Homozygotes*: failure to thrive, severe anaemia, splenomegaly, bone hypertrophy (secondary to extramedullary haemopoiesis)
  Heterozygotes: usually asymptomatic, mildly anaemic, ↓↓ MCV
- **Ix** Hb electrophoresis, blood film
- **Rx** Repeated blood transfusions
- **Cx** Secondary haemosiderosis, from repeated blood transfusions, endocrine disease

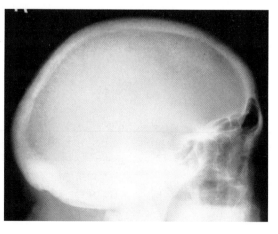

Figure 1.42 Expansion of the diploic space in thalassaemia due to extramedullary haemopoiesis

SICKLE CELL DISEASE

(A) Autosomal recessive genetic disease due to haemoglobin chain mutation

(P) Abnormal haemoglobin (HbS) has tendency to become rigid and sickle, causing occlusion of small vessels ('sickle cell crisis')
Crisis precipitated by infection, dehydration, hypoxia, cold

(S) Bone pain, pleuritic pain, priapism, jaundice and pigment gallstones secondary to chronic haemolysis, failure to thrive

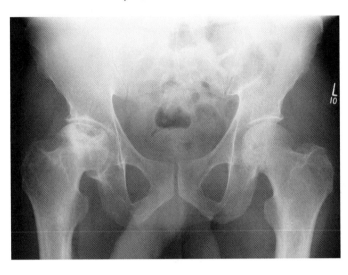

Figure 1.43 Avascular necrosis of the right femoral head due to sickle cell disease

(Ix) Blood film, Hb electrophoresis

(Rx) *Supportive*: aggressive analgesia, antibiotics and fluids when needed

(Cx) Gallstones, leg ulcers, avascular necrosis of femoral head, chronic renal disease

MACROCYTIC ANAEMIA (↑ MCV)

MEGALOBLASTIC ANAEMIA

(A) Vitamin B_{12}/folate deficiency

(P) Large erythroblasts in the bone marrow – faulty maturation due to defective DNA synthesis

VITAMIN B_{12} DEFICIENCY

(P) Vitamin B_{12} binds to IF (intrinsic factor) which is produced by the stomach parietal cells, and then is absorbed in the terminal ileum

(A) Pernicious anaemia deficiency (Ab against gastric parietal cells, IF), malabsorption (secondary to Crohn's disease affecting the terminal ileum, bacterial overgrowth) post-total gastrectomy, dietary

(Si) Pernicious anaemia can be associated with other autoimmune conditions, neurological manifestations (peripheral neuropathy, subacute combined degeneration of the cord, dementia), infertility

(Ix) ↑ MCV, ↓ B_{12}, ↓ platelets, ↓ WBC, IF antibodies, Schilling test, folate levels

(Rx) i.m. B_{12} injections

INFORMATION BOX: SCHILLING TEST

A Schilling test is performed to detect whether the body can absorb B_{12} normally.

A small dose of *radioactive* B_{12} is given orally with a large intramuscular dose of *normal* B_{12}. Urine is then collected to see if the radioactive B_{12} is excreted (and hence has been absorbed).

If negative, then the test can be repeated with the addition of oral IF. If the test becomes positive after this, then the diagnosis is pernicious anaemia (lack of IF). If the test is still negative, the diagnosis is small bowel disease.

FOLATE DEFICIENCY

(P) Folate is normally found in green vegetables, and absorbed in the upper part of the small intestine

(A) Dietary inadequacy, malabsorption, increased requirements (pregnancy, haemolysis), folate antagonists, e.g. methotrexate

(Ix) ↑MCV, ↓folate

(Rx) Folic acid supplements

NON-MEGALOBLASTIC ANAEMIA

(P) Normoblastic bone marrow
↑MCV

Box 1.28 NON-MEGALOBLASTIC CAUSES OF MACROCYTOSIS

- Alcohol excess (common)
- Reticulocytosis
- Hypothyroidism
- Physiological (pregnancy)
- Liver disease

(Rx) Treatment of underlying cause

NORMOCYTIC NORMOCHROMIC ANAEMIA (ANAEMIA OF CHRONIC DISEASE)

(A) Chronic renal failure, chronic infections, rheumatoid arthritis, connective tissue diseases, malignant diseases

(Ix) → ferritin, ↓serum iron, ↓total iron-binding capacity (TIBC)

(Rx) Treat underlying cause, erythropoietin injections in CRF

APLASTIC ANAEMIA

(A) Due to a decrease in pluripotential stem cells resulting in pancytopenia
Can be idiopathic, congenital or secondary: drugs (e.g. phenytoin, carbamazepine), parvovirus, viral hepatitis; ionizing radiation

(Sy) SOB, palpitations, chest pain, bleeding, easy bruising, recurrent infection

(Ix) FBC, blood film, bone marrow aspirate and trephine, LFT, viral titres

(Rx) Remove or treat precipitant, supportive (i.e. blood and platelet transfusions; G-CSF (granulocyte cell-stimulating factor)
Specific: immunosuppression, bone marrow transplantation

(Px) Relates to severity

HAEMOLYSIS

(P) Abnormal premature destruction of RBCs

Box 1.29 CAUSES OF HAEMOLYSIS

- *Congenital*:
  - hereditary spherocytosis
  - thalassaemia
  - sickle cell disease
  - G6PD (glucose-6-phosphate dehydrogenase) deficiency
- *Acquired*:
  - autoimmune haemolytic anaemia (AIHA)
  - microangiopathic haemolytic anaemia (MAHA)
  - infection

(Si) Pallor, jaundice, splenomegaly

(Ix) *Bloods*: ↑ unconjugated bilirubin, ↑ LDH, ↓ haptoglobins, ↑ reticulocyte count, Coombs' test
Blood film: polychromasia

HEREDITARY SPHEROCYTOSIS

(A) Autosomal dominant

(P) Defect in cell membrane, results in increased cell fragility

(Si) Splenomegaly, mild anaemia

(Ix) *Blood film*: spherocytes (small spherical darkly stained RBCs with no central pallor)

(Rx) Nil specific unless symptomatic → splenectomy

G6PD DEFICIENCY

(A) X-linked

(P) Normally G6PD generates NADPH, which is responsible for maintaining a healthy Hb so that it can withstand the stresses caused by drugs, sepsis
Deficiency of G6PD therefore means that Hb breaks down under stress resulting in haemolytic anaemia
Causes of haemolysis include analgesics, antimalarials and antibiotics

(Rx) Avoidance of drugs known to precipitate haemolysis

COAGULATION DISORDERS

AUTOIMMUNE THROMBOCYTOPENIC PURPURA (AITP)

(P) Due to antibodies against the antigens on the platelet surface resulting in removal via the reticuloendothelial system

(A) Affects middle-aged women and children

(Sy) Recurrent epistaxis, ecchymosis, gingival bleeding, menorrhagia

(Ix) FBC ($\downarrow$ platelets), blood film, bone marrow biopsy

(Rx) Only if platelets $<30 \times 10^9$/L, high dose of glucocorticoids, immunoglobulin infusion; if resistant consider splenectomy

HAEMOPHILIA A AND B

(A) Inherited disorders of coagulation, X-linked recessive (only males suffer from disease, females carry disease)

(P) Haemophilia A: deficiency of Factor VIIIc

Haemophilia B: deficiency of Factor IX

(Sy) Haemarthrosis, secondary arthritis, spontaneous soft tissue bleeds (i.e. psoas, gastrocnemius), GI bleeding, haematuria, loin pain

(Ix) $\uparrow$ APTT, $\rightarrow$ PT, $\rightarrow$ von Willebrand factor (vWF), platelets

Haemophilia A: $\downarrow$ factor VIII

Haemophilia B: $\downarrow$ factor IX

(Rx) *Haemophilia A*: purified factor VIIIc, desmopressin (increases factor VIII levels)

Haemophilia B: factor IX injections

VON WILLEBRAND'S DISEASE

(A) Most common inherited disorder of coagulation

Various subtypes, most common is autosomal dominant

(P) Associated with either low or abnormal vWF

(Sy) Mucosal/capillary bleeding, easy bruising

(Ix) FBC, $\uparrow$ APTT, $\rightarrow$ PT, $\downarrow$ factor VIIIc + vWF and $\uparrow$ bleeding time

(Rx) vWF concentrate, DDAVP (vasopressin) infusions, cryoprecipitate, fresh-frozen plasma (FFP)

DISSEMINATED INTRAVASCULAR COAGULATION (DIC)

(P) Pathological activation of coagulation resulting in bleeding and widespread microvascular thrombosis

Box 1.30 CAUSES OF DISSEMINATED INTRAVASCULAR COAGULATION
• *Infection*: Gram −ve, meningococcal, viral
• *Malignancy*: solid tumours, leukaemia
• *Obstetric*: eclampsia, retained placenta, amniotic fluid embolus
• *Immunological*: anaphylaxis
• *Liver disease*: acute liver disease, cirrhosis

(Sy) Haemorrhage, widespread microthrombi, large-vessel thrombosis, haemorrhagic tissue necrosis

(Ix) $\uparrow$ PT, $\uparrow$ APTT, $\uparrow$ thrombin time (TT), $\downarrow$ fibrinogen, $\uparrow$ fibrin degradation products (FDP)

(Rx) Treat underlying condition, FFP, platelets, cryoprecipitate

DEEP VEIN THROMBOSIS (DVT)

(P) Clot that occurs in a deep vein, most commonly in the lower limb

(A) Immobility (including long car/plane journeys), recent major operation/trauma, pregnancy, oral contraceptive pill (OCP)

Associated with malignancy, pro-coagulant states (see Thrombophilia below)

(Sy) Increased swelling, erythema, warm, tender over site of thrombosis

(Ix) Duplex USS of the affected limb, D-dimer

(Px) Anticoagulate, exclude underlying malignancy or possible thrombophilia (see below), TED (thromboembolic deterrent) stockings

(Cx) Pulmonary embolus, post-thrombotic limb

THROMBOPHILIA

(P) Conditions which induce a pro-coagulant state resulting in thrombosis, affects 5–7 per cent of the population

---

Box 1.31 CAUSES OF THROMBOPHILIA

- *Primary*:
  – protein C deficiency
  – protein S deficiency
  – antithrombin III deficiency
  – factor V Leiden
  – homocystinuria

- *Secondary*:
  – malignancy
  – immobility
  – major surgery (especially orthopaedic)
  – OCP
  – smoking
  – pregnancy
  – antiphospholipid syndrome

(Sy) Relate to the location of the clot
PE: SOB, haemoptysis, pleuritic chest pain
DVT: calf swelling, pain, tenderness, erythema

(Ix) Patients should be investigated if:
  – thromboembolism <45 years, or family history
  – recurrent thromboembolism/miscarriage
  – thrombosis at an unusual site
FBC (exclude polycythaemia, myelofibrosis), APTT, PT, fibrinogen, blood film

(Rx) Anticoagulation, avoid precipitants, e.g. OCP

PREMALIGNANT DISORDERS

POLYCYTHAEMIA

(P) $\uparrow$RCC, $\uparrow$PCV (haematocrit), $\uparrow$Hb

(A) $\male > \female$, mean age 50–60 years
Primary, due to a clonal stem cell disorder (polycythaemia rubra vera), or secondary (due to either hypoxia $\rightarrow$ high altitude, pulmonary disease or inappropriate erythropoietin secretion $\rightarrow$ cerebellar haemangioblastoma, renal tumour)

(Sy) Headaches, dizziness, pruritus after bathing, loss of consciousness, gout

(Si) Facial plethora, bleeding, splenomegaly, bruising

(Ix) FBC, nuclear medicine red cell mass, abdominal USS

(Rx) If primary: venesection, antiplatelet drugs for digital microvascular occlusion and TIA; if secondary treat underlying cause

(Cx) Transformation to myelofibrosis/acute myelogenous leukaemia (AML)

MYELOFIBROSIS

P Clonal proliferation of haemopoietic stem cells leading to bone marrow fibrosis

A Mean age 60 years

Si Pallor, bruising, oral thrush, massive splenomegaly, systemic symptoms

Ix FBC, blood film (leucoerythroblastic + tear-drop RBC), bone marrow trephine biopsy

Rx *Supportive*: blood transfusion
Specific: hydroxycarbamide, splenectomy, thalidomide

Cx DIC, transformation to AML, liver failure

Px Poor prognostic factors: ↑ age, anaemia, leucopenia, abnormal marrow karyotype

MYELODYSPLASIA

P Clonal disorder of bone marrow, produces morphological and functionally abnormal blood cells

Sy Features of anaemia, bacterial infections, bleeding

Ix FBC (↑ MCV, ↓ Hb, neutrophils, platelets); blood film, bone marrow biopsy

Rx *Supportive*: blood, platelet transfusions, antibiotics
Specific: treatment limited, in young patients allogeneic bone marrow transplantation may be curative

Px Poor, after 2–3 years one-third transform to AML
Median survival 3 years

MALIGNANCIES

ACUTE LYMPHOBLASTIC LEUKAEMIA

P Haematological malignancy resulting in ↑ production of lymphoblasts

A Commoner in children, peak age 4 years, bimodal in adults 15–25 years or >75 years

Sy Bleeding (bruising, menorrhagia, epistaxis), lethargy, SOB, arthralgia, malaise, recurrent infection, CNS infiltration, testicular disease

Ix FBC, clotting, blood film, cytochemistry, immunophenotyping, cytogenetics

Rx *Supportive*: treat infections, bleeding
Specific: chemotherapy, bone marrow transplant

Px Childhood good, adults poor

Cx Haemorrhage, thrombosis, tumour lysis syndrome (hyperuricaemia and renal failure) secondary to treatment

ACUTE MYELOGENOUS LEUKAEMIA

P Haematological malignancy resulting in the overproduction of immature myeloid WBCs

A Peak age of onset 70 years, rare under 20 years
Risk of transformation from chronic myeloid leukaemia (CML), myelodysplasia, myelofibrosis, polycythaemia rubra vera (PRV)

Sy Malaise, lethargy, anaemia, bleeding, recurrent infections

Si Purpura, organomegaly, lymphadenopathy, splenomegaly. DIC associated with M3 subtype.

Ix FBC ($\downarrow$ Hb, normal platelets), blood film, bone marrow trephine (Auer cells), lymph node biopsy, abdominal USS

Rx *Supportive*: blood transfusions, antibiotics
Specific: chemotherapy

Px Long-term survival 50 per cent

Cx Relapse of the disease, severe bleeding and infection, CNS infiltration

CHRONIC LYMPHOCYTIC LEUKAEMIA

P Monoclonal malignancy resulting in functionally incompetent lymphocytes

A Occurs in those aged over 60 years

Sy Recurrent infections, bleeding, anorexia, sweating, malaise, abdominal discomfort

Si Lymphadenopathy, splenomegaly, hepatomegaly, petechiae, pallor

Ix FBC (lymphocytosis, anaemia, thrombocytopenia), blood film (smudge cells), hypogammaglobulinaemia, bone marrow biopsy, lymph node biopsy

Rx *Supportive*: blood transfusions, antibiotics
Specific: chlorambucil $\pm$ prednisolone, splenectomy

Cx Increased risk of second malignancy, autoimmune haemolytic anaemia, idiopathic thrombocytopenic purpura (ITP)

CHRONIC MYELOID LEUKAEMIA

P Malignancy of granulocytes leads to $\uparrow$ production of myeloid precursors, with their differentiation ability still intact
Associated with the Philadelphia chromosome (translocation between 9 and 22 resulting in the *bcr-abl* gene that produces tyrosine kinase)

A Occurs in middle-aged and elderly

Sy Anaemia, weight loss, lassitude, anorexia, sweating, gout, bleeding, priapism, low-grade fever

Si Bruising, petechiae, splenomegaly, hepatomegaly

Ix FBC ($\uparrow$ WBC), clotting, blood film, cytochemistry, immunophenotyping, cytogenetics

Rx *Supportive*: blood transfusions, antibiotics
Specific: tyrosine kinase inhibitor (e.g. imatinib mesylate), alkylating agents, splenectomy, allogeneic bone marrow transplantation

HODGKIN'S LYMPHOMA

P Malignancy of the lymphatic system, involves clonal expansion of B and T white blood cells
Binucleate Reed–Sternberg cells ('owl's eye') are characteristic of Hodgkin's lymphoma

A Rare: <1500 new cases per annum in UK
Bimodal age distribution: peaks at 20–35 years and 50–60 years

S Painless lymphadenopathy – localized or generalized. Cervical chain is commonest site
Constitutional or 'B' symptoms are experienced in up to a quarter of patients: these include fever, weight loss (>10 per cent), pruritus, sweats

Ix *Bloods*: FBC, U&E, LFTs, LDH, ESR

Imaging: CXR, CT scan of the chest/abdomen/pelvis

Histology:
– Biopsy of lymph node
– Bone marrow aspirate and trephine

Box 1.32 ANN ARBOR STAGING SYSTEM FOR HODGKIN'S LYMPHOMA

- *Stage I*: confined to single lymph node group
- *Stage II*: two or more lymph node groups but confined to one side of the diaphragm
- *Stage III*: as for Stage II but both sides of diaphragm
- *Stage IV*: involvement of extralymphatic sites e.g. bone marrow

Staging includes absence (A) or presence (B) of systemic symptoms

---

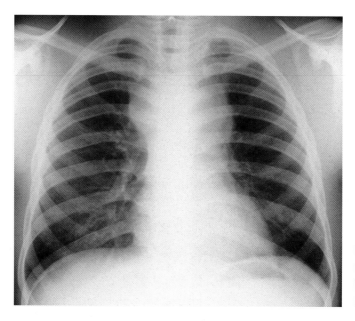

Figure 1.44 Anterior mediastinal mass due to lymphadenopathy from Hodgkin's lymphoma

Rx Localized disease (Stage IA and IIA): radiotherapy to involved and adjacent lymph node

Extensive disease (Stage III and IV): chemotherapy

If B symptoms are present: chemotherapy

Px 10-year survival rates vary from ~50 per cent for Stage IV to 80 per cent for Stage IA disease

NON-HODGKIN'S LYMPHOMA (NHL)

A 10 × more common than Hodgkin's lymphoma

Increases with age and slight male preponderance

Geographical variation: Burkitt's lymphoma common in Africa

Viruses are implicated, e.g. EBV, herpes simplex virus (HSV)

Immunosuppression is also a risk factor (including HIV/AIDS)

P   B-cell lymphoma (90 per cent of cases)
T-cell lymphoma (10 per cent of cases)
NHL can be classified as low, intermediate and high grade

S   Lymphadenopathy (60–70 per cent), hepatosplenomegaly, 'B' symptoms (as above)

Ix   As for Hodgkin's lymphoma
Staging: as for Hodgkin's lymphoma
Most patients present in Stage III or IV

Rx   *Stage I and II*: radiotherapy to the involved and adjacent lymph node or chemotherapy (depending on predominant cell subtype)
Stage III and IV: chemotherapy and interferon
Intermediate and high grade: high-dose chemotherapy
Consider autologous bone marrow transplantation in unresponsive or recurrent disease

Px   10-year survival rates vary from ~35 per cent for Stage IV to 80 per cent for Stage I disease

MULTIPLE MYELOMA

P   Malignancy of plasma cells resulting in abnormal plasma cells: ↑monoclonal antibodies

A   Peak age of incidence 60 years

Sy   Musculoskeletal (bone pain, pathological fractures, vertebral collapse, kyphosis), spinal cord compression, respiratory infections, anaemia (SOB, palpitations, lethargy), headaches + somnolence (due to ↑viscosity)

Si   Bleeding, bruising, purpura, pallor, bony tenderness

Ix   *Bloods*: FBC, blood film (leucoerythroblastic, rouleaux), bone marrow biopsy, ↑Ca^{2+}, ↑urea + creatinine, protein electrophoresis (shows monoclonal band), ↑↑ESR
Urine: Bence–Jones protein (immunoglobulin light chains in urine, not picked up on dipstick)
X-ray: skeletal survey looking for lytic lesions

Rx   Analgesia, radiotherapy to bony lesions, bisphosphonates, steroids, chemotherapy, plasmapheresis, thalidomide, bone marrow transplantation

Cx   Amyloidosis, renal failure, spinal cord compression, bone fractures

Px   Median survival 3 years

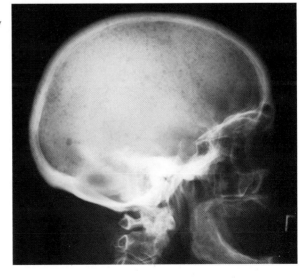

Figure 1.45 Widespread small lytic lesions in the cranial vault from multiple myeloma

INFECTIOUS DISEASES

AIDS (ACQUIRED IMMUNE DEFICIENCY SYNDROME)

(P) HIV (human immunodeficiency virus) infects CD4+ cells (T-helper cells) and destroys them; viral RNA is converted into DNA by reverse transcriptase; as the cell replicates protein it also replicates the HIV
When a patient's CD4 count is <200 cells/mm^3, the patient is said to have AIDS

(A) Transmitted by body secretions: intravenous drug use, sexual intercourse, vertical transmission, blood transfusions, tattoos

(S) Often there is a flu-like illness at the time of seroconversion; usually the first symptoms are due to opportunistic infections; common symptoms include fever, weight loss, lymphadenopathy, weakness

(Ix) HIV test, CD4 count, viral load

(Rx) *HAART (highly active anti-retroviral treatment)*
  – Nucleoside reverse transcriptase inhibitors (NRTI)
  – Non-nucleoside reverse transcriptase inhibitors (NNRTI)
  – Protease inhibitors
  New drugs: entry inhibitors, integrase inhibitors, assembly inhibitors, immunotherapy

(Cx) Drug resistance, opportunistic infections (see below), death

OPPORTUNISTIC INFECTIONS (OI)

(P) Infections which do not normally cause problems in a fully functioning immune system can cause fatal disease in AIDS. OIs occur when the CD4 count <200 cells/mm^3

There are multiple OIs, each which can present in different ways. Examples are shown in Box 1.33.

Box 1.33 DISEASES CAUSED BY OPPORTUNISTIC INFECTIONS

- *Fungal*: candidiasis, coccidioidomycosis, aspergillosis, cryptococcal meningitis
- *Bacterial*: *Mycobacterium avium* complex, tuberculosis
- *Protozoa*: *Pneumocystis carinii* pneumonia (PCP), cryptosporidiosis, toxoplasmosis
- *Viral*: CMV, HSV, human papilloma virus (HPV), herpes zoster virus (HZV), oral hairy leucoplakia, progressive multifocal leucoencephalopathy
- *Malignancy*: lymphoma (EBV), Kaposi's sarcoma (human herpesvirus-8), anal/cervical cancer (HPV)
- *Neurological*: AIDS dementia, peripheral neuropathy

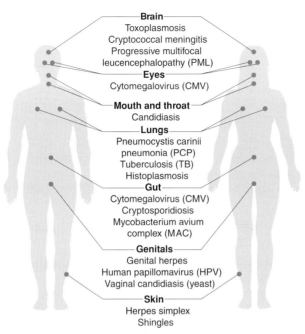

Brain
Toxoplasmosis
Cryptococcal meningitis
Progressive multifocal
leucencephalopathy (PML)
Eyes
Cytomegalovirus (CMV)
Mouth and throat
Candidiasis
Lungs
Pneumocystis carinii
pneumonia (PCP)
Tuberculosis (TB)
Histoplasmosis
Gut
Cytomegalovirus (CMV)
Cryptosporidiosis
Mycobacterium avium
complex (MAC)
Genitals
Genital herpes
Human papillomavirus (HPV)
Vaginal candidiasis (yeast)
Skin
Herpes simplex
Shingles

Figure 1.46 Opportunistic infections in AIDS

METHICILLIN-RESISTANT *STAPHYLOCOCCUS AUREUS* (MRSA)

(P) MRSA is commonly found on the skin or in the nose. Methicillin is the laboratory equivalent of flucloxacillin

(A) Usually occurs in hospitalized patients, at risk of cross-infection

(S) Dependent on the site of infection; it can range from asymptomatic colonization to bacteraemia

(Ix) Wound swabs

(Rx) Antibiotics (vancomycin/teicoplanin), isolation and barrier nursing to prevent cross-infection

VANCOMYCIN-RESISTANT ENTEROCOCCUS (VRE)

(P) Enterococci are part of the intestinal flora; spread by direct contact with the faeces of an infected patient; usually due to poor hygiene

(A) Hospitalized patients, chronic disease, immunosuppressed, previous antibiotic use

(S) Dependent on the site of infection: urinary tract infection (UTI), wound infections, endocarditis, bacteraemia, intra-abdominal infections

(Ix) FBC, septic screen

(Rx) Isolation and barrier nursing; combination of antibiotics is required – discuss with microbiologist as per regime

CLOSTRIDIUM DIFFICILE TOXIN

(P) *Clostridium difficile* is a Gram-positive anaerobe; it can colonize the colon and produce two toxins: A (enterotoxin) and B (cytotoxin)

(A) Antibiotic use, hospital stay, increased risk with older age

(S) Diarrhoea, fever, abdominal pain

(Ix) Stool MC&S, FBC ($\uparrow$WCC)

(Rx) Vancomycin, metronidazole, isolation and barrier nursing
(Cx) Pseudomembranous colitis, toxic megacolon, sepsis

BOTULISM

(P) *Clostridium botulinum* produces heat-resistant spores causing neuromuscular blockade
(A) Canned foods, inadequate cooking, wound contamination (e.g. injecting drugs into the skin)
(Si) Nausea, diarrhoea and vomiting, visual disturbance, descending paralysis
(Ix) Faecal analysis for toxin
(Px) Poor, >50 per cent mortality

INFECTIOUS MONONUCLEOSIS

(P) Caused by Epstein–Barr virus (EBV)
(A) EBV is spread by salivary secretions; has also been transmitted by blood transfusion and bone marrow transplant
(Sy) Fatigue, malaise, fever, myalgia
(Si) Papular rash, pharyngitis, lymphadenopathy, splenomegaly
(Ix) ↑WCC (lymphocytosis), ↓ platelets, ↑LFT, monospot, Paul Bunnell test, EBV titres
(Rx) Usually self-limiting and treatment is supportive;
(Cx) Bacterial superinfection, haemolytic anaemia, splenic rupture, myocarditis, pericarditis, meningitis, encephalitis, Guillain–Barré syndrome
EBV has also been associated with Burkitt's lymphoma, nasopharyngeal carcinoma, Hodgkin's disease and lymphoproliferative disease in immunosuppressed patients

HERPES SIMPLEX VIRUS (HSV)

(P) Double-stranded DNA virus, causes wide variety of syndromes
(A) Transmission via infected saliva, genital contact
(Sy) Cold sores (usually HSV-1), genital herpes (HSV-1 and -2)
(Si) Pyrexia, herpetic vesicles, cervicitis, urethritis
(Ix) Viral culture
(Rx) Aciclovir: topical for cold sores, systemic for genital herpes

CHICKENPOX

(P) Varicella zoster infection
(A) Usually affects children, person-to-person spread
(S) Fever, headache, vesicular rash
(Ix) Clinical, viral culture
(Rx) Supportive, aciclovir if immunocompromised or pregnant
(Cx) Pneumonia, shingles, birth defects if pregnant

MUMPS

(P) Parotitis as a result of infection with a paramyxovirus
(A) Droplet/direct contact transmission
Can be prevented by vaccination with MMR (measles mumps and rubella) vaccine
(S) Pyrexia, headache, parotid swelling

Ix   Clinical diagnosis

Rx   Supportive

Cx   Epididymo-orchitis, subfertility, meningitis, pancreatitis

MEASLES

P   Paramyxovirus infection

A   Droplet spread

     Can be prevented by vaccination with MMR

S   Pyrexia, Koplik spots (small grey lesions on buccal mucosa), maculopapular rash

Ix   Clinical

Rx   Supportive, analgesia

Cx   Common: pneumonia, gastroenteritis, subacute sclerosing panencephalitis (reactivation of virus in brain ~10 years after infection: almost universally fatal)

MALARIA

P   Transmitted by mosquito bites; four *Plasmodium* species: *falciparum*, *vivax*, *ovale*, and *malariae*; *vivax* and *ovale* species can remain dormant as hypnozoites and cause recurrent infections

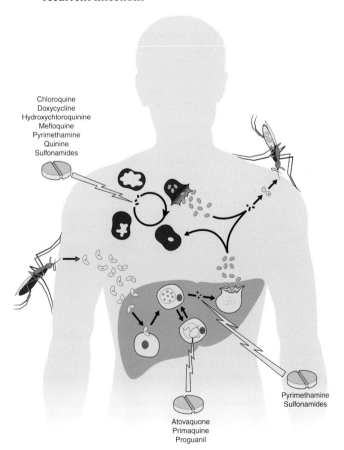

Figure 1.47 Life cycle of the malaria parasite (reproduced from Simonsen T, Aarbakke J, Kay I, Coleman I, Sinnot P and Lysaa R, *Illustrated Pharmacology For Nurses*, London: Hodder Arnold, 2006 with kind permission by the illustrator Roy A Lysaa)

(A) Occurs in tropical areas

(Sy) Fever, fatigue, myalgia, headache, nausea, vomiting

(Si) Tachycardia, anaemia, jaundice, splenomegaly,

(Ix) Blood smears, FBC (anaemia), ↑ESR, ↑CRP, U&E, LFT

(Rx) Quinine, mefloquine, doxycycline, chloroquine, artesunate (for severe falciparum malaria)

(Cx) Falciparum malaria: cerebral malaria, hypoglycaemia, renal impairment

TYPHOID

(P) Infection with *Salmonella typhi*

(A) Faecal–oral transmission via contaminated food or water
Preventable by vaccination

(S) Fever, headache, diarrhoea, rose spots (blanching maculopapular rash on trunk), splenomegaly

(Ix) Blood, urine, stool cultures, serology

(Rx) Third-generation cephalosporins (e.g. ceftriaxone), ciproflaxin (increasing resistance worldwide), fluids

(Cx) Pneumonia, haemolysis, meningitis, death

SEXUALLY TRANSMITTED INFECTIONS

SYPHILIS

(P) Caused by a spirochaete, *Treponema pallidum*

(A) Sexually transmitted infection

(S) *Primary syphilis*: primary lesion is the chancre, a raised painless papule with an ulcerated centre, usually found at the site of inoculation; lymphadenopathy
Secondary syphilis: widespread mucocutaneous lesions, fever, malaise, headache, lymphadenopathy, sore throat; other systems rarely involved
Tertiary syphilis: characterized by the **gumma**, usually found in the liver, bone and testes

(Ix) Microscopy of fluid from mucocutaneous lesions, VDRL (venereal diseases research laboratory), *Treponema pallidum* haemagglutination assay (TPHA)
Other investigations to assess for complications include CXR, CT/MRI, lumbar puncture

(Rx) Penicillin

(Cx) *Congenital syphilis*: spontaneous abortion, birth defects
Cardiovascular syphilis: aortic aneurysm, aortic regurgitation
Neurosyphilis: tabes dorsalis, brain atrophy, Argyll Robertson pupil

GONORRHOEA

(P) Bacterial infection caused by *Neisseria gonorrhoeae*

(A) Sexually transmitted infection

(Sy) Purulent penile discharge, often asymptomatic in women

(Ix) Microscopy of discharge reveals characteristic Gram-negative diplococci

(Rx) Cephalosporin, widespread antibiotic resistance

(Cx) Septic arthritis, most common cause of monoarthritis in sexually active adults

CHLAMYDIA

(P) Causative organism *Chlamydia trachomatis*

(A) Most common sexually transmitted infection in UK

(S) ♀ usually none, sometimes cervicitis/cystitis, lower abdominal pain, intermenstrual bleeding

♂ often asymptomatic, discharge, dysuria

(Ix) Urine testing for *Chlamydia*

(Rx) Azithromycin, widespread resistance

(Cx) Peri-hepatitis (Fitz-Hugh–Curtis syndrome)

GENITAL WARTS

(P) Infection with HPV causes warts

(A) Skin-to-skin contact during sexual contact

(Sy) Soft, fleshy warts anywhere in genital area

(Ix) Clinical

(Rx) No known cure, topical treatment with liquid nitrogen, podophyllin

(Cx) Implicated in pathogenesis of cervical cancer and anal cancer

DERMATOLOGY

DERMATOLOGICAL TERMS

- **Abscess:** a local accumulation of pus
- **Atrophy:** wasting away/diminution
- **Bulla:** blister >5 cm
- **Comedone:** plug of sebaceous and dead skin material stuck in the opening of a hair follicle: open (blackhead) or closed (whitehead)
- **Erosion:** loss of epithelium
- **Erythema:** redness of the skin
- **Hyperpigmentation:** increased pigmentation
- **Hypopigmentation:** decreased pigmentation
- **Macule:** a small, flat, distinct, coloured area of skin <10 mm in diameter
- **Nodule:** raised lesion >1 cm (an enlargement of a papule)
- **Papule:** small, circumscribed, palpable lesion
- **Plaque:** large elevated solid lesions
- **Purpura:** non-blanching, haemorrhagic lesions, >3 mm
- **Pustule:** blister containing pus
- **Scaling:** an increase in the dead cells on the surface of the skin (stratum corneum)
- **Telangiectasia:** prominent cutaneous dilated blood vessels
- **Ulcer:** full-thickness loss of epidermis or epithelium, may be covered with a dark-coloured crust (eschar)
- **Vesicle:** small, fluid-filled blister
- **Wheals:** cutaneous oedema due to leaking capillaries

ECZEMA

(P) *Atopic eczema*: begins in infancy. Occurs in 5 per cent of those <5 years old; 25 per cent of patients have a first-degree relative with atopy (an inherited altered immune reactivity, i.e. asthma, hay fever, conjunctivitis or eczema)

Exogenous eczema: irritant contact dermatitis, allergic contact dermatitis

(Sy) Itchy, ill-defined erythematous scaly patches on flexor surfaces

(Si) Erythematous scaly patches, oedema, vesicles

(Ix) Clinical diagnosis, can be associated with elevated IgE

Patch testing for contact dermatitis

(Rx) Atopic eczema:
- *topical*: emollients, tar, steroids, psoralen plus ultraviolet A (PUVA), sirolimus, tacrolimus
- *systemic*: oral antihistamines, antibiotics for infections, immunosuppressants (azathioprine)

Avoid irritants, if patients develop eczema herpeticum, i.e. secondary infection with HSV, then the patient needs to be admitted for i.v. aciclovir

(Px) Atopic eczema: 40 per cent resolve after 5 years, 90 per cent between 15 and 20 years

PSORIASIS

(A) Polygenic susceptibility

Arthropathy is associated with HLA B27

Exacerbating factors include drugs (antimalarials, β-blockers, alcohol, lithium), stress and infections, e.g. streptococcal sore throat can precipitate guttate psoriasis

(P) Several subtypes exist including stable chronic plaque, guttate, erythrodermic, and pustular psoriasis

(Si) Salmon-coloured silver scaly lesions often involving the scalp, behind the ear, predominantly on extensor surfaces but can occur anywhere

Lesions can be plaques, nummular (coin-shaped) or guttate (raindrop-shaped)

Exhibits the Koebner phenomenon (lesions occur over sites of trauma)

Nail signs: nail pitting, onycholysis, nail dystrophy, subungual hyperkeratosis

(Ix) Clinical diagnosis, but can do a biopsy

(Rx) *Supportive*: emollients

Topical: tar, topical steroids, dithranol, ultraviolet B (UVB), PUVA

Systemic: PUVA, methotrexate, ciclosporin, hydroxycarbamide, sulfasalazine

(Px) Only 1 per cent of patients with psoriasis develop psoriatic arthropathy

LICHEN PLANUS

(Si) *Skin*: pruritic eruption of violaceous, shiny, polygonal papules with Wickham's striae (characteristic white lines)

Mouth: oral involvement (white or grey streaks forming a linear or reticular pattern on a violaceous background)

Nails: onycholysis, dystrophy, longitudinal ridging, pterygium (scarring of the nail bed)

Scalp: alopecia

(Rx) Self-limiting, resolves within 8–12 months

URTICARIA

(A) Wide variety of causes (see Box 1.34)

Box 1.34 CAUSES OF URTICARIA

- *Recent illness*
- *Drugs*: ACE inhibitors, anaesthetics, antibiotics
- *Infection*: amoebiasis, malaria
- *Foods*: shellfish, fish, eggs, cheese, chocolate, nuts, berries, tomatoes
- *Synthetic products*: perfumes, creams, nail polish, nickel, rubber, latex, industrial chemicals, detergents
- *Pets*: exposure to new animals (dander)
- *Pregnancy*: usually occurs in last trimester and typically resolves spontaneously soon after delivery
- *Environmental*: dust, mould, chemicals or plants
- *Idiopathic*

(Si) Itchy blanching red wheals (circumscribed areas of raised erythema and oedema of the superficial dermis) in response to a precipitant

Acute form of urticaria lasts <4–6 weeks, and the chronic form lasts >4–6 weeks

(Ix) *Bloods*: ANA titres, hepatitis B + C, TFT

(Rx) Identify underlying cause, remove the precipitant and give symptomatic relief (antihistamines, steroids)

PEMPHIGUS

(A) Rare, most common at 45–50 years

(P) Direct action of an antibody attack on the intra-epidermal desmosomal structure

(Sy) Bullous lesions/blisters which may be confined to mucous membranes, but can occur on trunk, scalp and other parts of the body; the blisters rupture easily as they are intra-epithelial

(Ix) *Biopsy*: intra-epidermal blister with acantholysis

Immunology: direct immunofluorescence intercellular IgG and C3

(Rx) *Local*: wet dressings, lotions

Systemic: high-dose steroids, immunosuppressants, i.v. fluids

(Px) Prior to steroids, poor prognosis

(Cx) Secondary infection, sepsis, extensive loss of body fluids and electrolytes

PEMPHIGOID

(P) Autoimmune reaction against the basement membrane

(A) Most common in the elderly

(Si) Initially patients develop erythematous and eczematous areas on the trunk and limb, which then develop tense blisters; can be pruritic, rarely affects the mucosal membranes, bullae usually heal without scarring

(Ix) *Biopsy*: positive direct immunofluorescence demonstrating IgG and C3 at the basement membrane

(Rx) Steroids, azathioprine can be used as a steroid-sparing agent

ACNE VULGARIS

(A) Common skin disease that affects 85–100 per cent of people at some time during their lives

(Si) Characterized by non-inflammatory follicular papules or comedones, in severe cases inflammatory papules, pustules and nodules

Affects the areas of skin with the densest population of sebaceous follicles; include the face, the upper part of the chest and the back

(Rx) *Topical*: retinoids, antibiotics

Systemic: antibiotics (tetracyclines), OCP, isotretinoin

PITYRIASIS ROSEA

(Sy) May be prodromal symptoms prior to the development of the rash

(Si) Papular skin eruption that begins as a herald patch (pink oval patch 3–6 cm in diameter), normally initially found on the back before becoming distributed in a Christmas tree pattern

(Ix) Exclude treponemal infection

(Rx) Normally self-limiting, in very severe cases topical steroids

INFECTIONS

TINEA (DERMATOPHYTOSIS, RINGWORM)

(P) Dermatophytes are a group of fungi (ringworm) that invade the dead keratin of skin, hair and nails.

Box 1.35 SUBTYPES OF TINEA INFESTATION
• *Tinea capitis*: scalp hair
• *Tinea corporis*: trunk and extremities
• *Tinea manuum*: palms
• *Tinea pedis*: soles and interdigital webs
• *Tinea cruris*: groin
• *Tinea barbae*: beard area and neck
• *Tinea faciale*: face
• *Tinea unguium* (onychomycosis): nail

(Si) Pruritic lesions, classical lesion: central clearing surrounded by an advancing, red, scaly, elevated border. One or more lesions may appear, commonly in the groin, feet and axillae.

Nails: onychomycosis

(Ix) Microscopy of scrapings

(Rx) Topical imidazole, systemic terbinafine

(Px) Infection resolves within 1–2/52 with treatment (longer for onychomycosis)

(Cx) Secondary infection

PITYRIASIS VERSICOLOR

(P) Caused by yeasts of *Pityrosporum orbiculare* (can also be normal commensal)

(A) Occurs in hot, humid countries, or patients who sweat a lot

Si Flaky discoloured patches appear mainly on the chest and back, trunk and arms; the patches may be pink, coppery brown or paler than surrounding skin; mildly itchy

Ix Wood's light: yellow, green fluorescence, microscopy of scrapings

Rx Topical and systemic antifungal agents used

CELLULITIS

P Superficial skin infection due to either staphylococcal or streptococcal subgroups

A Predisposed by trauma, oedema or tinea pedis

Si Painful, swelling, warmth and erythema over affected site, pyrexia

Ix FBC, blood cultures, swabs over affected area

Rx Antibiotics (penicillin and flucloxacillin)

Cx Sepsis

SCABIES

P Infestation of the skin with the microscopic mite *Sarcoptes scabiei*; very contagious
May take up to 4–6 weeks before symptoms occur

Sy Severe itchiness

Si Symmetrical rash affecting fingers, backs of hands, axillae, breasts and buttock
Excoriated papules and nodules; occasionally burrows are seen

Ix Skin scraping: under microscope can see burrow contents

Rx Topical insecticides (e.g. permethrin, malathion), imperative to also treat partners and cohabitants

CUTANEOUS MANIFESTATIONS OF SYSTEMIC DISEASE

DERMATITIS HERPETIFORMIS

P Strong association with HLA B8, DR3, DQw2 haplotype

A Associated with gluten-sensitive enteropathy (coeliac disease)

Sy Itchy small blisters on extensor surfaces, buttocks or face

Ix *Histology*: subepidermal blisters and microabscesses in the dermal papillae
Immunology: direct immunofluorescence IgA in the papillary tips

Rx Dapsone, gluten-free diet

ERYTHEMA NODOSUM

Si Tender, erythematous nodules which resolve after 6/52, occur on shins and not associated with scarring

Rx Treat underlying cause, supportive treatment of skin lesions

Box 1.36 CAUSES OF ERYTHEMA NODOSUM
• Infection: *Streptococcus*, tuberculosis
• Sarcoidosis
• Inflammatory bowel disease: Crohn's disease, ulcerative colitis
• Drugs, e.g. sulfonamides, OCP
• Idiopathic

ERYTHEMA MULTIFORME

(Si) Symmetrical eruption of raised target lesions, may be associated with pyrexia
If associated with mucosal involvement known as Stevens–Johnson syndrome

---

Box 1.37 CAUSES OF ERYTHEMA MULTIFORME

- Infection: herpes simplex, *Mycoplasma*, psittacosis, hepatitis B, EBV, histoplasmosis
- Lupus
- Drugs, e.g. sulfonamides, antibiotics
- Malignancy including leukaemia
- Pregnancy
- Pre-menstrual
- Sarcoid

(Rx) Steroids, symptomatic treatment

PYODERMA GANGRENOSUM

(A) Inflammatory bowel disease, seronegative rheumatoid arthritis, myeloma
(Si) Painful, rapidly growing ulcerated nodules
(Rx) Oral steroids
(Px) Heals with scarring

LUPUS PERNIO

(P) Cutaneous manifestation characteristic of chronic sarcoidosis
(Si) Chronic, indurated violaceous papules or plaques that affect the mid-face, particularly the alar rim of the nose

LUPUS VULGARIS

(P) Cutaneous tuberculosis affecting the face
(Si) Brownish tubercles that often heal slowly and leave scars. The lesion spreads with a hyperpigmented margin and a hypopigmented core, often with ulceration

ACANTHOSIS NIGRICANS

(A) Associated with numerous conditions including malignancy, acromegaly, dermatomyositis, scleroderma and Wilson's disease
(Si) Lesions begin as hyperpigmented macules/papules and progress on to velvety plaques with associated skin tags. Most commonly occur in axilla, groin and posterior neck
(Ix) Need to exclude a possible underlying malignancy, diabetes and insulin resistance
(Rx) None

THROMBOPHLEBITIS MIGRANS

(A) Associated with stomach and other intra-abdominal malignancies
(Si) Occurrence of inflammation and thrombosis of veins occurring sequentially at multiple sites

NECROBIOSIS LIPOIDICA

(A) Associated with diabetes

(Si) Asymptomatic shiny patches that slowly enlarge over months to years, patches are initially red–brown and progress to yellow, depressed atrophic plaques; most commonly occurs over pre-tibial areas; Koebner phenomenon (i.e. occurs at site of trauma)

(Rx) Limited, but topical and intra-lesion steroids may slow progression

GRANULOMA ANNULARE

(A) Associated with trauma, diabetes

(Si) Erythematous, firm, ring-shaped lesions with an elevated edge (diameter 1–5 mm)

(Rx) Usually self-limiting, but can use topical steroids

XANTHELASMA

(A) Frequently occur in patients with Type II + IV hyperlipidaemia

(Si) Yellow plaques that occur most commonly near the inner canthus of the eyelid

(Rx) Control of hypercholesterolaemia

Surgery

Gareth Jones

GENERAL SURGERY

SALIVARY GLANDS

INFLAMMATION AND CALCULI

(P) Inflammation of one or more of the paired salivary glands – parotid, submandibular and sublingual

(A) Calculi (causing obstruction) or infection (bacterial, mumps or HIV)

(Sy) Lumps, pain and swelling – exacerbated by eating when due to calculus

(Si) External swellings, erythema ± purulent discharge from duct openings in mouth, bimanual palpation of calculi, lymph node enlargement

(Ix) X-ray or sialogram (contrast injected into duct) to reveal calculi

(Rx) *Calculi*: removed via mouth if distal, or gland excision
Bacterial infection: hydration and antibiotics
Mumps: rest and antipyretics

MALIGNANCY

(A) 80 per cent of tumours involve the parotid gland (80 per cent in the superficial lobe)

(P) Benign (80 per cent pleomorphic adenoma) or malignant (commonly adenocarcinoma)

(Sy) Salivary gland lump, pain

(Si) Palpable swelling, may have evidence of facial nerve (VII) involvement (as nerve VII passes through the parotid)

(Ix) Computed tomography (CT), magnetic resonance imaging (MRI) or sialogram (injection of contrast into salivary duct – now rarely used). Fine-needle aspiration (FNA)

Rx *Benign*: wide excision of tumour with preservation of facial nerve
Malignant: radical parotidectomy (facial nerve sacrificed if adherent to tumour) and
radiotherapy ± lymph node dissection

Cx Post-operative: facial nerve injury, Frey's syndrome (facial sweating while eating due
to abnormal connection between autonomic and facial nerve fibres)

Px Poor prognosis in malignant tumours (5-year survival ~50 per cent)

OESOPHAGUS

GASTRO-OESOPHAGEAL REFLUX DISEASE (GORD)

Please refer to section in Chapter 1 (p. 34)

PERFORATION

This is a **surgical emergency**

A Oesophagogastroduodenoscopy (OGD) (increased risk if dilatation or biopsy
performed), foreign body, external trauma, post-emesis (Boerhaave's syndrome),
carcinoma

Sy Chest pain, odynophagia

Si Shock (tachycardia, tachypnoea, hypotension),
surgical emphysema of neck/chest (air in tissues
– produces a 'crackling' sensation on palpation
and is visible on X-ray). Fever/signs of systemic
sepsis will rapidly develop if undiagnosed

Ix Chest X-ray (CXR): mediastinal surgical
emphysema, air/fluid level in pleural cavity.
Water-soluble contrast swallow (e.g.
Gastrografin)

Rx Small perforation may be managed
conservatively: nil by mouth (NBM), i.v.
(intravenous) fluids, antibiotics
Larger perforations require urgent surgical
repair

Px If operation (when indicated) is delayed >48 h,
mortality is >50 per cent

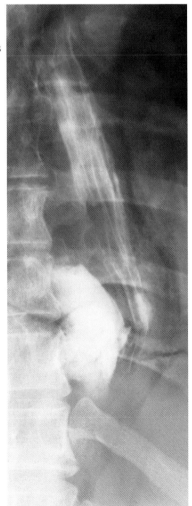

Figure 2.1 Oesophageal perforation: water soluble
contrast examination showing contrast leakage at the
lower end of the oesophagus

STRICTURES

P Narrowing of any tubular structure, e.g. oesophagus

A *Benign*: ingestion of corrosives, GORD, trauma (e.g. OGD), foreign body
Malignant: See p. 109

Sy Dysphagia (initially food > fluid)

Si May be malnourished/cachectic

Ix OGD, barium swallow

Rx Endoscopic dilatation (if unsuccessful or frequently required, may consider surgical resection of stricture)

HIATUS HERNIA

P Herniation of the gastro-oesophageal junction (GOJ) and/or proximal part of stomach through diaphragm into the thorax
Three types:
– sliding (80 per cent): GOJ enters thorax (disturbs lower oesophageal sphincter mechanism)
– rolling (5 per cent): proximal part of stomach herniates into thorax
– mixed (15 per cent): combination of rolling and sliding

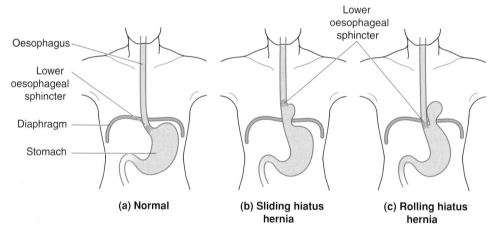

Figure 2.2 Hiatus hernia. (a) Normal oesophagus and stomach; (b) sliding hiatus hernia; (c) rolling/para-oesophageal hiatus hernia

A Classically obese, >50 years, women

Sy Asymptomatic, GORD (in sliding variety)

Ix Barium swallow. OGD to assess oesophagitis

Rx *Conservative* : ↓ weight, lifestyle changes and medical treatment as per GORD
Surgical : Open/laparoscopic Nissen's fundoplication (wrap fundus of stomach around lower oesophagus). Indicated in rolling hiatus hernias due to risk of volvulus, and when symptoms/sequelae of GORD are not controlled conservatively

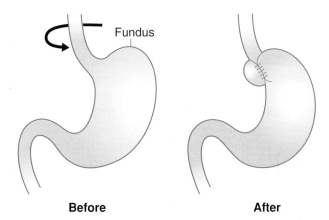

Figure 2.3 Nissen fundoplication

MALIGNANCY

A   Incidence : ↑ China, ↑↑ Iran versus UK

Associated with smoking, alcohol, diet, Barrett's oesophagus, achalasia

P   Upper two-thirds squamous carcinoma, lower one-third adenocarcinoma (Barrett's oesophagus associated)

Site: 20 per cent upper one-third, 50 per cent middle one-third, 30 per cent lower one-third (increasing due to Barrett's oesophagus)

Sy   Progressive dysphagia, general symptoms of malignant disease (i.e. weight loss, anaemia, etc.)

Si   Hoarse voice indicating possible invasion of recurrent laryngeal nerve

Ix   CXR, barium swallow, OGD + biopsy/brushings, CT and PET scans to stage

Rx   An attempt at curative oesophagectomy (e.g. Ivor–Lewis) is appropriate in <50 per cent

Palliative treatment includes stenting, radiotherapy, chemotherapy, laser therapy

Px   Overall 5 year survival ~17%

VARICES

P   Portal hypertension results in dilatation of veins at sites of porto-systemic anastomosis, i.e. lower oesophagus, rectum, umbilicus (caput medusae)

Dilated veins project into lumen of oesophagus and are liable to haemorrhage

Sy   Upper gastrointestinal (GI) haemorrhage, therefore haematemesis, melaena

Si   Evidence of chronic liver disease (is there a history of alcohol abuse or cirrhosis?)

Ix   OGD

Rx   *Acute bleeding*:

- resuscitate and correct possible clotting abnormalities
- i.v. terlipressin (or somatostatin analogue) reduces bleeding
- OGD + sclerotherapy/banding of varices
- if unsuccessful, pass a Sengstaken–Blakemore tube (contains an inflatable balloon used to compress varices)
- continued bleeding requires surgical decompression

Prophylaxis:

- β-blockers to reduce portal pressure
- OGD + sclerotherapy/banding of varices
- transjugular intra-hepatic portosystemic shunting (TIPSS)

Px   Each bleeding episode has a mortality of ~20 per cent

ACHALASIA

P Neuromuscular disorder characterized by failure of relaxation of the lower oesophageal sphincter (LOS), together with absence of oesophageal peristalsis. May be mimicked by Chagas' disease (*Trypanosoma cruzi* infection in South America)

A Typically aged 25–60 years

Sy Dysphagia > regurgitation, chest pain, weight loss

Ix *Barium swallow*: tapering of lower oesophagus described as a 'bird's beak', together with proximal dilatation
Oesophageal manometry: reveals incomplete relaxation of LOS
OGD: exclude malignancy

Rx *Endoscopy*: pneumatic dilatation or botulinum toxin injection at OGD
Surgery: Heller's operation whereby the muscle of the LOS and proximal stomach is divided down to the mucosa (open or laparoscopic)

Cx Associated with malignant change in the distal oesophagus

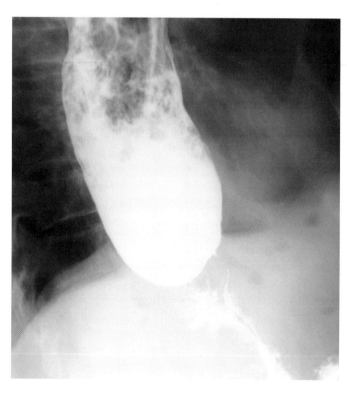

Figure 2.4 Achalasia of the oesophagus: grossly dilated oesophagus with a smooth narrowing at its lower end

PHARYNGEAL POUCH/ZENKER'S DIVERTICULUM

P Protrusion of mucosa and submucosa between two parts of the inferior pharyngeal constrictor muscle (this area of weakness is called Killian's dehiscence)

Sy Dysphagia, regurgitation, bulging or gurgling of the neck, halitosis

Si Neck swelling, halitosis, signs of aspiration pneumonia may be present

Ix Barium swallow

Rx Surgical excision of pouch, plus repair of defect in inferior constrictor

PLUMMER–VINSON/PATERSON–BROWN KELLY SYNDROME

(P) Web: thin eccentric extension of normal oesophageal tissue
(A) Upper oesophageal web in association with iron deficiency anaemia and dysphagia
(Sy) Dysphagia
(Si) Those of iron deficiency anaemia, i.e. koilonychia and glossitis
(Ix) Investigation with barium swallow, OGD
(Cx) Associated with malignant change
(Rx) Iron replacement; dilatation of web if required

STOMACH

PEPTIC ULCERS

This is covered in detail in Chapter 1 (p. 35)
Indications for surgery:

- *haemorrhage not controlled with medical therapy*:
  - duodenal ulcers – suture ligation of ulcer ± vagotomy and pyloroplasty
  - gastric ulcers – oversewing of ulcer (sometimes require resection)
- *ulcer perforation*:
  - closure with an omental patch followed by peritoneal lavage
- *ulcer producing gastric outlet obstruction*
- *malignant change*:
  - distal gastrectomy – either Billroth 1 (gastroduodenostomy) or Billroth 2 (gastrojejunostomy)

UPPER GI BLEED

This is a **surgical emergency**

(P) Bleeding proximal to the ligament of Treitz (marks duodenojejunal flexure)
(A) Peptic ulcer, gastritis, oesophageal varices, Mallory–Weiss tear (mucosal tear in oesophagus due to vomiting) and malignancy
(Sy) Haematemesis (bright red or coffee-ground appearance), melaena (black motions), fresh blood per rectum (PR) (very rapid bleed)
(Si) Assess state of shock (i.e. urine output, pulse, blood pressure [BP], conscious level). Be alert to signs of chronic liver disease. PR for melaena. Epigastric tenderness
(Ix) *Initially*: bloods (full blood count (FBC), urea and electrolytes (U&E), coagulation, cross-match 4–6 units), urine output, electrocardiogram (ECG)
Once stabilized: OGD to identify, treat and assess prognosis of bleeding
(Rx) Resuscitate. Correct clotting abnormalities
OGD allows adrenaline or sclerosant injection/diathermy/laser phototherapy/variceal banding
Indications for surgery are Hospital Trust dependent, they include: bleeding vessel not controlled at endoscopy, continued bleeding, rebleeding and patients >60 years
(Px) Rockall Risk Score is used to predict mortality
Overall mortality rate: 6–10 per cent

PYLORIC STENOSIS

(P) Hypertrophy of smooth muscle in the antrum and pylorus of the stomach

(A) Typically presents ~4 weeks of age

(Sy) Non-bilious vomiting after feeding, which becomes projectile

(Si) Pylorus palpable as an 'olive' in epigastrium/right upper quadrant (RUQ)

(Ix) Ultrasound scan (USS), U&E (loss of H_2O and H^+Cl^- during vomiting)

(Rx) Correct dehydration and electrolyte disturbances prior to definitive treatment with Ramstedt's pyloromyotomy (incision of pylorus muscle)

GASTRIC CARCINOMA

(A) Incidence declining in the UK, although it remains second most common cause of cancer-related death in the world (highest incidence: Japan)

Box 2.1 RISK FACTORS FOR GASTRIC CARCINOMA
• Diet (pickled/smoked foods)
• Achlorhydria, e.g. atrophic gastritis, pernicious anaemia
• Blood group A
• Low social class
• Smoking
• *H. pylori*
• Previous gastric surgery

(Sy) Anorexia, weight loss, nausea, dyspepsia, dysphagia and epigastric pain, among others, are late symptoms

(Si) Cachexia, epigastric mass. Metastases may present with hepatomegaly or classically, a palpable Virchow's node (located in the left supraclavicular fossa)

(Ix) FBC may reveal anaemia

Barium meal

OGD + multiple biopsies

CT/MRI to assess metastatic disease

(Rx) Total or partial gastrectomy plus lymph node resection is potentially curative. Palliative procedures centre on relieving gastric obstruction

(Px) 5-year survival ~15 per cent (improved in countries employing screening programmes)

SMALL INTESTINE

MECKEL'S DIVERTICULUM

(P) Persistence of a segment of the vitello-intestinal duct

(A) Rule of 2s:
  − ~2 per cent population affected
  − ~2 inches long
  − ~2 feet proximal to ileocaecal valve

  None of the above is 2 accurate!

  Frequently contains ectopic tissue – gastric (50 per cent), pancreatic, colonic, etc.

(S) Asymptomatic finding at laparotomy (most common)

  Ulceration (due to presence of gastric mucosa), haemorrhage, small bowel obstruction, perforation and diverticulitis

(Ix) Barium follow-through, technetium nuclear medicine scan, laparoscopy

Rx Resection of diverticulum (resection of asymptomatic Meckel's is controversial)

Px Lifetime risk of requiring surgery ~4 per cent

LARGE INTESTINE

APPENDICITIS

P Inflammation of the vermiform appendix (arises from caecum)

A Lifetime incidence ~7 per cent (rare in very young/old)

Due to bacterial infection secondary to luminal obstruction (most often a faecalith or lymphoid hyperplasia)

Sy Anorexia. Classically, colicky central abdominal pain (inflammation of appendix) followed by localization of pain to right iliac fossa (inflammation of overlying peritoneum)

Nausea, vomiting and constipation/diarrhoea are more variable

Si Low grade pyrexia, patient tries to minimize movements. Right iliac fossa (RIF) tenderness, guarding and rebound/percussion tenderness. Right-sided tenderness on PR

Rovsing's sign: RIF pain on palpation of left iliac fossa (LIF)

Differential diagnosis: ectopic pregnancy, ovarian torsion, diverticulitis, pelvic inflammatory disease, Crohn's disease, mesenteric adenitis

Ix Commonly ↑ white cell count (WCC) (neutrophilia) and ↑ C-reactive protein (CRP). USS and CT if uncertain of diagnosis. β-human chorionic gonadotrophin (β-HCG) to exclude ectopic pregnancy in females. Laparoscopy can be diagnostic and therapeutic

Cx Perforation leading to either generalized peritonitis or a localized appendix abscess. Omentum may cover inflammation resulting in an appendix mass

Rx Laparoscopic/open appendicectomy (prophylactic cefuroxime and metronidazole continued if evidence of perforation)

Px Mortality rate <1 per cent

DIVERTICULAR DISEASE OF THE COLON

P Acquired outpouchings of bowel mucosa secondary to high intraluminal pressures

Most commonly affects sigmoid colon

A Postulated to be secondary to low-fibre Western diets

Box 2.2 IMPORTANT DEFINITIONS

- *Diverticulosis*: existence of diverticula with no inflammation
- *Diverticulitis*: inflammation of a diverticulum
- *Diverticular disease*: diverticula associated with abdominal pain and disturbed bowel habit

---

Sy Depend on site, severity and presence of complications

Abdominal pain (usually in LIF), fever, altered bowel habit, nausea and PR bleeding

Si Pyrexia. Localized tenderness, guarding and rebound/percussion tenderness (often LIF). PR for tenderness/blood

Ix Gastrografin enema, CT scan, sigmoidoscopy and colonoscopy

℞   *Diverticular disease*: high-fibre diet (ensure carcinoma has been excluded)
       Diverticulitis:
       – mild disease treated as an outpatient with liquid diet and broad-spectrum
         antibiotics
       – if unable to tolerate fluids or inadequate analgesia, then admit; NBM, i.v. fluids
         and i.v. broad-spectrum antibiotics
       – failure to respond to medical therapy/perforation/obstruction will generally
         require a Hartmann's procedure, with colostomy reversal 3–6 months later

Cx   Perforation, obstruction, haemorrhage, fistulae, abscess formation

STOMAS

- Surgically created opening of a tube (bowel or urinary tract) to a body surface (usually the abdomen)
- Collecting bag attaches over stoma
- Profound psychological implications for patient – involve stoma nurse early
- Stoma position decided pre-operatively (avoid umbilicus, scars and bony prominences)
- Defunctioning stomas aim to prevent digested products reaching a distal section of bowel – allow healing of an anastomosis, or resolution of infection prior to reversal
- *End ileostomy/colostomy*: single lumen of bowel
- *Loop ileostomy/colostomy*: section of bowel incised ~250° of its circumference to create two lumens
- *Double-barrel colostomy*: proximal and distal sections of bowel brought out as separate single lumens

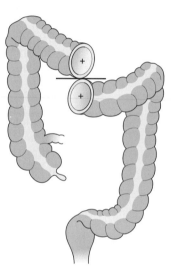

(a)   **Loop colostomy**

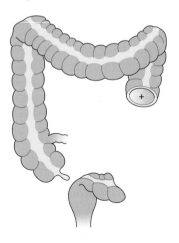

(b)   **End colostomy**

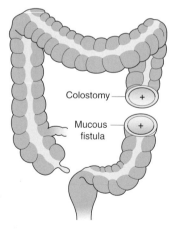

(c)   **Double-barrel colostomy**

Figure 2.5 Colostomies: (a) loop colostomy; (b) end colostomy; (c) double-barrel colostomy

Ileostomy

- Stoma involving ileum
- Usually located in right lower quadrant
- Spout to prevent their irritant liquid effluent from contacting skin
  - *end ileostomy* – e.g. after total colectomy
  - *defunctioning loop ileostomy* – e.g. if concerned regarding a colonic anastomosis

Colostomy

- Stoma involving colon
- Usually located in left lower quadrant
- Flush with skin
  - *end colostomy* – e.g. after abdominoperineal resection (removal of anus and rectum for low rectal cancer)
  - *Hartmann's procedure* – distal segment of colon is left *in situ* and closed with sutures. The proximal segment is exteriorized as an end colostomy. This offers the possibility of reversal at a later date

(Cx) Diarrhoea and constipation

Ileostomies can result in electrolyte imbalances due to large fluid losses

Necrosis, prolapse and stenosis of stoma

Parastomal hernia

MALIGNANCY

(A) Second commonest cause of cancer-related deaths in the UK

Incidence ↑ with age

Risk factors:
- environmental: ? diet high in fat, ? alcohol, red meat
- inflammatory bowel disease
- familial adenomatous polyposis coli syndrome (FAP) and hereditary non-polyposis colon cancer (HNPCC) (see p. 117)

(P) Majority located in rectum and sigmoid colon (left side of colon)

Adenoma → carcinoma theory

(Sy) Weight loss, anorexia, change in bowel habit, blood PR, tenesmus, or abdominal pain. Symptoms of anaemia, perforation or obstruction. In general:
- *right-sided lesions*: weight loss, anaemia
- *left-sided lesions*: change of bowel habit, tenesmus, obstruction, blood PR

(Si) Anaemia, cachexia, palpable mass in abdomen/PR, disseminated malignancy (e.g. hepatomegaly, jaundice, lymphadenopathy). Signs of obstruction

(Ix) FBC: ↓ haemoglobin (Hb), ↓ mean corpuscular volume (MCV), liver function tests (LFTs) and coagulation (derangement suggests hepatic metastases), tumour markers (CEA, CA19–9), faecal occult blood (used in the NHS Bowel Cancer Screening Programme for those aged 60–69)

Sigmoidoscopy, colonoscopy, CT scan, barium enema

(Rx) Aim is open/laparoscopic surgical resection of tumour ± chemotherapy

Palliative procedures centre on relieving obstruction (e.g. stents or bypass operations)

Adjuvant radiotherapy may be employed with rectal carcinomas

(a) (b)

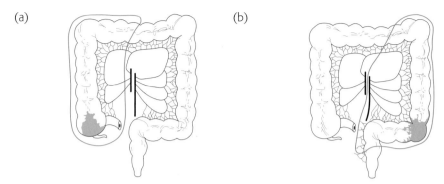

Figure 2.6 (a) Right hemicolectomy; (b) left hemicolectomy (reproduced with permission from Mortensen NJMcC in Russell RCG, Williams NS and Bulstrode CJK (eds), *Bailey & Love's Short Practice of Surgery*, 24th edn, London: Hodder Education, 2004)

Px Depends on the stage of disease (see Table 2.1)

Table 2.1 Modified Dukes' classification of colorectal carcinoma

Stage	Pathology	5-year survival (%)
A	Confined to bowel wall (mucosa)	90
B	Growth through bowel wall (muscle)	60
C	Regional lymph node involvement	30
D	Distant metastases	5

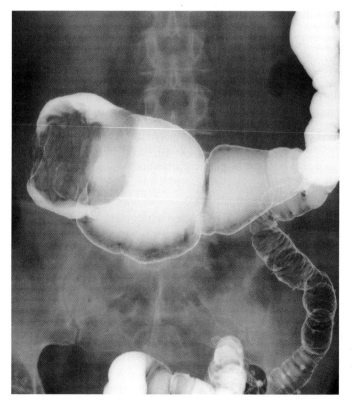

Figure 2.7 Barium enema: large polypoidal filling defect in the transverse colon due to a colonic carcinoma

FAMILIAL ADENOMATOUS POLYPOSIS COLI SYNDROME (FAP)

(A) Autosomal dominant disorder of tumour suppressor *APC* gene
Colorectal cancer develops in all patients if no treatment
(P) Characterized by hundreds/thousands adenomatous polyps throughout the colon
(Rx) Prophylactic total colectomy, excision of rectum and formation of ileoanal pouch

HEREDITARY NON-POLYPOSIS COLON CANCER (HNPCC)

- Autosomal dominant disorder of DNA mismatch repair system
- Develop mainly right-sided carcinomas
- Very few colorectal polyps develop (hence the name)

SURGICAL ASPECTS OF INFLAMMATORY BOWEL DISEASE

Ulcerative colitis

- Surgically curable disease (it is limited to the colon)
- *Operations*: proctocolectomy and ileostomy versus total colectomy and ileoanal pouch
- *Indications*: failure to control disease with medication, unacceptable drug side-effects, evidence of dysplasia or strictures, toxic megacolon

Crohn's disease

- Surgery is not curative – aim to avoid surgical intervention
- *Operations*: segmental resection, temporary colostomy/ileostomy
- *Indications*:
  - failure to control disease with medication, strictures and perforation, perianal fistulae and abscesses.
  - temporary colostomy/ileostomy may allow healing of perianal fistulae/abscesses

ANAL AND PERIANAL DISEASE

HAEMORRHOIDS

(A) Affect 50 per cent of population aged over 50 years
Predisposing conditions: straining with defaecation, pregnancy
(P) Displacement and dilatation of one or more anal cushions (vascular tissue)
Classified into grades I–IV:

Box 2.3 CLASSIFICATION OF HAEMORRHOIDS
• *Grade I*: bleed only
• *Grade II*: prolapse but spontaneously reduce
• *Grade III*: prolapse and require manual replacement
• *Grade IV*: permanently prolapsed

(Sy) Painless bright red PR bleeding, perianal lump, pruritus ani
(Si) Visible prolapsed haemorrhoids and anaemia (if bleeding is brisk)
Examine abdomen for masses

(Ix) PR (haemorrhoids are not palpable), proctoscopy (visualize haemorrhoids), sigmoidoscopy (to exclude higher pathology)

(Rx) Increase dietary fibre and fluid intake + stop straining at stool

Grade I–III: sclerosant injection/banding/cryotherapy/infrared coagulation in outpatients

Grade IV: haemorrhoidectomy (also indicated if above measures fail)

(Cx) Strangulation; blood supply to a prolapsed haemorrhoid is restricted due to contraction of the anal sphincter, resulting in pain and swelling. May become thrombosed (extremely painful)

PERIANAL HAEMATOMA

(P) Rupture of a perianal subcutaneous blood vessel

(Sy) Acute onset of perianal pain after straining at stool

(Si) Blue/black bulge at the anal margin

(Rx) Resolves spontaneously. Incision indicated only for pain relief

FISSURE IN ANO

(P) Painful tear in the anal epithelium ± mucosa

Associated with hypertonicity of internal sphincter

Majority occur in posterior midline

(A) Thought to be secondary to passage of a hard stool

(Sy) Severe pain during and after bowel motions, bright red PR bleeding

(Si) Fissure ± sentinel pile (skin tag at external aspect of fissure)

(Ix) PR may be impossible due to pain

(Rx) *Conservative*: dietary fibre and stool softeners

Medical: glyceryl trinitrate (GTN) cream (relaxes internal sphincter), botox

Surgery: indicated for failed medical treatment or chronic fissure – anal stretch (now rarely performed), lateral sphincterotomy

(Cx) If fissure occurs off midline or suspicious history, exclude other diagnoses, e.g. Crohn's disease, AIDS, carcinoma

ANORECTAL ABSCESS

(P) Infection originating in cryptoglandular epithelium lining the anal canal spreads to surrounding soft tissues, with subsequent abscess formation

Location: perianal 60 per cent, ischiorectal 20 per cent, intersphincteric 5 per cent, supralevator 4 per cent (see Fig. 2.8)

(A) Predisposing factors to exclude: Crohn's, diabetes, immunosuppression, TB, cancer

(Sy) Anal or rectal pain, often worse on defecation. Fevers/rigors

(Si) Erythematous, indurated or fluctuant mass

(Ix) Fluctuant tender mass on PR. Examination under anaesthesia (EUA). May require CT/MRI of intersphincteric and supralevator abscesses

(Rx) Early surgical drainage with healing by secondary intention

(Cx) Fistula formation in 7–40 per cent of patients

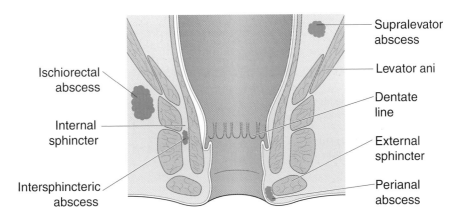

Figure 2.8 Locations of peri-anal abscesses

FISTULA IN ANO

P An abnormal connection between a primary opening inside the anal canal and a secondary opening in the perianal skin

A Majority form secondary to a perianal abscess (again remember to rule out Crohn's, carcinoma, TB, etc.)
Parks' classification: intersphincteric 70 per cent, trans-sphincteric 25 per cent, suprasphincteric 5 per cent and extrasphincteric <1 per cent
Goodsall's rule: imagine a transverse line through the anus in the lithotomy position. Fistulae with an external opening anterior to this line will follow a straight line to the anus. Fistulae with an opening posterior to this line follow a curved course to open in the midline

Sy History of anorectal abscess. Perianal discharge and pain persist

Si External opening on perineum ± visible discharge

Ix PR (may palpate primary opening). MRI to evaluate complex fistulae. EUA

Rx Laying open of fistula in intersphincteric and low trans-sphincteric fistulae (do not involve internal/external sphincters)
High fistulae require placement of a seton (a suture) through the fistula which is progressively tightened over 6–8 weeks to promote scar tissue whilst maintaining sphincter integrity

Cx Recurrence. Faecal incontinence post-operatively

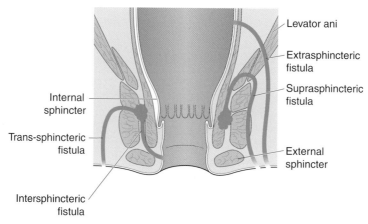

Figure 2.9 Parks' classification of anal fistulae (reproduced with kind permission from Parker S, http://www.sugical-tutor.org.uk/pictures/diagrams/fistulae.gif, accessed on 18 May 2006)

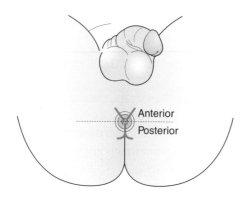

Figure 2.10 Goodsall's rule

PILONIDAL SINUS

P Hair-containing sinus in the sacro-coccygeal area (majority in natal cleft)

A Controversial: hair follicle inflammation with subsequent trapping of hairs, which act as foreign bodies, thus producing chronic inflammation

Risk factors: male, hirsute, obese, occupations involving prolonged sitting (classically taxi/lorry drivers)

Sy Asymptomatic, or pain, purulent discharge

Si Visible tracts ± purulent discharge, tenderness, fluctuance

Rx *Prophylactic*:
   – local hygiene and shaving

   Surgery:
   – incision and drainage of abscess/sinus
   – recurrence may require wide skin excision + skin flap

RECTAL PROLAPSE

(P) Two distinct clinical entities:
- *full-thickness* – prolapse of all layers of rectal wall through anus
- *mucosal* – prolapse of rectal mucosa through anus

(A) Majority of patients are women (often multiparous). Also children <3 years

(Sy) Palpable mass, faecal incontinence, PR bleeding

(Si) Protruding rectal mass (ask patient to bear down), reduced sphincter tone on PR, evidence of ulceration

(Ix) Sweat test to exclude cystic fibrosis in children
Sigmoidoscopy to examine rectal mucosa for ulceration or other contributing disease

(Rx) Acutely, reduce with gentle digital pressure
Definitive surgical repair is either via a perineal (e.g. Delorme's procedure) or abdominal (open or laparoscopic rectopexy) approach

ANAL CARCINOMA

(A) Uncommon tumour (incidence ~300 per year)
Increased risk: anal warts (human papillomavirus [HPV]), and receptive anal intercourse

(P) 80 per cent are squamous cell carcinomas

(Sy) Change in bowel habit, pain, bleeding, palpable mass

(Rx) Radiotherapy ± chemotherapy is now the mainstay of treatment

HIRSCHSPRUNG'S DISEASE

(P) Absence of parasympathetic ganglion cells in the rectum or colon

(A) Commonly males

(S) Presents as acute obstruction with failure to pass meconium in the neonate, or chronic constipation in older children

BOWEL OBSTRUCTION

(P) *Simple obstruction*: occlusion of bowel without vascular compromise
Strangulation: occlusion of bowel with vascular compromise

(Si) Absent bowel sounds, constant localized pain and peritonism, ↑WCC

Box 2.4 GENERAL CLASSIFICATION OF CAUSES OF BOWEL OBSTRUCTION

- *Intraluminal*:
  - foreign body
  - impacted faeces/food
  - intussusception
  - gallstones
- *Bowel wall lesions*:
  - tumours
  - strictures
  - Crohn's disease
  - diverticulitis

- *Extrinsic*:
  - adhesions
  - hernias
  - volvulus
  - external compression

LARGE INTESTINE

Ⓐ Commonly carcinoma, sigmoid/caecal volvulus (twisting of bowel around its mesenteric attachment)

Box 2.5 THE FOUR CLASSIC SIGNS OF COMPLETE BOWEL OBSTRUCTION
1   Absolute constipation (no passage of flatus or faeces)
2   Colicky abdominal pain
3   Abdominal distension
4   Vomiting (often late or absent)

Ⓢ As in Box 2.5; note that passage of flatus suggests partial obstruction
Discomfort, dehydration and tachycardia
Abdomen:
– distended, generalized tenderness, evidence of scars or masses
– tinkling bowel sounds.
PR: empty rectum, faecal impaction, mass, blood

Ⓘⓧ *Bloods*: minor ↑WCC, dehydration on U&Es (third space losses)
Erect CXR: air under the diaphragm indicates perforation
AXR (abdominal X-ray): distended large bowel (>5 cm diameter), identified by its peripheral position and haustral folds (partially cross lumen)
Gastrografin enema: to identify level/cause of obstruction
CT scan: to identify level/cause of obstruction

Ⓡⓧ NBM, nasogastric tube (NGT) insertion and i.v. fluid resuscitation – 'drip and suck'
Endoscopic reduction of sigmoid volvulus (allows planned definitive surgical procedure)
Removal of obstruction and resection of accompanying non-viable bowel, followed by delayed anastomosis due to invariable faecal contamination (i.e. temporary colostomy)

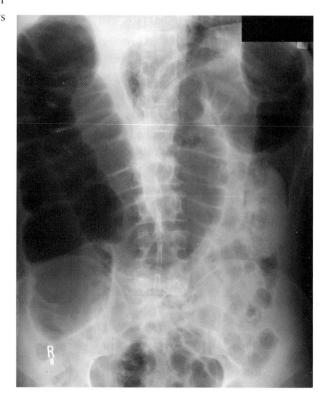

Figure 2.11 Large bowel obstruction: gas is seen in the large bowel up to the mid-descending colon

SMALL INTESTINE

A *Common causes*:
- adhesions (fibrous bands between loops of bowel secondary to previous abdominal surgery)
- hernias

Sy Absolute constipation may be a late feature
Vomiting (occurs early), periumbilical colicky pain, distension (less than large bowel)

Si Discomfort, dehydration and tachycardia
Abdomen : distended, generalized tenderness, evidence of scars, hernias or masses
Tinkling bowel sounds
PR: empty rectum, blood

Ix *Bloods*: minor ↑ WCC, dehydration on U&Es
Erect CXR: air under the diaphragm indicates perforation
AXR : distended small bowel (>2.5 cm diameter), identified by its central position and valvulae conniventes (completely cross lumen)
CT scan: identify level/cause of obstruction
Gastrografin follow-through: to identify level/cause of obstruction

Rx Trial of NBM, NGT insertion and i.v. fluid resuscitation
Evidence of strangulation, or failure of conservative measures requires laparotomy to remove the cause of obstruction and resect non-viable bowel (usually with primary anastomosis)

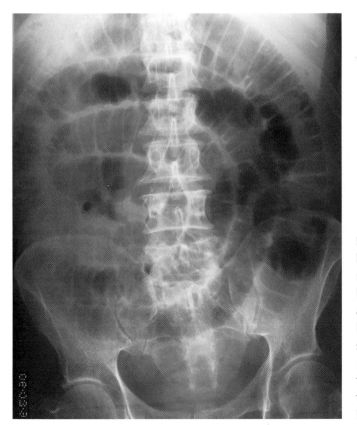

Figure 2.12 Small bowel obstruction: multiple dilated small bowel loops with absence of gas in the large bowel; note the small bowel folds (valvulae conniventes) traverse the entire thickness of the small bowel

INTUSSUSCEPTION

P   Telescoping of one portion of bowel into an immediately adjacent segment. Subsequent restriction of blood supply and oedema of bowel wall rapidly leads to obstruction and potentially gangrene/perforation

A   Most common in those aged 3–12 months

Sy Paroxysmal colicky abdominal pain, vomiting and redcurrant jelly stools

Si Shock. Palpable sausage-shaped mass, redcurrant jelly on PR

Rx Reduction with air enema. If this fails, reduction at laparotomy is required

(a)
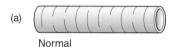
Normal

(b)
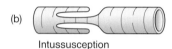
Intussusception

Figure 2.13 Intussusception: (a) normal intestine; (b) intussusception

PSEUDO-OBSTRUCTION/ILEUS

P   Functional bowel obstruction due to reduced motility

A   Metabolic disturbances, anticholinergics, intra-operative bowel manipulation

Sy As per large/small bowel obstruction

Si As per large/small bowel obstruction *except* bowel sounds are absent

Ix U&Es. AXR and Gastrografin swallow/enema reveal dilated bowel with no evidence of mechanical obstruction

Rx Withhold drugs which inhibit GI mobility. Correct electrolyte abnormalities with i.v. fluids. NGT. Analgesia
Pro-kinetics such as oral metoclopramide and erythromycin, or i.v. neostigmine may be effective
Decompression may be attempted via colonoscopy

HERNIAS

P   Protrusion of a viscus or part of a viscus through its containing cavity into an abnormal position

---

Box 2.6 COMMON TERMS USED TO DESCRIBE HERNIAS

- *Reducible*: can push back into original cavity
- *Irreducible/incarcerated*: unable to push back into original cavity
- *Obstructed*: bowel contents unable to pass through hernia
- *Strangulated*: blood supply of contents is occluded

A   Abdominal wall hernias occur at sites of inherent weakness. Operations, advancing age, obesity and malnutrition result in further loss of muscular strength

Raised intra-abdominal pressure is also a risk factor, e.g. chronic cough or constipation, urinary obstruction, heavy lifting

(Sy) Lump, pain or symptoms of complication i.e. obstruction or strangulation

(Si) Lump at recognized site with an expansile cough impulse

Scars

A tense, tender and erythematous lump together with signs of intestinal obstruction suggests strangulation

(Ix) USS if unsure of diagnosis

(Rx) Surgical repair unless risk of strangulation is low (e.g. large defect in containing cavity). In general, surgery involves excision of the hernial sac (herniotomy) and repair of the hernial defect (herniorrhaphy)

(Cx) Obstruction and strangulation

INGUINAL HERNIA

(P) Protrusion of a viscus through the inguinal canal

(A) ♂ > ♀

The inguinal canal is an oblique passage through the inferior part of the anterior abdominal wall. Contents – spermatic cord (♂), round ligament (♀) and ilioinguinal nerve (♂♀)

Table 2.2 Borders of the inguinal canal

	Lateral	Medial
Floor	Inguinal ligament	Inguinal ligament and lacunar ligament
Roof	Internal oblique and transversus abdominis	Internal oblique and transversus abdominis
Anterior wall	External oblique aponeurosis and internal oblique	External oblique aponeurosis
Posterior wall	Transversalis fascia	Transversalis fascia

Internal ring:
  – U-shaped condensation of transversalis fascia which allows passage of cord from abdomen into inguinal canal
  – lies at midpoint of inguinal ligament (halfway between pubic tubercle and anterior superior iliac spine [ASIS]), lateral to inferior epigastric vessels
External ring:
  – formed by two crura of external oblique which allows spermatic cord to leave the inguinal canal and enter the scrotum
  – lies just above and medial to the pubic tubercle
Indirect inguinal hernias enter canal via the internal ring (65 per cent)
Direct inguinal hernias enter canal via a defect in the posterior wall medial to the internal ring (35 per cent)

(Si) Hernia originates above and medial to the pubic tubercle

Once reduced, digital pressure over the internal ring will prevent an indirect hernia from reappearing when the patient is asked to cough. Reappearance of the hernia during this manoeuvre suggests a direct hernia (NB this is not an accurate test – accurate determination can only be made operatively)

(Rx)   *Conservative*: truss (like a corset) is prescribed in patients whose comorbidity excludes them from operative repair
Surgery: laparoscopic or open repair of defect with mesh

FEMORAL HERNIA

(P)   Protrusion of a viscus through the femoral canal
Canal connects superiorly with abdomen via femoral ring

(A)   ♀ > ♂ (NB overall inguinal hernias > femoral hernias in women)

(Si)   Hernia originates below and lateral to the pubic tubercle

(Rx)   Always require surgical repair as hernia is prone to obstruction and strangulation against the sharp lacunar ligament (medial border of canal)

INCISIONAL HERNIA

(P)   Protrusion of a viscus through the scar of a previous operation/injury
Skin remains intact

(A)   *Pre-operative*: elderly, respiratory disease, anaemia, obesity, uraemia, jaundice, diabetes, malnutrition, malignancy, steroids or cytotoxics
Intra-operative: type of incision/sutures, surgical technique
Post-operative: wound infection, ischaemia, abdominal distension, chronic cough

(Sy)   Cosmetic appearance (usually have a large neck, therefore low risk of strangulation)

(Si)   Hernia with overlying scar

(Rx)   Truss if unsuitable (or unwilling) to have surgery
Surgical closure of defect with sutures ± mesh

(Cx)   Recurrence of hernia after repair

GALLSTONES AND RELATED DISORDERS

(A)   Present in ~12 per cent of men and 24 per cent of women

(P)   Bile contains cholesterol, bile salts and lecithin
Three main types of stone: cholesterol, pigment and mixed

(Rx)   May be asymptomatic

(Cx)   Complications best considered in relation to position (see Fig. 2.14)

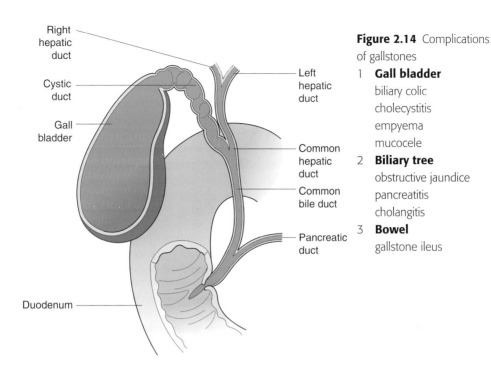

Right hepatic duct

Cystic duct

Gall bladder

Duodenum

Left hepatic duct

Common hepatic duct

Common bile duct

Pancreatic duct

Figure 2.14 Complications of gallstones

1 **Gall bladder**
biliary colic
cholecystitis
empyema
mucocele

2 **Biliary tree**
obstructive jaundice
pancreatitis
cholangitis

3 **Bowel**
gallstone ileus

BILIARY COLIC

P Due to impaction of stone in gall bladder neck or cystic duct

Sy RUQ colicky pain (± radiation to tip of right scapula), vomiting

Si Tender RUQ

Ix Bloods (FBC, LFTs, U&Es, amylase), USS

Rx *Conservative*: NBM, i.v. fluids, opiate analgesia
Surgery: laparoscopic (rarely open) cholecystectomy at 6–12 weeks when biliary tree less inflamed

CHOLECYSTITIS

P An impacted stone obstructing the gall bladder outlet may result in infection of the accumulating bile

Sy Constant RUQ pain (± referred pain radiating to tip of right scapula)
Fever and vomiting

Si Pyrexia, tenderness, rebound and guarding in RUQ
Murphy's sign: patient catches breath on inspiration when two fingers are placed in RUQ (valid if negative in left upper quadrant [LUQ])

Ix FBC (↑WCC), USS (gallstones, thickened gall bladder wall, pericholecystic fluid)

Rx *Conservative*: NBM, analgesia, i.v. fluids and antibiotics (e.g. cefuroxime and metronidazole)
Surgery: laparoscopic (rarely open) cholecystectomy (72 h or 6–12 weeks)

Cx Chronic cholecystitis, mucocele (distends with bile), empyema (distends with pus), gangrene and perforation

GALLSTONE OBSTRUCTIVE JAUNDICE

(P) Gallstone impacts in, and obstructs common bile duct

(Sy) Jaundice, pale stools, dark urine, pruritus
Symptoms of biliary colic or painless

(Si) Jaundice ± tenderness RUQ

(Ix) Bloods ($\uparrow$ alkaline phosphatase [ALP], gamma glutamyl transferase [GGT], unconjugated bilirubin)
USS, endoscopic retrograde cholangiopancreatography (ERCP), magnetic resonance cholangiopancreatography (MRCP) to image biliary tree

(Rx) *Endoscopy*: ERCP allows stone removal/sphincterotomy/stent placement
Surgery: open bile duct exploration, cholecystectomy 6–12 weeks

(Cx) Ascending cholangitis

ASCENDING CHOLANGITIS

(P) Gallstone impacted in the common bile duct (CBD) results in infection of the biliary system

(Sy) Pale stools, dark urine and pruritus
Charcot's triad:
1. jaundice
2. fever
3. RUQ pain

(Si) Pyrexia, RUQ tenderness and rigors

(Ix) Bloods ($\uparrow$ WCC in addition to a picture of obstructive jaundice), USS, ERCP, MRCP

(Rx) *Conservative*: NBM, analgesia, i.v. fluids and antibiotics (e.g. cefuroxime and metronidazole)
Endoscopy: ERCP allows stone removal/sphincterotomy/stent placement
Surgery: open bile duct exploration, cholecystectomy 6–12 weeks

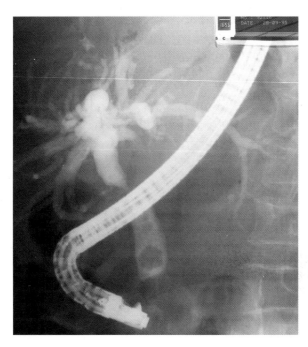

Figure 2.15 ERCP showing a lobulated filling defect in the common bile duct from a calculus

GALLSTONE ILEUS

P   Gallstone erodes through into the duodenum

May cause a mechanical bowel obstruction

GALL BLADDER CARCINOMA

A   Rare, 80 per cent have gallstones

Sy   Abdominal pain, nausea and vomiting, weight loss

Rx   If possible, operative resection

Px   Very poor

CHOLANGIOCARCINOMA

P   Malignancy of the biliary tree

Intra- or extra-hepatic

A   Associated with primary sclerosing cholangitis (and hence inflammatory bowel disease [IBD])

Sy   As with obstructive jaundice + dull abdominal pain, weight loss

Si   Palpable gall bladder, abdominal mass, hepatomegaly

Ix   USS, MRI, CT, ERCP

Rx   *Palliation*: stents, radiotherapy and chemotherapy

Surgery: 10 per cent may be suitable for curative resection

PANCREAS

ACUTE PANCREATITIS

P   Inflammation of exocrine pancreas

A   Most common (>95 per cent): gallstones/alcohol

Other causes: tumours, viruses (mumps), drugs (e.g. thiazide diuretics), hyperlipidaemia, hypercalcaemia, ERCP (iatrogenic)

Sy   Severe epigastric pain (radiates to back), nausea, vomiting

Si   ↑ heart rate (HR), ↑ temperature, ↓ BP, abdominal tenderness, ↓ bowel sounds (secondary to ileus)

Generalized tenderness and guarding

Grey–Turner's sign: flank discolouration

Cullen's sign: periumbilical discolouration

Ix   Serum amylase >1000 IU/ml, FBC, U&E, LFT, arterial blood gases (ABG), USS, CT, MRCP

Rx   Analgesia, i.v. fluids, O_2, urinary catheter, naso-jejunal feeding (to avoid pancreatic stimulation), consider CVP monitoring, ERCP if gallstone obstructing bile duct

Cx   Pseudocyst (fluid collection in lesser sac), abscess, adult respiratory distress syndrome, renal failure, chronic pancreatitis

Px   Depends on severity of attack (see Box 2.7, Ranson criteria)

Box 2.7 MODIFIED GLASGOW CRITERIA IN ACUTE PANCREATITIS

- PaO$_2$ <60 mmHg/7.9 kPa
- Age >55 years
- Neutrophils: WBC >15
- Calcium >2 mmol/L
- Renal function: urea >16 mmol/L
- Enzymes: LDH >600 iu/L, AST >200 iu/L
- Albumin <32 g/L
- Sugar: glucose >10 mmol/L

Three or more positive factors detected within 48 hours of onset suggest severe pancreatitis (refer to HDU/ITU)

CHRONIC PANCREATITIS

(P) Long-term pathological process of pancreatic fibrosis + calcification

(A) Majority due to chronic alcohol use

(Sy) Chronic abdominal pain relieved by opiates, fat malabsorption → steatorrhoea

(Ix) Serum amylase (may be normal)

CT: pancreatic calcification

Pancreatic function tests: endocrine/exocrine insufficiency

(Rx) Stop alcohol consumption

Pancreatic enzyme supplementation for malabsorption

Analgesia (may require coeliac plexus block)

Surgical resection if pain refractory to opioid analgesics

PANCREATIC CARCINOMA

(A) Incidence ↑ in UK

Associated with chronic pancreatitis, diabetes and smoking

Patients are typically 50–70 years of age

(P) Mostly ductal adenocarcinomas, occurring in head of pancreas

(Sy) Abdominal/back pain, weight loss, anorexia

(Si) Painless jaundice, thrombophlebitis migrans (tender nodules in blood vessels), palpable gall bladder, ascites

Courvoisier's Law: 'if in the presence of jaundice the gall bladder is palpable, then the jaundice is unlikely to be due to stones'

(Ix) Bloods (obstructive jaundice, ↑ CA19–9), USS, CT, ERCP (plus cytological brushings)

(Rx) *Palliative*: analgesia, biliary stents, bypass surgery (for bowel obstruction)

Curative: <10 per cent suitable for Whipple's pancreatoduodenectomy

(Px) Poor, ~16 per cent 1-year survival

Rare hormone-secreting pancreatic tumours

- *Insulinoma*: recurrent hypoglycaemic attacks
- *Glucagonoma*: diabetes, dermatitis
- VIPoma (vasoactive intestinal peptide-oma): watery diarrhoea
- *Gastrinoma*: recurrent GI ulceration (Zollinger–Ellison syndrome)

SPLEEN

SPLENIC RUPTURE

P Highly vascular organ

A Most commonly injured organ in blunt abdominal trauma
Risk of rupture increased in splenomegaly

Sy *Stable patients*: asymptomatic or LUQ pain
Unstable patients: abdominal distension, tenderness and shock

Ix USS, CT, angiography

Rx Conservative non-operative management is preferable
Ongoing haemorrhage requires angiographic embolization of vessels, or splenectomy (immunize against haemophilus, meningococcus and pneumococcus infection prior to discharge)

SKIN

SEBORRHOEIC KERATOSIS

A Common benign tumour in elderly

Sy Cosmetic, catch on clothing

Si Brown/yellow round to oval lesion ± greasy with well-demarcated border

Rx Shave biopsy to exclude melanoma or for cosmetic reasons

SOLAR KERATOSIS

A Most common sun-related growth
Fair/blonde/red haired are at most risk

Sy Single lesion in sun-exposed skin (typically face, ears, dorsum of hands) which progresses/becomes multiple

Si Generally a flat lesion with a rough/scaly surface

Ix Biopsy suspicious/non-responding lesions

Rx Educate about minimizing sun exposure and sunscreen
Cryotherapy. For large areas use topical 5-fluorouracil (5-FU)

Cx Potential to undergo malignant change

KERATOACANTHOMA

P Low-grade malignancy

Sy Rapidly growing nodule with central crateriform ulceration

Rx Will resolve spontaneously (residual scarring)
Excision biopsy to exclude squamous cell carcinoma (SCC) and minimize scarring

SEBACEOUS CYST (EPIDERMOID CYST)

P Mostly found in hair-bearing areas

Sy Asymptomatic, mobile, firm to fluctuant dome shaped lesion ± central punctum
Foul-smelling, toothpaste-like discharge

Si Tethered to overlying skin

Rx Excision (failure to completely remove sac may result in recurrence)

DERMOID CYST

P Cystic swellings

A *Inclusion dermoids*: embryological origin
Implantation dermoids: secondary to penetrating injury (introduces epidermal cells subcutaneously)

Rx Excision

LIPOMA

A Most common benign soft tissue tumour in adults

Sy Cosmetic. Multiple and tender lipomas – Dercum's disease

Si Smooth and fluctuant

Rx Excision for cosmetic reasons – no malignant transformation risk

NECROTIZING FASCIITIS

P Infection spreads from subcutaneous tissue along fascial planes
Involvement of scrotum and penis: Fournier's gangrene

A Usually polymicrobial infection (classically involves group A β-haemolytic streptococcus)
Infected needle, abscesses, open fractures, surgery or idiopathic

Sy Fever, erythema ± vesicle formation

Si Initially similar to cellulitis, septic, rapidly advancing erythema ± painless ulcers

Ix Bloods ($\uparrow$ WCC, $\downarrow$ Na$^+$), CT

Rx Intensive therapy unit (ITU)
Broad-spectrum i.v. antibiotics. Bold surgical resection down to healthy tissue – reassess daily

Px Mortality ~25 per cent

MALIGNANT SKIN LESIONS

BASAL CELL CARCINOMA (BCC)

A Most common skin cancer, caused by sun exposure, radiation

P Typically occur on head and neck
Slow growing and locally destructive (does not metastasize)

Sy Non-healing skin lesion which may bleed

Si Raised pearly nodule with rolled edge. Often crossed by fine blood vessels

Ix Biopsy

Rx Radiotherapy/curettage/excision depending on characteristics

Cx Increased risk of developing further BCC. Metastasis extremely unusual

SQUAMOUS CELL CARCINOMA

(A) Second most common skin cancer
Arises in sun-exposed skin
More common in fair/blonde/red hair types
If arising in area of chronic inflammation – Marjolin's ulcer

(Sy) New skin lesion: asymptomatic/itch/bleed/pain

(Si) Ulcerated firm pink/flesh-coloured irregular lesion. May be a background of multiple solar keratoses

(Ix) Biopsy

(Rx) Resection

(Cx) 2–6 per cent metastasize

BOWEN'S DISEASE

(P) SCC *in situ*

(A) Sun exposure, arsenic, HPV 16

(S) Asymptomatic, enlarging, scaly erythematous plaque

(Sy) Cryotherapy, topical 5-FU, or surgical excision

(Cx) 5 per cent progress to invasive SCC

MALIGNANT MELANOMA

(P) Malignancy of melanocytes
Four main subtypes: superficial spreading, nodular, lentigo maligna and acral lentiginous

(A) 4 per cent of skin cancers but causes most skin cancer-related deaths
Arise *de novo* or in pre-existing melanocytic naevi (moles)
Risk factors: fair skin, sun exposure (legs ♀, arms and trunk ♂)

(S) Changing mole. Remember **ABCD**:

Box 2.8 WORRYING FEATURES OF A MOLE

- **A**symmetry
- **B**order irregularity
- **C**olour variation
- **D**iameter >6 mm
- **E**volving over time

(Ix) Excisional biopsy to stage tumour → Breslow depth (or Clark level)

(Rx) Primary prevention with sun exposure avoidance and sunscreen
Surgical resection ± lymph node dissection

(Cx) Metastases

(Px) Correlates with Breslow depth (i.e. depth of invasion)
   – <0.75 mm: 5-year survival 95%
   – >4 mm: 5-year survival 45%

VASCULAR SURGERY

ARTERIAL OCCLUSIVE DISEASE

LOWER LIMB

(P) Most common cause atherosclerosis

Sudden onset suggests embolic disease

(A) *Fixed risk factors:* age, male sex, diabetes, family history of early atherosclerosis

Modifiable risk factors: smoking, hyperlipidaemia, hypertension

(Sy) Intermittent claudication, rest pain, ulcers

(Si) Cold limb, pallor, absent/weak pulses, muscle weakness, reduced sensation

---

Box 2.9 SIX 'P'S OF CRITICAL ISCHAEMIA

- Pain
- Pallor
- Perishing with cold
- Pulselessness
- Paraesthesiae
- Paralysis

(Ix) ECG (atrial fibrillation), urinalysis, FBC, lipid profile, USS, arteriography, magnetic resonance angiography (MRA)

Ankle-brachial pressure index (ABPI):

- ≥ 1 = normal,
- 0.9–0.6 = claudication,
- 0.6–0.3 = rest pain,
- <0.3 = critical ischaemia

(Rx) *Conservative:* smoking cessation, control of diabetes, hypertension and hyperlipidaemia, aspirin, exercise programme

Operative: angioplasty ± stent, open endarterectomy, bypass

Embolus: anticoagulation, thrombolysis, embolectomy

(Cx) Gangrene, renal failure, compartment syndrome

(Px) Variable, poor if risk factors not modified

Embolism: good if treated within 24 h of onset; source of embolus must be sought

---

INFORMATION BOX: ABPI

- ABPI: ankle brachial pressure index is measured by taking blood pressures from the ankle and arm and calculating the ratio.
- Usually BP is higher in the leg than the arm.
- If blood flow to the leg is impaired, leg BP drops below arm BP: the greater the drop the worse the blood flow.
- Caution is needed in diabetes where calcification of vessels can give falsely high readings.

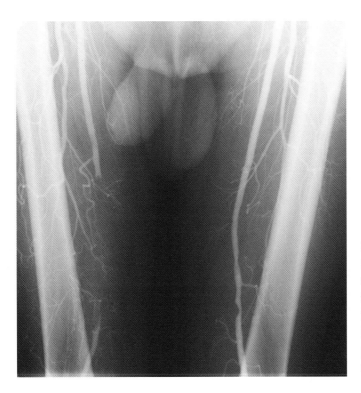

Figure 2.16 Angiogram showing a femoral artery embolus: filling defect in the right superficial femoral artery, its upper border having a convex protrusion on the contrast column

INTERMITTENT CLAUDICATION

P Ischaemic muscle pain brought on by exercise and relieved by rest
Most common site is the calf

S Aorto-iliac disease causes thigh/buttock pain
Rest pain occurs in the foot when perfusion is inadequate for basal metabolic needs
Rest pain most common at night due to elevated feet and ↓ BP during sleep

LERICHE'S SYNDROME

P Combination of buttock claudication and impotence – caused by aorto-iliac disease

Rx As above, with conservative or operative therapy depending on patient choice, fitness and overall prognosis

BUERGER'S DISEASE

P Also known as thromboangiitis obliterans
Inflammation and occlusion of medium-sized arteries

A Common in male smokers, much younger age of onset than atherosclerosis

Rx Patients must give up smoking or risk developing irreversible damage to arterial tree

Px Worse prognosis than atherosclerosis

CAROTID DISEASE

P Atherosclerosis common at bifurcation/internal carotid artery origin
Stroke is third commonest cause of death in UK
80 per cent of strokes are ischaemic

Sy Amaurosis fugax (temporary unilateral blindness), transient ischaemic attack (TIA), stroke

(Si) Carotid bruit

(Ix) FBC, U&E, glucose, lipid profile, duplex USS, MRA, carotid angiography (less common recently)

(Rx) *All patients*: smoking cessation, control of diabetes, hypertension and hyperlipidaemia, aspirin

Symptomatic patients with 70–99 per cent stenosis: carotid endarterectomy under local anaesthetic (LA) or general anaesthetic (GA)

Important complications of endarterectomy include stroke and death

(Px) Surgical benefit proven for those with symptomatic/severe stenosis

MESENTERIC DISEASE

(P) Due to either atherosclerosis or embolus

(Sy) *Ischaemia*: mesenteric angina (abdominal pain after eating), fear of eating

Infarction: abdominal pain, shock, rectal bleeding

(Si) Weight loss, abdominal tenderness, mass if bowel infarcted

(Ix) FBC, U&E, glucose, ABG, erect CXR, mesenteric angiography

(Rx) *Ischaemia*: arterial bypass sometimes possible

Infarction: bowel resection

(Px) Depends on extent of affected bowel; total mesenteric infarction usually fatal

UPPER LIMB

(P) Atherosclerosis uncommon, embolus more common

Buerger's disease may affect upper limbs

(S) As for lower limb acute ischaemia

(Ix) Often clinical diagnosis, may use duplex USS, arteriography

(Rx) Anticoagulation, thrombolysis, embolectomy

(Px) Good if treated within 24 h of onset, source of embolus must be sought

RAYNAUD'S PHENOMENON/DISEASE

(A) Common

(P) Intermittent spasm of small arteries and arterioles of hands and feet

Raynaud's *disease* is idiopathic and occurs in females

Raynaud's *phenomenon* is due to a range of causes, e.g. connective tissue disorder

(Sy) Characteristic colour changes in hands, often triggered by cold exposure

Classically occur in the following stages:

1. white (ischaemic)
2. blue (cyanosed), and finally
3. red (hyperaemic)

(Si) May be none, necrotic areas on digits

(Ix) Exclude other causes of ischaemia, e.g. cervical rib, subclavian stenosis, Buerger's disease

(Rx) *Supportive*: smoking cessation, keep hands and feet warm

Medical: vasodilator drugs (rarely successful)

Surgery: sympathectomy (good result but usually short-lived), amputation of necrotic digits if disease is severe

ULCERS

ARTERIAL

P Caused by chronic ischaemia
Large vessel disease (e.g. atherosclerosis) or small vessel (e.g. diabetes)
Usually on toes or over pressure areas

Sy Pain at rest (venous ulcers are classically painless)

Si Punched-out edge, sloughy base, may be very deep, poor peripheral pulses, other signs of ischaemia in affected limb (pallor, cyanosis)

Ix As for ischaemic limb, biopsy

Rx As for ischaemic limb. May need debridement and skin grafting after revascularization of limb. Amputation for uncontrollable pain

Px Poor as often a sign of end-stage vascular disease

VENOUS

A Common in patients with venous reflux disease
May be a history of deep vein thrombosis (DVT) (so called post-thrombotic limb)

P Occurs with both deep and superficial reflux
Usually preceded by chronic venous skin changes e.g. venous eczema, lipodermatosclerosis (chronic fibrosis of skin/fat secondary to extravasation of red blood cells)
Usually in the gaiter area (see Fig. 2.17)

Sy Pain, mainly when dressings are applied, little pain at rest

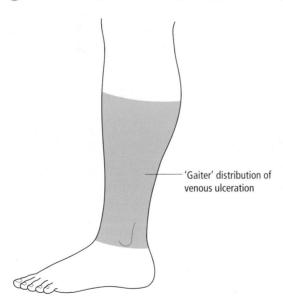

'Gaiter' distribution of venous ulceration

Figure 2.17 Gaiter distribution of venous ulceration

Si Sloping edge, granulation tissue and fibrotic tissue in base, usually shallow, usually venous skin changes in surrounding tissue, often varicose veins in affected limb

(Ix)   Exclude ischaemia, venous duplex USS, biopsy
(Rx)   *Conservative*: 4-layer compression bandaging and/or hosiery
       Surgical: correction of superficial venous reflux, debridement and skin grafting
(Px)   Good, may require lifelong compression hosiery

MARJOLIN'S ULCER

(P)   Squamous cell carcinoma in a chronic ulcer
(Sy)   Chronic venous ulcer
(Si)   Ulcer with raised edge or any other atypical feature, local lymphadenopathy
(Ix)   Biopsy
(Rx)   Wide excision, skin graft may be necessary once margins are clear
(Px)   Long-term follow-up necessary as recurrence is possible

ANEURYSMS

TRUE ANEURYSM

(P)   Abnormal dilatation of an artery or the heart involving all layers of vessel wall
       May be saccular (protrudes from one side of vessel) or fusiform (generalized dilatation of vessel)
(A)   Many causes: atherosclerotic most common

Box 2.10 AETIOLOGY OF ANEURYSMS
• *Congenital weakness*: berry aneurysm in circle of Willis artery, Marfan's syndrome
• *Degenerative*: abdominal aortic aneurysm due to atherosclerosis
• *Trauma*: injury to vessel wall can cause weakness leading to true aneurysm formation
• *Infection*: bacterial arteritis
• *Inflammatory*: inflammatory process within arterial wall causes aneurysm formation (e.g. Kawasaki disease)

FALSE ANEURYSM (PSEUDOANEURYSM)

(P)   Haematoma containing liquid blood in contact with blood in arterial lumen
(A)   Due to trauma, e.g. iatrogenic arterial puncture for angiography
(Si)   Pulsatile mass with history of trauma or arterial puncture (commonly in groin post-angioplasty)
(Ix)   Duplex USS
(Rx)   Direct pressure with USS probe, surgical repair of defect

ABDOMINAL AORTIC ANEURYSM (AAA)

(A)   Common in patients aged >60 years, more common in males
       May have a family history
(P)   May be atherosclerotic or inflammatory
       95 per cent are infrarenal
       Major risk is rupture; risk increases exponentially with aneurysm diameter

Sy Back or loin pain; may be asymptomatic. Rupture causes severe pain and collapse

Si Pulsatile mass, rupture causes hypovolaemic shock

Ix USS, CT, rupture often clinical diagnosis requiring immediate surgery

Rx Consider repair when diameter ≥5.5 cm

Regular USS surveillance if diameter <5 cm

Open repair with synthetic graft for elective and emergency cases, endovascular stent graft in selected patients

Modification of risk factors (BP/diabetic control) in patients with small aneurysms

Cx Death, renal failure (if renal arteries involved), ischaemic bowel (inferior mesenteric involvement common), limb loss, paralysis, myocardial infarction, stroke, graft infection

Px Elective operative mortality ~5 per cent

Rupture mortality ~75 per cent

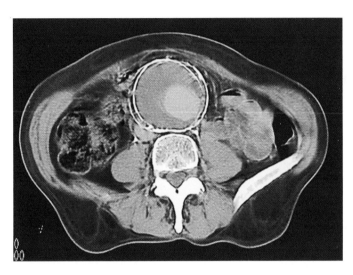

Figure 2.18 Calcified abdominal aortic aneurysm; the lumen of the aorta is surrounded by haematoma

AORTOENTERIC FISTULA

P Abnormal communication between aorta and GI tract, usually duodenum/jejunum

A Potentially life-threatening complication in patients who have had aortic surgery

Si Brisk GI bleed with melaena, hypotension

Ix Upper GI endoscopy, CT

Rx Emergency surgery, graft replacement

Px Poor

POPLITEAL ANEURYSM

A Commonest peripheral aneurysm

Occurs in 10 per cent of patients with AAA, commonly bilateral

Sy Often asymptomatic

Si Pulsatile mass possibly bilateral, distal ischaemia following thrombosis or embolization

Ix Duplex USS, angiography to assess distal vessels

Rx Surgical bypass with ligation of popliteal artery

Cx Thrombosis, distal embolization, rupture

Px Good if treated electively

AORTIC DISSECTION

(P) Blood tracks through breach in intima creating parallel true and false lumens
Type A involves ascending aorta, Type B starts at origin of left subclavian artery

(A) Major risk factor is chronic hypertension

(Sy) Tearing chest pain radiating to back, hemiplegia, paraplegia, mesenteric or limb ischaemia

(Si) Shock, aortic regurgitation if aortic valve involved, unequal pulses or blood pressure unilaterally

(Ix) ECG, CXR shows widened mediastinum, CT, echocardiography

(Rx) *Type A:* surgical emergency requiring replacement of affected aorta using cardiopulmonary bypass
Type B: medical treatment of hypertension, may require surgical repair with graft if distal ischaemia occurs

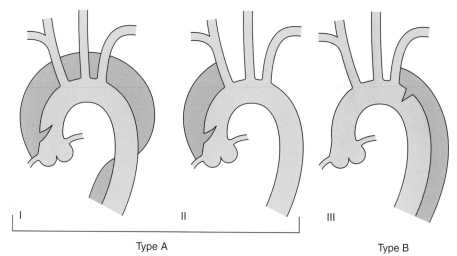

I   II   III

Type A   Type B

Figure 2.19 Classification of aortic dissection (reproduced with kind permission from Parker S, http://www.surgical-tutor.org.uk/default-home.htm?system/vascular/dissection.htm~right, accessed on 18 May 2006)

(Cx) Sudden death, stroke, mesenteric infarction, ischaemic limb, paralysis

(Px) Type A mortality high, Type B better prognosis

VENOUS REFLUX DISEASE

(P) Due to incompetence of venous valves
May occur in superficial, deep or perforating veins of legs
Superficial reflux may cause varicose veins

(A) Usually idiopathic, may be due to previous DVT (post-thrombotic limb) or raised venous pressure

(Sy) Leg swelling, aching, burning, cosmetic appearance

(Si) Deep and superficial reflux may cause leg swelling and skin changes including ulcers
Dilated tortuous superficial veins, palpable saphena varix, leg oedema, venous skin changes (venous eczema, venous flares, lipodermatosclerosis, atrophy blanche and ulceration)

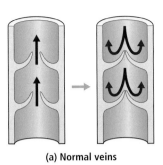

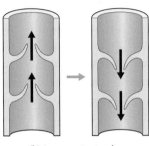

(a) Normal veins

(b) Incompetent veins

Figure 2.20 Mechanism of venous reflux disease: (a) healthy venous valves; (b) varicose veins

Ix Venous duplex USS, venography

Rx *Conservative*: compression hosiery, injection sclerotherapy (high recurrence rate)
Surgery: only if deep venous incompetence is excluded. Ligation and stripping, endoluminal endothelial radiofrequency or laser ablation of incompetent veins accompanied by superficial avulsions. Ligation or endothelial ablation of incompetent perforator veins

Cx Venous ulcers cause disability and are costly to treat in the community

Px Recurrence after ligation and stripping remains common. Due to failure of surgical technique (e.g. failure to ligate all groin tributaries) or growth of neovascular tissue. Re-do surgery possible, but it has a higher complication rate than primary surgery

VENOUS THROMBOEMBOLISM

P Virchow's triad of predisposing conditions:
1. altered thrombotic tendency
2. altered blood flow
3. alteration to vessel wall

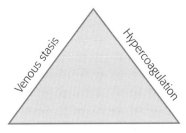

Figure 2.21 Virchow's triad

(A)   Surgery may induce all three

Peri-operative prevention is critical: early mobilization, compression hosiery, intermittent pneumatic pump, low-molecular weight heparin (LMWH, e.g. enoxaparin)

Box 2.11 COMMON CAUSES OF VENOUS THROMBOSIS

- Increasing age
- Thrombophilia
- Immobility
- Hormone replacement therapy (HRT)
- Surgery (especially pelvic/lower limb)
- Oral contraceptive pill (OCP)
- Malignancy
- Obesity

(Sy)   Painful, swollen leg or arm

(Si)   Variably swollen, tender, warm limb

(Ix)   Duplex USS, D-dimer (excludes thrombosis if –ve), venography (rarely performed nowadays, but still considered 'gold standard')

(Rx)   Anticoagulation, compression hosiery

(Cx)   Pulmonary embolism – may be fatal, post-thrombotic limb

(Px)   Good if treated promptly

LYMPHOEDEMA

(P)   Failure of lymphatic drainage causes oedema

(A)   Primary lymphoedema due to congenital lymphatic abnormality, onset may be at any age, more common in females

Secondary lymphoedema due to infection (e.g. recurrent cellulitis, filariasis), malignancy (e.g. axillary metastases from breast cancer), surgery (e.g. axillary clearance), radiotherapy or trauma causing lymphatic damage

(Sy)   Swelling of limb, episodes of cellulitis

(Si)   Swollen limb (foot typically affected), thick, scaly skin, lymphadenopathy if lymphoedema secondary to malignancy

(Ix)   Lymphoscintigraphy compares uptake of isotope on each side

(Rx)   *Conservative*: manual lymphatic drainage, pneumatic compression pump, compression hosiery

Surgery: severe cases only, removal of subcutaneous tissue and skin graft or lymphatic bypass, results often poor

(Cx)   Recurrent cellulitis

(Px)   Condition not curable, treatment aims to control symptoms

BREAST DISEASE

BENIGN BREAST DISEASE

LUMPS

Aetiology, treatment and prognosis are considered under individual headings

Ix Triple assessment is the cornerstone of diagnosis:
1. clinical examination
2. radiological investigation (mammography, USS)
3. biopsy (fine needle aspiration for cytology, core biopsy for histology)

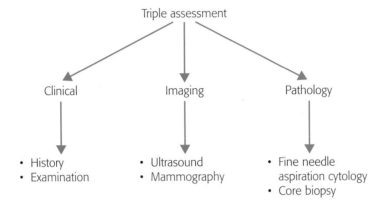

Figure 2.22 Triple assessment of breast lumps

FIBROADENOMA

P Aberration of normal development, arise from whole lobule
A Peak incidence in third decade, may occur at any age
Sy Lump(s) usually painless
Si Firm, highly mobile lump, may be multiple
Rx *Conservative*: age <40 years, biopsy-proven diagnosis
Excision: age >40 years, size >4 cm or increasing, patient choice
Px Usually remain unchanged, one-third resolve spontaneously

CYST

P Enlarged, involuted lobule
A Common in perimenopausal women
Sy Lump(s) which may be painful
Si Fluctuant or solid lump, may be tender, may be multiple
Rx Aspiration, cytology of fluid only if bloody, biopsy of any residual lump after aspiration
Px Commonly recur, slightly increased risk of breast cancer with cystic disease

PHYLLODES TUMOUR

(P) Uncommon fibroepithelial neoplasm
Majority are benign but may recur after excision
May be malignant but metastasis uncommon

(S) Firm lump, size may increase rapidly

(Rx) Wide excision, mastectomy for large tumours

DUCT PAPILLOMA

(P) Common benign neoplasm
Often occurs in subareolar ducts

(S) Single or multiple lump(s), nipple discharge which may be bloodstained

(Rx) Conservative or surgical excision of duct (microdochectomy)

FAT NECROSIS

(A) Often due to trauma

(S) History of trauma, firm lump, associated haematoma may be present
Clinically difficult to differentiate from carcinoma

(Rx) Conservative once diagnosis proven on biopsy

(Px) Usually resolves spontaneously

DUCT ECTASIA

(P) Normal changes in which ducts shorten and widen during breast involution in later life

(S) Lump, nipple discharge (may be bloody), nipple retraction (usually slit-like)

(Rx) Conservative, surgery for excessive discharge

LIPOMA

(A) Common benign neoplasm, may occur in breast

(Ix) May require excision to confirm diagnosis

BREAST PAIN (MASTALGIA)

(A) Very common, not associated with carcinoma

(P) Cyclical or non-cyclical

CYCLICAL BREAST PAIN

(A) Occurs in response to hormonal changes of menstrual cycle

(Sy) Pain from mid-cycle to menstruation, breast heaviness and lumpiness

(Si) Premenopausal woman, breast tenderness typically affects lateral half

(Rx) Reassurance, gamolenic acid (evening primrose oil – slow response, few side-effects), danazol and bromocriptine (side-effects common)

NON-CYCLICAL BREAST PAIN

(A) Pain may arise in the breast or chest wall
Usually postmenopausal women

(Sy) Pain may be continuous or intermittent

(Ix) Exclude referred pain, e.g. arthritis of chest wall, lung disease

(Rx) Reassurance, simple measures, e.g. ensure correctly fitted bra, non-steroidal anti-inflammatory medications, gamolenic acid, surgery not indicated

INFECTION

LACTATING

(P) *Staphylococcus aureus* most common pathogen
(Sy) Pain, tenderness, swelling, redness
(Si) Pyrexia, erythema, tenderness, fluctuance indicates abscess
(Rx) Antibiotics, aspiration or incision and drainage of abscess, continue breast feeding

NON-LACTATING

(P) Caused by aerobic and anaerobic bacteria
(A) Smoking is a risk factor
(Sy) Pain, tenderness, redness, may have lump
(Si) Pyrexia, erythema, tenderness, inflammatory mass or abscess may occur
(Rx) Antibiotics, aspiration or incision and drainage of abscess, investigation of any residual lump after treatment
(Cx) Mammary duct fistula requires surgical excision

GYNAECOMASTIA

(P) Benign breast tissue growth in males (carcinoma must be excluded)
(A) Occurs at any age, common in elderly and at puberty

Box 2.12 CAUSES OF GYNAECOMASTIA

- Idiopathic
- Digoxin
- Cimetidine
- Spironolactone
- Cannabis
- Cirrhosis
- Renal failure
- Testicular tumours

(S) Unilateral or bilateral soft, diffuse lump, may be painful
(Ix) Mammography if any suspicious signs (1 per cent of all breast cancer occurs in males)
(Rx) *Conservative*: withdrawal of drugs, danazol, tamoxifen
Surgery: occasionally indicated
(Px) Usually responds to conservative treatment

MALIGNANT BREAST DISEASE

DUCTAL CARCINOMA *IN SITU* (DCIS)

(P) Carcinoma which has not penetrated basement membrane
DCIS most common form of breast carcinoma *in situ*
Graded as low- to high-grade lesions on histology

(S) Lump, nipple discharge, asymptomatic screening detected

(Ix) Triple assessment (see p. 143)

(Rx) According to size of lesion, wide local excision (WLE) and radiotherapy, mastectomy, consider tamoxifen

(Px) Follow up with regular mammography to detect recurrence

Risk of progression to invasive carcinoma, highest risk for high-grade DCIS

LOBULAR CARCINOMA *IN SITU*

(A) Rare condition

(Rx) Treatment by observation, tamoxifen or bilateral mastectomy ($\uparrow$ risk of carcinoma in contralateral breast)

(Px) Risk of progression to invasive carcinoma

INVASIVE CARCINOMA

(A) Most common cancer in females

Lifetime risk approximately 1 in 10 (increasing)

Occurs at any age, rare under 30 years

Box 2.13 RISK FACTORS FOR BREAST CANCER

- Female sex (1 per cent of cancers in males)
- Age
- Family history: genes include *BRCA1* and *BRCA2*
- Early menarche, late menopause
- Nulliparity, higher age at first pregnancy
- Higher socioeconomic group
- HRT: small effect

Assessment and treatment should be in a specialist breast unit

Treatment is multimodality involving surgery, radiotherapy and chemotherapy

Diagnosis and assessment

- Presentation with palpable lump or screening-detected abnormality
- Triple assessment of any breast lump: clinical examination, radiological investigation (mammography/ultrasound) and biopsy
- Histological grading 1, 2 or 3 according to differentiation
- TNM (tumour, node, metastasis) staging according to tumour size, lymph node involvement and metastases
- Staging involves examination, radiological investigation (e.g. CXR, abdominal USS or CT) and surgery

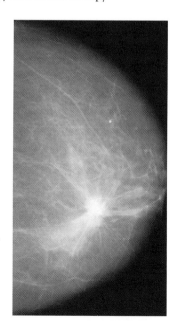

Figure 2.23 Breast carcinoma: spiculated mass on mammography

Breast surgery

- According to size of tumour and size of breast
- Breast-conserving surgery involves WLE followed by radiotherapy
- Clear resection margins are important
- Mastectomy if tumour too large for breast-conserving surgery or for patient choice
- Reconstructive surgery can be simultaneous with mastectomy or delayed
- Reconstruction is by myocutaneous flap based on the latissimus dorsi or rectus abdominis

Axillary surgery

- Performed for almost all invasive cancers
  Axillary clearance can be level 2 (includes nodes lateral and deep to the pectoralis minor) or level 3 (also includes apical nodes)
- For smaller tumours, axillary node sampling or sentinel node biopsy are options
- Sampling requires at least four random nodes for examination
- Positive node sampling or biopsy requires further axillary treatment by clearance or radiotherapy
- Axillary clearance and radiotherapy carry risk of arm lymphoedema

INFORMATION BOX: SENTINEL NODE BIOPSY

Sentinel node biopsy involves identification of the first node draining the tumour by injecting radioactive isotope and coloured dye. Sampling this node indicates whether lymphatic spread has occurred, and saves some women the need for extensive axillary surgery.

Adjuvant therapy

- Tamoxifen or anastrozole (Arimidex, AstraZeneca) for oestrogen receptor-positive tumours
- Cytotoxic chemotherapy for patients at high risk of recurrence, e.g. node-positive disease
- Radiotherapy to the breast following breast-conserving surgery
- Radiotherapy to the chest wall following mastectomy in those at high risk of recurrence
- Radiotherapy to axilla in selected cases, e.g. positive node sample

Paget's disease of the nipple

(P) Eczematous skin change to the nipple due to underlying malignancy
(Si) May have associated lump
(Ix) Triple assessment (see p. 143) including incisional skin biopsy
(Rx) Mastectomy and axillary clearance if separate mass present
WLE and radiotherapy possible if mass lies behind nipple

SCREENING

- Self-examination
- Two-view mammography offered every three years to UK women aged 50 to 64 years
- After age of 64 years, women can self-refer for mammograms if they wish
- Suspicious mammographic sign prompts recall
- Screen-detected cancers generally smaller and lower grade than symptomatic lesions
- Drawbacks include cost and potential psychological morbidity of false positives

ENDOCRINE SURGERY

THYROID GLAND

CONGENITAL ANOMALIES

Box 2.14 CONGENITAL THYROID ABNORMALITIES

- *Lingual thyroid*
  - failure of descent of part or all of the thyroid into the neck
  - presents with a lump at the back of the tongue
- *Thyroglossal cyst*:
  - thyroglossal duct sometimes remains along the tract of the thyroid descent from the tongue to the neck
  - cyst may develop in a persistent duct
  - presents with a midline neck lump which moves up on protrusion of the tongue
  - treatment is surgical excision of the lump and duct remnant, may require excision of part of the hyoid bone
- *Thyroglossal fistula*
  - patent thyroglossal duct remnant opening onto the skin
  - presents with a fluid discharge from fistula
  - treatment is surgical excision of fistula, duct remnant and part of the hyoid bone

---

THYROTOXICOSIS (GRAVES' DISEASE)

This is covered in detail on p. 67.

Rx Thyroidectomy is often needed for disease refractory to medical therapy

Cx See Box 2.15

Box 2.15 COMPLICATIONS OF THYROIDECTOMY

- Haemorrhage causing airway compression
- Recurrent laryngeal nerve injury (hoarse voice)
- Thyroid crisis
- Injury to parathyroids (hypoparathyroidism + hypocalcaemia)
- Hypothyroidism

Px Good after surgery, relapse frequent with medical therapy

GOITRE

P Defined as enlargement of the thyroid gland

A See Box 2.16

Box 2.16 CAUSES OF GOITRE

- *Physiological*:
  - due to puberty, pregnancy or iodine deficiency
  - iodine replacement may be required
- *Nodular*:
  - commonest cause in Western world
  - gland diffusely enlarged and irregular
  - patient usually euthyroid but may be thyrotoxic if dominant nodule is overactive
  - treatment indicated for thyrotoxicosis, compression of adjacent structures or suspicion of malignant change
- *Toxic goitre*:
  - Graves' disease
- *Hashimoto's disease*:
  - antithyroid autoantibodies produced
  - gland diffusely enlarged
  - patient usually hypothyroid
  - treatment with thyroxine
- *de Quervain's thyroiditis*:
  - gland inflammation due to viral infection
  - thyroid enlarged and tender
  - classically causes hyper- and then hypothyroidism
  - usually resolves spontaneously
- *Riedel's thyroiditis*:
  - gland infiltration with scar tissue
  - biopsy to differentiate from carcinoma
  - usually causes hypothyroidism
  - conservative treatment, thyroxine may be required

Ix TFT, thyroid antibodies, radio-isotope scan, USS, FNA for cytology

Rx See under individual causes

BENIGN NEOPLASMS

- Thyroid cysts may be aspirated, may require excision as recurrence is common
- Follicular adenoma can only be differentiated from carcinoma on histology, excision is therefore required
- Dominant nodule in nodular goitre: no treatment required but may need excision to prove diagnosis

THYROID CANCER

See Box 2.17

Box 2.17 SUBTYPES OF THYROID CANCER

- *Papillary carcinoma*:
  commonest
  age 10–40 years, ♀ > ♂
  slow growing, spread to lymph nodes occurs late
- *Follicular carcinoma*:
  age 40–60 years, ♀ > ♂
  may arise in nodular goitre
  spread is by blood
- *Medullary carcinoma*:
  any age, ♀ = ♂
  arises in parafollicular C cells and secretes calcitonin
  associated with multiple endocrine neoplasia
- *Anaplastic carcinoma*:
  elderly patients, ♀ > ♂
  rapid growth
  early local invasion and spread by lymphatics
- *Lymphoma*:
  uncommon

Sy   Lump, sometimes pain, dysphagia, hoarse voice

Si   Lump, sometimes cervical lymphadenopathy

Ix   TFT, radio-isotope scan, USS, fine needle aspiration (FNA)

Rx   *Papillary*:
- thyroid lobectomy or total thyroidectomy
- block dissection of involved nodes
- long-term thyroxine to suppress remaining thyroid

Follicular:
- thyroid lobectomy or total thyroidectomy
- block dissection of involved nodes
- long-term thyroxine replacement
- radioactive iodine may be used to supplement surgery or for secondary disease

Medullary:
- total thyroidectomy
- block dissection of involved nodes
- calcitonin used as marker for recurrence

Anaplastic:
- frequently inoperable
- palliative radiotherapy often given

Px   Good for papillary, follicular and medullary cancer, very poor for anaplastic carcinoma

OTHER NECK LUMPS

- *Lymph node*: common, reactive or due to tumour deposit, investigation for associated malignancy, e.g. head and neck, lymphoma
- *Cystic hygroma*: congenital cystic mass developing in remnant of jugular lymph sac, usually seen in children, transilluminates, treatment by surgical excision

- *Branchial cyst*: remnant of branchial arch, lies anterior and deep to sternocleidomastoid, may form abscess, treatment by surgical excision
- *Carotid body tumour*: tumour of chemoreceptor cells, slow growing, may metastasize late, may be pulsatile, treatment surgical or conservative (in the elderly)
- *Carotid aneurysm*: pulsatile, expansile mass

MISCELLANEOUS

CARCINOID TUMOUR

(P) Tumour arising from amine precursor uptake and decarboxylation (APUD) cells
Secretes 5-hydroxytryptamine (5-HT)
May occur anywhere in the gastrointestinal tract or lung
Site: appendix 35 per cent, ileum 28 per cent, rectum 13 per cent and bronchi 13 per cent

(A) Most common neuroendocrine tumour (incidence 2–7 per million)
♀ = ♂, tends to occur in those aged over 30 years

(S) *Carcinoid tumour*: few initially. May present as appendicitis or obstruction
Carcinoid syndrome: hepatomegaly, profuse colicky diarrhoea, cutaneous flushing, abdominal pain, right-sided cardiac valve disease and bronchoconstriction

(Ix) *Urine*: 24-h urine collection for 5-hydroxyindoleacetic acid (5-HIAA) which is a metabolite of 5-HT
Imaging: CT/USS of liver. MIBG (metaiodobenzylguanidine) nuclear medicine scan to localize primary tumour

(Rx) Resection of tumour and possibly liver secondaries, chemotherapy, sometimes only symptomatic treatment with 5-HT antagonists, somatostatin analogues

(Px) Slow-growing tumour, patients commonly survive many years
Median survival ~ 5–8 years

MULTIPLE ENDOCRINE NEOPLASIA (MEN)

(P) Rare syndromes involving endocrine adenomas or adenocarcinomas
MEN 1:
  - autosomal dominant inheritance
  - parathyroid tumour
  - pancreatic islet cell tumour
  - pituitary tumour
MEN 2a:
  - autosomal dominant inheritance
  - thyroid medullary carcinoma
  - phaeochromocytoma
  - parathyroid tumour
MEN 2b:
  - thyroid medullary carcinoma
  - phaeochromocytoma
  - mucocutaneous ganglioneuromas

BURNS

A Thermal, electrical, chemical or irradiation
P Tissue damage related to temperature and duration of burn
Assessment: airway, breathing, circulation (ABC)
Use the Wallace 'rule of nines' chart (see Box 2.18 and Figure 2.24)

Box 2.18 THE WALLACE 'RULE OF NINES'	
● Head and neck	9%
● Each arm	9%
● Anterior trunk	18%
● Posterior trunk	18%
● Each leg	18%
● Perineum	1%
● Total	100%

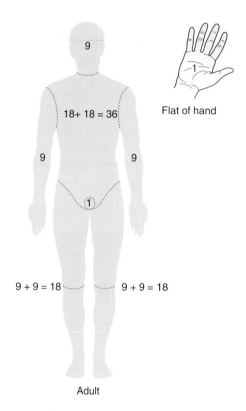

Flat of hand

Adult

Figure 2.24 Wallace 'rule of nines' chart

Lund and Browder charts are more accurate and take account of patient age
Classified as full or partial thickness depending on how much epithelium has been lost

Table 2.3 Differentiation of full- and partial-thickness burns

Full thickness	Partial thickness
May be painless	Painful
Sloughy	Reddened, may blister
Heals by granulation tissue and scarring	Heals by growth of new epithelium

A:
- may require intubation

B:
- 100 per cent O_2
- measure carboxyhaemoglobin if carbon monoxide poisoning suspected. May require hyperbaric oxygen
- may require escharotomy if thoracic burns limit chest movement

C:
- *Fluid replacement:* according to formula such as Muir and Barclay: give (weight in kg $\times$ per cent burn $\times$ 0.5) mls of colloid over each time period (4, 4, 4, 6, 6 and 12 h)
- *Analgesia:* opiates often required
- *Escharotomy:* full-thickness circumferential burns to limb or thorax may restrict blood flow or breathing. Performed to save life or limb

Refer to specialist burns unit if burns >10 per cent in children or elderly and >20 per cent at other ages

FLUID BALANCE

70KG MAN

- 60 per cent water = 42 L
- Extracellular fluid (ECF) = 14 L
  - plasma: 3 L
  - interstitial fluid: 11 L
  - transcellular fluid: small amount
- Intracellular fluid (ICF) = 28 L
- Transcellular fluid includes cerebrospinal, intraocular, pericardial, pleural and peritoneal fluid

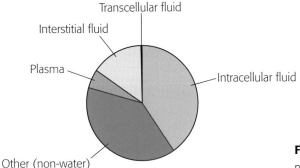

Figure 2.25 Pie chart showing proportions of fluid in an adult

NORMAL DAILY REQUIREMENT

- *Replacement of*:
  - insensible loss, e.g. faeces, lungs – 500 mL
  - urine – 1000 mL
  - insensible loss from skin – 500–2000 mL
- *Basic regime each 24 h*:
  - 3000 mL water
  - 100 mmol sodium
  - 60 mmol potassium
- *This can be achieved with*:
  - 1000 mL normal saline
  - 2000 mL 5 per cent dextrose
  - 20 mmol potassium with each 1000 mL of fluid

ASSESSMENT OF FLUID STATUS

- Thirst
- Skin turgor, tongue, mucous membranes
- Pulse, blood pressure, jugular venous pressure (JVP)
- Urine output (should be at least 0.5 mL/kg/h)
- Input/output charts with overall 24-h fluid balance
- Blood urea and electrolyte measurement
- Central venous pressure: absolute value less useful than trend following intravenous fluid administration
- Fluid replacement: maintenance fluids + replacement of abnormal losses, such as vomit, blood and third space fluid, e.g. in pancreatitis

Table 2.4 Types of intravenous fluid

Crystalloid	Colloid
Electrolytes in solution in water	Contain high-molecular weight particles
Distribute rapidly through ECF volume	Remain in circulation and exert oncotic pressure, drawing interstitial fluid into plasma
Include normal saline, Hartmann's solution, 5% dextrose	Include blood, Haemaccel (Syner-Med), Gelofusine (Braun)

PARENTERAL NUTRITION

- Intravenous nutrition
- Given until enteral feeding is possible
- *Indications*:
  - enteral feeding not possible for >4 days
  - multiple injuries
  - malabsorption
  - intestinal fistulae
- Administered in co-operation with dietitian/nutritionist

- Usually administered via central vein as solutions are hypertonic and damage smaller veins
- *Composition*:
  - carbohydrate and lipid provide calories
  - protein
  - trace elements and vitamins
- *Monitoring*:
  - daily weight
  - blood tests for electrolytes and albumin

NEUROSURGERY

HEAD INJURY

 Common at all ages

 May lead to skull fractures and brain injuries

Skull fractures:
- facial bones
- base of skull
- skull vault

Brain injuries: primary due to direct trauma
- Coup: at site of impact
- Contre-coup: brain impacts skull on opposite side to that of trauma
- Shear: causes diffuse axonal injury

Secondary brain injury due to delayed effects of injury, e.g. hypoxia, intracranial haemorrhage

Cerebral perfusion depends on cerebral perfusion pressure = blood pressure – intracranial pressure (ICP)

Head injury can cause ↑ICP which ↓ cerebral perfusion pressure

Classification:
- minor (Glasgow Coma Score (GCS) 13–15)
- moderate (GCS 9–12)
- severe (GCS <9)

INFORMATION BOX: GLASGOW COMA SCORE

- Standardized means of assessing and describing conscious level
- Possible score from 3 to 15
- GCS ≤ 8 is defined as coma (see Table 2.5)

Rx Airway with cervical spine immobilization
Breathing
Circulation
Specialist treatment depends on extent and type of injuries and is discussed later

Table 2.5 Glasgow Coma Scale

Observation	Score
Eye opening	
Spontaneous	4
To speech	3
To pain	2
None	1
Best verbal response	
Orientated	5
Confused	4
Inappropriate words	3
Incomprehensible sounds	2
None	1
Best motor response	
Obeys commands	6
Localizes to pain	5
Withdraws from pain	4
Abnormal flexion	3
Extension	2
None	1
Total	/15

INTRACRANIAL HAEMORRHAGE

SUBARACHNOID HAEMORRHAGE

- **P** Traumatic or secondary to leaking aneurysm
- **Sy** Sudden-onset headache, 'the worst headache of my life, doctor'
- **Si** Neck stiffness, photophobia
- **Ix** CT, cerebral angiography
- **Rx** *Conservative*
  Surgery: clipping or embolization of aneurysm

SUBDURAL HAEMORRHAGE

- **P** Tear of venous bridging veins between cortex and venous sinuses
- **A** Acute due to severe head injury
  Chronic common in alcoholics and elderly, often due to minor head injury, especially if anticoagulated
- **S** Headache, weakness, numbness, slurred speech, nausea/vomiting, lethargy, seizures
- **Ix** CT
- **Rx** Surgical evacuation of haematoma
- **Px** Related to severity of head injury

EXTRADURAL HAEMORRHAGE

(P) Trauma causes damage to extradural vessel

(Si) ICP rises causing decreasing GCS

Compression of 3rd cranial nerve (false localizing sign) causes ipsilateral pupil dilatation

(Rx) Immediate surgical decompression to prevent death

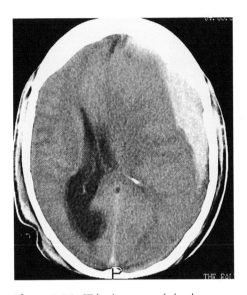

Figure 2.26 CT brain scan: subdural haemorrhage

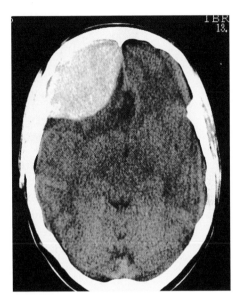

Figure 2.27 CT brain scan: extradural haemorrhage

NEUROLOGICAL TUMOURS

GLIOMA

(A) Arise from glial cells in the brain

(P) Divided into astrocytomas (most common), medulloblastomas, ependymomas and oligodendrogliomas according to the cell type of origin

(Rx) Surgical excision where possible

Palliative treatment is often the only option and includes surgery, chemotherapy and radiotherapy

MENINGIOMA

(A) Arise from arachnoid cells in the meninges

(P) Usually benign and slow growing

(Rx) Surgical excision

ACOUSTIC NEUROMA

(A) Arise from Schwann cells of cranial nerve 8 (associated with neurofibromatosis)

(P) Presses on 5th, 7th, 9th, 10th and 12th cranial nerves as tumour expands

(Sy) Unilateral deafness, facial numbness and weakness

(Rx) Surgical excision but risks nerve damage

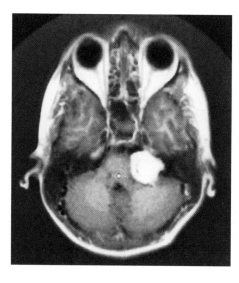

Figure 2.28 Acoustic neuroma: mass of increased signal at the cerebellopontine angle

PITUITARY TUMOURS

P   Usually adenomas
        May cause endocrine abnormalities, e.g. hypopituitarism, Cushing's syndrome
Si May compress optic chiasm causing bitemporal hemianopia
Rx Surgical excision or hormonal manipulation

LYMPHOMA

A   Uncommon, occurs with increased frequency in AIDS
Rx Radiotherapy
Px Poor, survival often <1 year

METASTASES

A   Common
P   Principally from primaries in breast, lung, kidney and malignant melanoma
Rx Supportive, steroids

OTHER CNS DISORDERS

SPINAL CORD COMPRESSION

P   Compression of the spinal cord is an emergency
A   Vertebral metastases, abscess, disc prolapse, cord tumour, trauma
Sy Sudden-onset leg weakness, leg pain, sensory loss, painless urinary retention
Si Sensory level, motor weakness, hyperreflexia
Ix MRI
Rx *Metastases*: steroids, radiotherapy, surgical decompression
        Abscess: drainage, antibiotics
        Disc prolapse: surgical decompression
Cx Paralysis, neurogenic bladder
Px Depends on cause. Best chance of recovery with early treatment

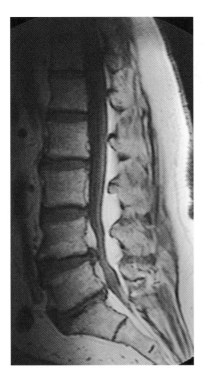

Figure 2.29 Lumbar disc prolapse: the MRI scan shows a L4/5 disc protrusion extending up to the theca

CAUDA EQUINA SYNDROME

(A) Compression of the cauda equina has the same causes as cord compression
(S) Commonly causes back pain, bladder and bowel sphincter dysfunction
Leg weakness occurs together with absent reflexes
(Rx) Treatment varies with cause as for cord compression

HYDROCEPHALUS

(P) Raised cerebrospinal fluid (CSF) pressure in the ventricular system of the brain
(A) Obstruction of the normal production, circulation and reabsorption pathway of CSF within the ventricles
May be congenital or acquired

INFORMATION BOX: HYDROCEPHALUS

- *Non-communicating hydrocephalus* is due to obstruction of CSF flow from the brain to the subarachnoid space – may be due to congenital malformation or development of a tumour.
- *Communicating hydrocephalus* is due to failure of CSF reabsorption from the subarachnoid space – may be due to congenital abnormality in arachnoid villi, meningitis or subarachnoid haemorrhage.

(Rx) Treatment is by relief of pressure with a shunt or resection of any obstructing lesion

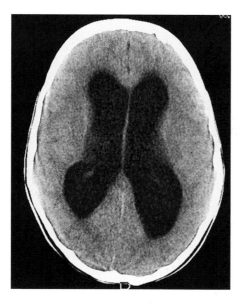

Figure 2.30 Hydrocephalus: dilatation of the ventricles without enlargement of the sulci

PERIPHERAL NERVOUS SYSTEM DISORDERS

SCIATICA

P Sciatic nerve originates from L4–5 and S1–3 nerve roots
Compression of nerve root by prolapsed intervertebral disc causes leg pain

Sy Pain typically shoots down leg to below knee

Si Limited straight leg raise due to pain, decreased sensation over relevant dermatome, muscle weakness (weak hallux extension in L5 compression, foot plantar flexion in S1)

Ix MRI

Rx Conservative treatment usually effective, surgical discectomy in selected cases

Px Complete resolution may take months

MERALGIA PARAESTHETICA

P Compression of the lateral cutaneous nerve of the thigh
Occurs as nerve exits beneath inguinal ligament

A Caused by obesity and extrinsic compression from overly tight belts/clothing

S Causes pain and altered sensation over anterior and lateral part of thigh which is relieved by hip flexion

Rx *Conservative*: weight loss, loose clothing
Surgery: decompression may be effective in difficult cases

CARPAL TUNNEL SYNDROME

P Compression of the median nerve within the carpal tunnel (deep to the flexor retinaculum)

A Associated with pregnancy, rheumatoid arthritis, acromegaly, hypothyroidism

Si Pain and paraesthesia in radial three digits
Wasting of thenar muscles

Rx *Conservative*: splinting
Surgery: steroid injection, surgical carpal tunnel decompression (division of flexor retinaculum)

BRACHIAL PLEXUS LESIONS

- *Upper trunk lesion: Erb's palsy*
  - occurs with forced contralateral neck abduction
  - C5 and 6 nerve roots injured
  - arm internally rotated with extended elbow (waiter's tip position)
  - decreased sensation over C5 and 6 dermatomes
- *T1 lesion: Klumpke's palsy*
  - occurs with shoulder dislocation or cervical rib
  - wasting of intrinsic muscles of hand
  - decreased sensation over T1 dermatome

RADIAL NERVE LESIONS

A Commonly injured in fractures of spiral groove of humerus
Si Wrist drop
Decreased sensation over dorsum of first webspace

ULNAR NERVE LESIONS

A Commonly injured in fractures around elbow and lacerations
Si Causes clawing of the 4th and 5th digits (*main en griffe*)
Decreased sensation over ulnar one-and-a-half digits

CHAPTER 3

Orthopaedics

Gareth Jones and Julian Leong

FRACTURE

P A fracture is a break in the continuity of the cortex of a bone (with an associated soft tissue injury)

CLASSIFICATIONS

- Closed – overlying skin intact
- Open fractures (previously called compound fractures)
  - a break in the overlying skin which communicates with the fracture and/or the fracture haematoma. The Gustilo–Anderson classification grades severity according to soft-tissue injury

Table 3.1 Gustilo–Anderson classification of open fractures

Grade	Characteristics
Type I	Low-energy clean wound <1 cm with minimal soft tissue injury and fracture comminution
Type II	Wound 1–10 cm with moderate soft tissue damage and fracture comminution
Type III	High energy, wound >10 cm (IIIA no periosteal stripping, IIIB periosteal stripping, IIIC major vascular injury)

- *Simple*: single fracture line producing two fracture fragments (transverse, oblique, spiral)
- *Comminuted*: more than two fragments
- Intra- or extra-articular: does the fracture involve the joint surface (intra-articular)?
- Undisplaced or displaced: bone fragments remain in alignment v. loss of alignment
- Pathological: a fracture through abnormal bone (e.g. tumour)
- Salter–Harris: classified children's fractures involving the growth plate (epiphysis).

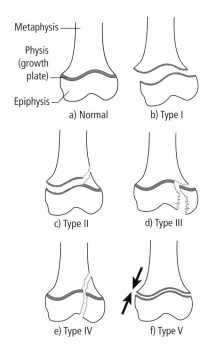

Figure 3.1 Salter–Harris classification of epiphyseal injuries (a) Normal (note that the growth plate is radiolucent); (b) Type I: epiphyseal slip only; (c) Type II: fracture through the growth plate with a segment of metaphysis attached; (d) Type III: fracture through the epiphysis extending into the growth plate; (e) Type IV: fracture of the epiphysis, crossing the growth plate; (f) Type V: crush injury to the epiphyseal plate

COMPLICATIONS

IMMEDIATE (MINUTES TO HOURS)

- Pain
- Nerve, blood vessel, skin and muscle damage
- Fat embolism
- Visceral damage (pneumothorax in rib fracture, etc.)
- Disruption to overlying soft tissues

EARLY (HOURS TO DAYS)

- Compartment syndrome (see p. 164)
- Immobility
- Wound infection (if open injury)
- Deep venous thrombosis and pulmonary embolism

LATE (WEEKS TO MONTHS)

- Stiffness
- Sudek's atrophy (complex regional pain syndrome/regional sympathetic dystrophy/ reflex osteodystrophy)
- Malunion (fracture heals in abnormal position), delayed union (slower than expected fracture healing), non-union (the fracture is still present and healing has stopped)
- Pseudoarthrosis ('false joint' due to a persistent non-union)
- Secondary osteoarthritis (secondary to intra-articular fractures)
- Chronic osteomyelitis (open fractures or postoperative)

PRINCIPLES OF FRACTURE MANAGEMENT

- Fractures can vary in severity from insignificant occurrences not warranting any treatment to life- or limb-threatening episodes
- For serious/multiple fractures use advanced trauma life support (ATLS) guidelines (ABC – airway, breathing, circulation)
- The history should reveal the mechanism of injury, premorbid conditions and fitness for surgery
- *Examination*: general and specific to reveal any occult injuries
- *Investigations*: baseline pre-operative investigations and radiographs for suspected fracture sites

GENERAL TREATMENT

- Analgesia
- Assess risk of venous thromboembolism (VTE) and implement prophylaxis with low-molecular weight heparin (LMWH) plus anti-embolism stockings (TEDS) if appropriate, e.g. hip fractures
- Identify and treat other injuries

FRACTURE-SPECIFIC TREATMENT

1. *Reduce*:
    – for displaced fractures
2. *Hold*:
- Non-operative:
    – *simple splinting*: neighbouring strap (e.g. metacarpal fractures)
    – *plaster of Paris (POP)*: easily moulded, cheap. Often applied acutely as a backslab (i.e. POP on one side only) to allow for swelling
    – *Fibreglass cast*: lighter, less bulky, more rigid (a disadvantage if swelling occurs) and more durable than POP
- Operative:
    – *internal fixation*: Kirschner wire (K wire); screws and plate; intramedullary device
    – *external fixation*: uniplanar or ring (e.g. Ilizarov frame)
3. *Rehabilitate*:
    – physiotherapy, occupational therapy

OTHER EMERGENCY TREATMENTS

- *Dislocation*: reduction – closed (without a skin incision) if possible
- *Open fracture*: tetanus, i.v. antibiotics, photograph of wound (prevents repeated removal of dressings), saline-soaked gauze, immobilise. Combined orthopaedic and plastic surgery operation ASAP
- *Compartment syndrome*: emergency fasciotomy
- *Vascular compromise*: angiography ± vascular repair ± fasciotomy

COMPARTMENT SYNDROME

- **A** Increased pressure in a closed fascial compartment, usually secondary to trauma
- **P** Osseofascial compartments have a fixed volume. Adding to this volume (e.g. blood, traumatic exudate) will increase the compartment pressure. If compartment

pressure exceeds capillary pressure, ischaemia results. Ischaemia initiates a vicious cycle of more fluid exudate, and increasing compartment pressures. Irreversible muscle necrosis will occur if not treated.

(Si) Pain out of proportion to the injury
Pain on passive stretching of muscles in the compartment
Palpable tense compartment and paraesthesia
Pulselessness is a late (and often terminal) sign

(Rx) If suspected: emergency fasciotomy (division of fascia to relieve pressure)

COMMON TRAUMA

UPPER LIMB

PROXIMAL HUMERUS

(A) Most common in elderly osteoporotic patients
Fall onto outstretched hand (usually higher energy trauma in young patients)

(P) Can be comminuted (Neer's classification)

(Rx) Majority can be treated conservatively with a collar and cuff
Physiotherapy
Displaced comminuted fractures may need open reduction and internal fixation (ORIF) or shoulder hemiarthroplasty

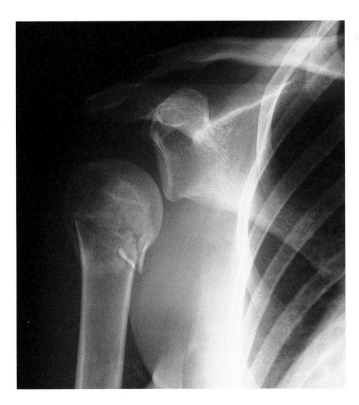

Figure 3.2 Humeral neck fracture with downward subluxation of the humeral head secondary to blood in joint (haemarthrosis)

SHOULDER DISLOCATION

(P) Most commonly dislocates antero-inferiorly

(A) First episodes are often traumatic

Posterior dislocations are often secondary to epileptic seizure

(Sy) Pain, decreased movement

(Si) Loss of deltoid contour, arm held internally rotated and adducted

Must examine and document axillary nerve function (sensation to the regimental arm badge area) and presence of radial pulse before attempting reduction

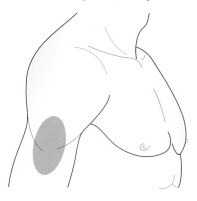

Figure 3.3 Region of the arm supplied by the sensory branch of the axillary nerve

(Ix) X-rays: anteroposterior (AP) and axillary (or scapular Y view)

(Rx) Reduction as soon as possible – sedation or formal anaesthesia

Number of closed reduction techniques exist (e.g. Kocher's)

Open reduction if closed techniques fail

Immobilize in broad-arm sling for approximately 3 weeks

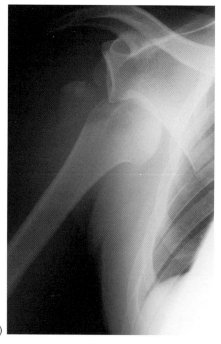
(a)

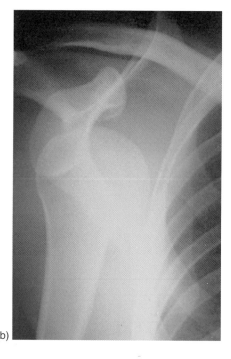
(b)

Figure 3.4 Anterior dislocation of the shoulder

ROTATOR CUFF DISORDERS

Rotator cuff consists of:

- *inserting into the greater tuberosity:* supraspinatus (abduction), infraspinatus (external rotation), teres minor (external rotation)
- *insertion into the lesser tuberosity:* subscapularis (internal rotation)
- **(P)** Chronic degenerative changes or trauma result in tendonitis (acute or chronic) ± tears (complete or partial)

Calcifying tendonitis

- **(P)** Most commonly involves the supraspinatus tendon
- **(A)** Asymptomatic, acute or chronically painful shoulder; exacerbated by activity
- **(Ix)** X-ray reveals calcific deposits within the tendon
- **(Rx)** Majority resolve with non-operative treatment

Chronic tendonitis

- **(P)** Otherwise known as impingement syndrome (tendon is compressed against the coracoacromial arch)
- **(A)** Gradual onset of pain with overhead activities
- **(Ix)** Dynamic USS or MRI
- **(Rx)** *Non-operative*: physiotherapy, NSAIDs and subacromial injection (steroid + local anaesthetic)
  Operative: subacromial decompression ± tendon repair

Tendon tears

- **(P)** Complete tears abolish active movement of the particular muscle involved, while partial tears present as pain and weakness.

BICEPS TENDON RUPTURE

- **(P)** Usually a rupture of the long head of biceps tendon. Classically have 'Popeye' sign with muscle contraction (visible bulge in middle of biceps because of retraction of ruptured tendon)

FROZEN SHOULDER (ADHESIVE CAPSULITIS)

- **(A)** Three recognized stages. Total duration about 1–3 years
  Painful phase: gradual onset of predominantly night pain
  Frozen phase: progressive reduction in range of movement (especially external rotation)
  Thawing phase: progressive improvement in pain and ROM
- **(Si)** Reduced range of active and passive movement (especially external rotation)
- **(Ix)** X-ray to exclude other diagnoses
- **(Rx)** Analgesia, steroid injections and physiotherapy. Consider MUA or arthroscopy for resistant cases

(a)

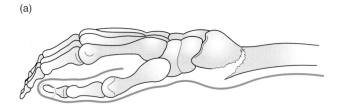

(b)

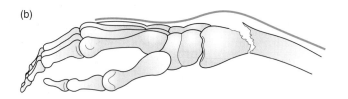

Figure 3.5 (a) Fracture of the distal radius with dorsal angulation; (b) fracture of the distal radius with volar (palmar) angulation

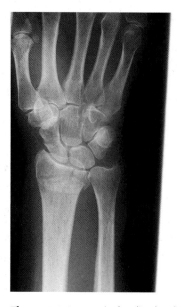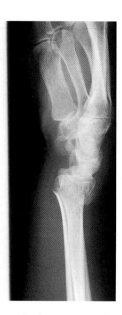

Figure 3.6 Intra-articular distal radius fracture with shortening and dorsal angulation

DISTAL RADIUS

- Two main types
  - Dorsal angulation and shortening of distal fragment
  - Volar (palmar) angulation and shortening of distal fragment
- Two eponymous radio-ulna injuries to know:
  Galeazzi fracture: fracture of radial shaft with dislocation of the distal radio-ulna joint
  Monteggia fracture: fracture of the proximal ulna with dislocation of the radial head

SCAPHOID FRACTURE

Sy Wrist pain and swelling following fall onto outstretched hand

Si Tenderness in the anatomical snuff box and pain on telescoping the thumb

Ix Scaphoid view X-rays (taken from four different angles)

If X-rays are equivocal, repeat clinical and radiographic examinations at 7–14 days. Bone scan or MRI if diagnosis remains uncertain

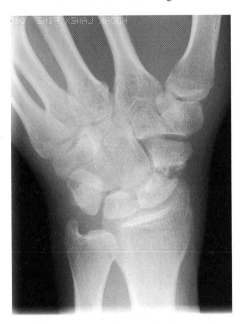

Figure 3.7 Scaphoid wrist fracture

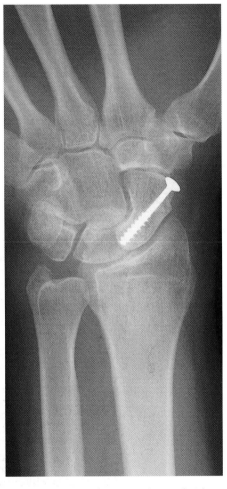

Rx Scaphoid plaster if any suspicion of injury (anatomical snuff box tenderness), and re-examine at 7–14 days

Displaced fractures require internal screw fixation

Cx Blood supply to the scaphoid enters distally; hence the risk of avascular necrosis (and non-union) of the proximal scaphoid following fracture

Figure 3.8 Internal fixation of a scaphoid fracture

BENNETT'S FRACTURE

A Most common thumb injury

P Intra-articular fracture of the base of the first metacarpal ± CMC joint subluxation

Rx Failure of closed manipulation and thumb immobilization necessitates K-wire or screw fixation

LITTLE FINGER METACARPAL NECK FRACTURE (BOXER'S FRACTURE)

(A) Classically caused by striking a solid object with a closed fist

(P) Volar (palmar) angulation of the distal fragment

(Rx) Temporary splinting for most. Operative intervention if rotation (fingers overlap when making a fist), significant volar angulation (greater than 45°), or shortening

LOWER LIMB

FRACTURED NECK OF FEMUR

(A) In the UK about 70 000 people over 60 years old suffer a hip fracture (the number rises approximately 2 per cent each year)

Patients often elderly and osteoporotic, with multiple co-morbidities

(Sy) Pain in the hip after fall, unable to weight-bear

(Si) Affected leg is shortened and externally rotated

(Ix) AP pelvic X-ray and lateral of affected hip (full length femur if pathological fracture suspected)

CT, MRI or bone isotope scan if diagnosis is uncertain e.g. minimally displaced fractures

---

Box 3.1 CLASSIFICATION OF FRACTURES OF THE FEMORAL NECK

- *Intracapsular fracture*:
  - blood supply to femoral head (via retinacular vessels) disrupted, hence risk of femoral head avascular necrosis and fracture non-union. Be aware of Garden classification (although it is now preferable to divide intracapsular fractures into undisplaced and displaced)
- *Extracapsular fracture*:
  - blood supply to femoral head intact

(Rx) All patients require adequate rehydration and preparation for theatre (blood tests, ECG, etc). Early involvement of orthogeriatricians recommended

Operative fixation should not be delayed for more than 48 hours unless there are recognized reversible medical conditions.

Non-operative: only if moribund and not fit for an anaesthetic

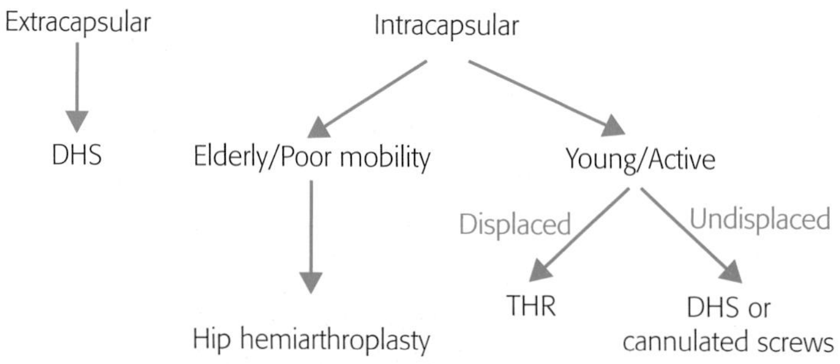

Figure 3.9 Hip fracture treatment summary

Internal fixation:

Post-operative: multidisciplinary approach (i.e. orthopaedic team, orthogeriatrician, physiotherapist, occupational therapist, social worker and family)

Mortality 10 per cent at 30 days, 30 per cent at 1 year

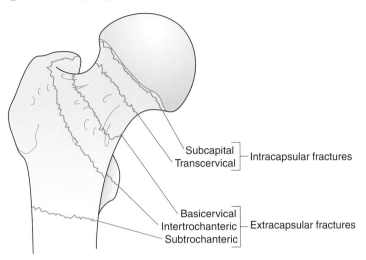

Figure 3.10 Common sites of fracture of the femoral neck

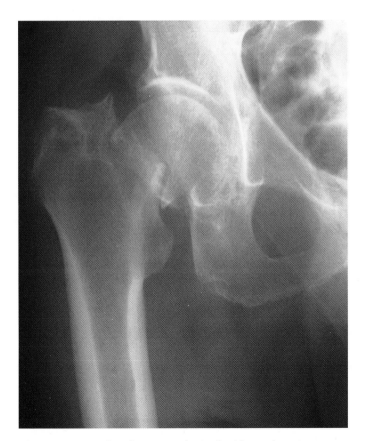

Figure 3.11 Displaced intracapsular neck of femur fracture

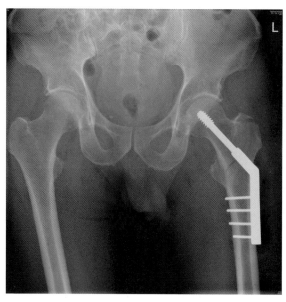

Figure 3.12 Dynamic hip screw

ANTERIOR CRUCIATE LIGAMENT RUPTURE

(A) Contact or non-contact injury, often occurs when changing direction

(Sy) Audible pop. Significant knee swelling (haemarthrosis) within a few hours

(Si) Positive anterior draw, Lachman's test ± pivot shift – difficult to assess acutely due to pain
Long-term: knee instability with changes in direction or rotation

(Ix) *X-ray*: occasionally patient may have avulsion fracture of tibial spine rather than ligament rupture
MRI: investigation of choice to confirm rupture and identify associated injuries, e.g. meniscal tears
Examination under anaesthesia (EUA) and arthroscopy: only if diagnosis is in doubt (e.g. MRI reveals partial tear)

(Rx) *Non-operative*:
– may be suitable for patients not involved in activities which involve pivoting, e.g. cycling, running
– physiotherapy for ROM and strengthening
Operative:
– indicated if symptomatic knee instability
– arthroscopic anterior cruciate reconstruction with hamstring, or patellar tendon graft

TIBIAL PLATEAU FRACTURE

● Low energy (osteoporotic bone) or high energy (often RTA or sports-related injuries)
● Schatzker classification: Type I–VI
● Displacement or articular depression >5 mm are indications for internal/external fixation

TIBIAL SHAFT FRACTURE

(P) Most commonly injured long bone – often high-energy injuries

(Rx) Plaster, intramedullary nail, or external fixation depending on fracture pattern and soft tissue damage

Cx Beware compartment syndrome (patients should be admitted overnight for observation)
Check and document neurovascular status

ACHILLES TENDON RUPTURE

A Sudden plantar flexion of the foot, or forced dorsiflexion.
Typically occurs in intermittently active individuals
Systemic steroids increase risk

Sy Loud 'pop' and feeling of 'kicked in the back of the leg'
Tender, swelling and palpable gap in the Achilles tendon

Si Simmonds/Thompson test – absence of foot plantar flexion on squeezing calf

Ix Ultrasound scan

Rx *Non-operative*: serial plasters starting with foot in full equinus
Operative: tendon repair and serial plasters. Thought to reduce risk of re-rupture.

ANKLE FRACTURES

A Common orthopaedic presentation to the emergency department

Ix Radiographs: AP, mortise and lateral views of the ankle

Box 3.2 DANIS–WEBER CLASSIFICATION OF ANKLE FRACTURES

There are three types depending on the level of fracture of the fibula
- *Type A*: below the syndesmosis
- *Type B*: at the level of the syndesmosis
- *Type C*: above the syndesmosis

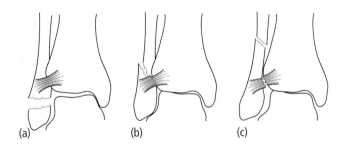

(a)   (b)   (c)

Figure 3.13 Danis–Weber classification of ankle fractures. There are three types depending on the level of the fracture of the fibula (a) Type A: below the syndesmosis (b) Type B: at the level of the syndesmosis (c) Type C: above the syndesmosis (reproduced with kind permission from Solomon L, Warwick DJ, Nayagam S. *Apley's Concise System of Orthopaedics and Fractures*, 3rd edn, London: Arnold, 2005)

Rx Fracture dislocation of the ankle requires emergency reduction and immobilization in plaster backslab, usually under sedation in the emergency department
Danis-Weber A: most can be treated with an ankle support brace
Danis–Weber B: operative fixation if evidence of talar shift (talus no longer perfectly aligns with tibial articular surface – best appreciated on mortise view)
Danis–Weber C: suggests syndesmotic injury and requires operative fixation

ELECTIVE ORTHOPAEDICS

OSTEOARTHRITIS

(P) Most common articular disease worldwide.

Traditionally considered a degenerative joint disease of articular cartilage (new evidence points towards an inflammatory component, and that the disease involves the entire joint, i.e. synovium, cartilage and subchondral bone).

Characterized by progressive cartilage loss, subchondral bone formation and bony osteophytes

May be secondary to trauma, infection, congenital conditions (e.g. developmental dysplasia of the hip)

(Sy) Pain after exertion, stiffness (morning stiffness classically < 30 min), reduced range of movement and deformity

---

Box 3.3 RADIOGRAPHIC FEATURES OF OSTEOARTHRITIS

- **L**oss of joint space
- **O**steophytes
- **S**ubchondral sclerosis
- **S**ubchondral cysts

(Rx) *Non-operative*:
  - analgesia
  - lifestyle changes (especially weight loss)
  - physiotherapy
  - occupational therapy
  - walking aids
  - intra-articular steroid injection
- *Operative*:
  - arthroscopy (NICE advise only if symptoms of mechanical locking)
  - osteotomy (aims to correct malaligned joint)
  - arthroplasty (joint replacement, e.g. total hip replacement)
  - arthrodesis (joint fusion)

LOWER LIMB ORTHOPAEDIC COMPLICATIONS

For clarity, the complications of total hip replacement are shown in Box 3.4.

Box 3.4 SPECIFIC COMPLICATIONS OF TOTAL HIP REPLACEMENT

- *Immediate*:
  - fat embolism
  - fracture of the femur or acetabulum
  - nerve damage (e.g. sciatic)
  - haemorrhage
  - leg length discrepancy
  - vascular injury

- *Early*:
  - infection (superficial and deep)
  - DVT/pulmonary embolism (PE)
  - dislocation
- *Late*:
  - aseptic loosening
  - periprosthetic fracture
  - loss of bone stock
  - component failure
  - heterotopic ossification
  - infection

BAKER'S/POPLITEAL CYST

(P) Distension of a normal bursa, or posterior herniation of knee joint capsule. Often secondary to OA or other intra-articular pathology

(Si) Painless swelling in popliteal fossa. Beware expansile pulsatile swellings (popliteal aneurysm) Rupture results in calf swelling and pain (similar presentation to DVT, which must be excluded)

(Ix) USS

(Rx) Aspiration occasionally for symptom relief Treat underlying intra-articular pathology

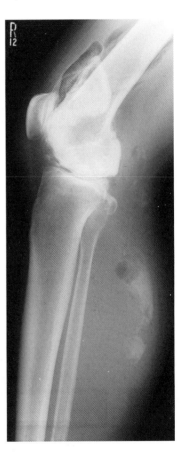

Figure 3.14 Ruptured Baker's cyst: arthrography with injection of contrast and air into the knee joint; extravasation into the upper calf

LOWER BACK PAIN

(A) Common presentation to general practitioner (GP) and emergency department

(Sy) Sciatica pain: lower back pain radiating down leg(s) in a dermatomal distribution Paraesthesiae to a dermatome

(Si) Straight leg raise (SLR) – reproduces pain. Further exacerbated by forced dorsiflexion of the foot (sciatic stretch test)
May present with other neurology
Number of differential diagnoses (see Box 3.5).
- Low back pain + unilateral/bilateral leg motor/sensory abnormality + bowel and/or bladder dysfunction = urgent MRI to exclude cauda equina syndrome (see p. 159)

> **Box 3.5 CAUSES OF LOWER BACK PAIN**
>
> - *From the bone*:
>   - mechanical back pain
>   - spinal stenosis ('spinal claudication')
>   - instability (spondylolisthesis)
>   - infection (Potts' disease – TB of the spine)
>   - tumour (primary, secondary)
>   - multiple myeloma
>   - referred pain from the hip
> - *From the nerve*:
>   - nerve root compression (radiculopathy)
> - *From the intervertebral disc*:
>   - spinal stenosis
>   - prolapsed disc
>   - infection (discitis)
>   - degenerative disc
> - *Connective tissue disease:*
>   - ankylosing spondylitis
> - *From the abdomen*:
>   - abdominal aortic aneurysm
>   - pancreatitis
>   - renal stone

Ix According to suspected diagnosis
MRI is most useful for spinal pathology
Urgent computed tomography (CT) for suspected AAA

Rx *Conservative*:
- most mechanical back pain and disc prolapse can be treated conservatively
- physiotherapy, analgesia

Operative treatment
- epidural, facet joint injections
- discectomy
- spinal decompression
- spinal fusion
- intervertebral disc replacement

COMMON PAEDIATRIC CONDITIONS

DEVELOPMENTAL DYSPLASIA OF THE HIP (DDH)

P Congenital dislocation or instability of the hip resulting in abnormal hip joint development

Sy Usually identified during newborn, 6-week, or 8-month baby checks. If missed, late presentation as pain/limp/abnormal gait

Si Asymmetrical thigh ± skin creases. Ortolani test (hip joint reduces with clunk when abducted) and Barlow test (gentle posterior pressure with legs adducted results in hip dislocation)

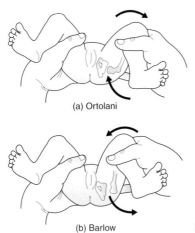

(a) Ortolani

(b) Barlow

Figure 3.15 (a) Ortolani test (b) Barlow test

Ix   USS, X-ray (>6 months), MRI
X-ray – AP pelvis and frog lateral (>5 months)

Rx   Pavlik harness if identified <6 months of age
Manipulation under anaesthetic + hip spica plaster
Open reduction (if older)
Complex pelvic and femoral osteotomies if late presentation

SEPTIC ARTHRITIS

A   Surgical emergency. Can affect children of any age, but most common <3 years

P   Most commonly *Staphylococcus*

S   Pain, reluctance to move leg (often held flexed and abducted), limp, systemic sepsis

Ix   WBC, CRP, ESR, blood cultures. X-ray, USS ± aspiration

Rx   If any doubt proceed to joint aspiration ± washout in theatre
Systemic antibiotics

LEGG–CALVE–PERTHES' DISEASE

P   Avascular necrosis of the femoral head of unknown aetiology

A   Affects children from 3–12 years

Sy   Hip/groin pain, limp and referred knee pain

Ix   X-ray, MRI

Rx   Treatment depends on severity of disease

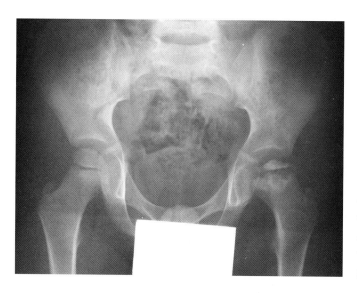

Figure 3.16 Perthes' disease: well established with flattening of the left femoral ossific nucleus and thickening of the femoral neck. A lead genital shield is in place

SLIPPED UPPER FEMORAL EPIPHYSIS

Ⓐ 10–15 years, often obese males
Sy Hip pain, limp and referred knee pain
Ix X-ray: femoral epiphysis in abnormal 'slipped' position in relation to femoral neck
Rx In general, screw fixation to stabilize slip

BONE TUMOURS

See Table 3.3

Table 3.3 Examples of bone tumours

Origin	Benign	Malignant
Primary		
Cartilage	Chondroma	Chondrosarcoma
Bone	Osteochondroma	Osteosarcoma
Fibrous tissue	Fibroma	Fibrosarcoma
	Myxoid fibroma	
Plasma cells		Multiple myeloma
Secondary		
Breast		
Bronchus		
Prostate		
Kidney		
Thyroid		

Ear, nose and throat

Irfan Syed

EARS

OTITIS EXTERNA

- **P** Inflammation of the skin of the external auditory meatus (ear canal)
- **A** May be caused by bacteria (commonly *Staphylococcus* or *Pseudomonas*) or fungi
- **Sy** Irritation, pain, discharge and deafness (canal becomes blocked with debris)
- **Si** Tenderness upon moving the ear, moist debris, which when removed reveals an erythematous canal
- **Rx** Microsuction and topical antibiotic and steroid drops. If the canal is very oedematous, insert wick to splint open canal and allow drops into ear

ACUTE OTITIS MEDIA

- **P** Acute inflammation of the middle ear cavity, highest incidence in children (3–7 years old)
- **A** May be primary infection or secondary following an upper respiratory tract infection (common)
  Causative organisms *Streptococcus pneumoniae*, *Haemophilus influenza* and *Moraxella catarrhalis*
- **Sy** Otalgia (sudden relief if tympanic membrane perforates with release of pus), decreased hearing in affected ear
- **Si** Fever, bulging, red tympanic membrane, sometimes fluid level visible behind membrane
- **Ix** Full blood count (FBC)
- **Rx** Antibiotics and analgesia
- **Cx** Mastoiditis, meningitis, intracranial abscesses, lateral sinus thrombosis

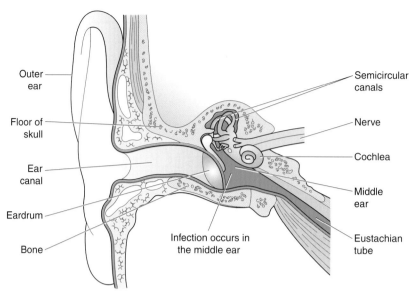

Figure 4.1 Otitis media (diagram source copyright EMIS and PiP as distributed on http://www. patient.co.uk)

MASTOIDITIS

(P)   Follows acute otitis media

(Si)   Tenderness ± erythema overlying mastoid, displacement of the ear forward and a red or bulging tympanic membrane

(Rx)   Antibiotics and if evidence of an abscess or no response with antibiotics, then surgery, i.e. mastoidectomy

OTITIS MEDIA WITH EFFUSION ('GLUE EAR')

(P)   Characterized by fluid in the middle ear resulting in conductive deafness
Underlying cause: Eustachian tube dysfunction, e.g. secondary to large adenoids. Middle ear pressure falls, inflammation results and copious, tenacious mucus forms

(A)   Vast majority of cases occur in children, most present between 3 and 6 years old and are worse during the winter

(Sy)   Deafness. Less commonly speech and language delay, otalgia and recurrent infections

(Si)   Dull, retracted tympanic membrane

(Ix)   Audiogram and tympanogram (compliance falls with middle ear fluid). In adults, the post-nasal space should be visualized to exclude a tumour obstructing the Eustachian tube orifice, especially if unilateral

(Rx)   Grommet insertion (ventilation tubes) if spontaneous resolution does not occur. Adenoidectomy may also be performed if there are significant nasal symptoms

INFORMATION BOX: TYMPANOGRAM

A tympanogram is a specialist investigation used to look at the movement of the tympanic membrane when a blast of air hits it. A graph is produced of the movement – this can show decreased compliance in diseases such as glue ear where fluid prevents proper movement of the membrane (see Fig. 4.2)

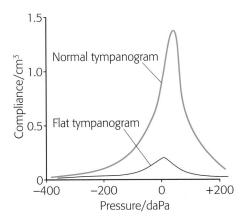

Figure 4.2 Normal and flat tympanogram, demonstrating reduced tympanic membrane compliance in otitis media with effusion

CHOLESTEATOMA

P Stratified squamous epithelial cells within the middle ear cleft, independently growing and causing local destruction often with superadded infection

A May be congenital or acquired

Sy Foul-smelling discharge; presentation is usually with recurrent ear infections. Associated progressive conductive hearing loss, vertigo, etc., arouses suspicion

Si Otoscopy reveals congenital cholesteatoma – pearly white mass, acquired (this is by far most common type) retracted/perforated TM, granulation tissue

Ix Audiogram and computed tomography (CT) scan

Rx Surgical excision

Cx Facial nerve (VII) palsy, hearing loss (conductive/sensory), vertigo, meningitis and cerebral abscess formation

Px Surgery is usually curative but long term follow up is required because of the risk of recurrence

MÉNIÈRE'S DISEASE

P Also known as cochleo-vestibular disorder that may be caused by endolymphatic hydrops (dilated labyrinth in inner ear)

A ♀ = ♂; occurs in early to late adulthood

Sy Episodes of severe disabling vertigo, which are closely associated with tinnitus, deafness and aural fullness (pressure in ear)

Si Vertigo, usually associated with vomiting; nystagmus during attacks only

Ix Audiogram may show low-frequency hearing loss after repeated attacks

Rx *Medical*: labyrinthine vasodilator e.g. betahistine, vestibular sedatives e.g. prochlorperazine for acute attacks only, intratympanic steroids/gentamicin
Surgery: ventilation tube insertion, vestibular nerve section, labyrinthectomy, endolymphatic sac decompression

PINNA HAEMATOMA

(P) Traumatic collection of blood between the cartilage and the perichondrium, from which it takes its blood supply

(A) Prompt treatment is needed to prevent permanent deformity ('cauliflower ear' – common in boxers)

(S) Swollen, painful ear with fluctuant collection

(Rx) Aseptic evacuation of the haematoma with subsequent compression to prevent recollection

OTALGIA

If the ears look normal consider referred pain from the following:

- *teeth* (auriculo-temporal branch of the trigeminal nerve)
- *herpes zoster*, i.e. Ramsay–Hunt syndrome (sensory branch of facial nerve), pain
- *throat*, e.g. tonsillitis or base of tongue (tympanic branch of glossopharyngeal)
- *larynx*, e.g. carcinoma (auricular branch of the vagus)
- *neck and cervical discs* (great auricular nerve [C2–3] and lesser occipital nerve [C2])

NOSE

EPISTAXIS

(P) Haemorrhage from the nose

Most recurrent epistaxis is from the anterior part of the septum (Little's area)

(A) Anterior bleeding is more common

Box 4.1 CAUSES OF EPISTAXIS

- *Local*:
  - idiopathic
  - trauma
  - tumours

- *Systemic*:
  - anticoagulants
  - bleeding disorders
  - hypertension
  - Osler–Weber–Rendu disease/ hereditary haemorrhagic telangiectasia (rare)

(S) Nose bleed (occasionally shock or haematemesis)

(Ix) Direct inspection of nose ± blood tests (haemoglobin, clotting screen, group and save)

(Rx) Cautery (with silver nitrate), nasal packing. For refractory bleeding surgery with artery ligation or radiological embolization may be required

(Cx) Hypotension, shock

SINUSITIS

(P) Inflammation and infection of the sinuses, maybe acute or chronic. Any one or all of the four pairs may be affected

(A) Usually secondary to viral upper respiratory tract infection (URTI). Maxillary sinusitis may be dental in origin, e.g. dental root abscess

Sy Facial pain over sinuses, nasal obstruction, preceding URTI

Si Fever, tenderness over sinuses, mucopus in middle meatus; NB swelling over the cheek is rare in maxillary sinusitis, swelling over the frontal sinus may be secondary to frontal osteomyelitis

Ix CT scan if planning surgery or if there is atypical presentation

Rx Antibiotics, nasal vasoconstrictors. In chronic disease, surgery involves operative enlargement of sinus drainage opening when maximal medical therapy has failed

Cx Orbital cellulitis or abscess, meningitis, intracranial abscess, osteomyelitis of the frontal bone ('Potts puffy tumour')

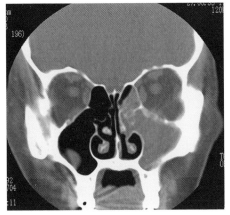

Figure 4.3 Coronal CT with polypoidal mucosal thickening in the right maxillary antrum and complete opacification on the left

RHINITIS

P Inflammation of the nasal mucosa

A Either allergic or non-allergic

Sy Rhinorrhoea, nasal obstruction, sneezing

Si Copious mucous, oedematous nasal mucosa, transverse nasal skin crease (in children who continuously rub their nose)

Ix Skin prick testing, radioallergosorbent test (RAST) (allergy testing)

Rx Avoid allergen, antihistamines (cetirizine/chlorphenamine), topical steroid spray, vasoconstrictor nasal drops (short term only)

NASAL POLYPS

P Abnormal lesions from the nasal mucosa or paranasal sinuses

A May be associated with asthma and aspirin sensitivity
If present in children, a diagnosis of cystic fibrosis must be considered

Sy Asymptomatic, nasal obstruction, rhinorrhoea, post-nasal drip, hyposmia

Si Pale fleshy polyps seen usually arising from the middle meatus (may need nasendoscopy). If large they may protrude out of the nose

Rx *Medical*: topical ± oral steroids
Surgery: endoscopic sinus surgery and polypectomy

THROAT

TONSILLITIS

P Inflammation of the tonsils (pharyngeal), part of Waldeyer's lymphoid tissue ring

A Causative organisms:

– *bacterial*: β-haemolytic *Streptococcus, S. pneumoniae, H. influenzae*
– *viral*: influenza, parainfluenza, adenovirus

(Sy)   Malaise and sore throat with odynophagia (pain on swallowing) with or without otalgia (ear ache)

(Si)   Fever, inflamed and enlarged tonsils with exudate, cervical lymphadenopathy
Differential diagnosis: glandular fever, caused by Epstein–Barr virus has similar presentation

(Ix)   Full blood count ± Monospot test (for glandular fever)

(Rx)   Analgesia, penicillin (treats bacterial infection and prevents superadded infection with viral tonsillitis), may require intravenous (i.v.) fluids if unable to swallow
Careful with amoxicillin – if patient has glandular fever the drug causes a widespread maculopapular rash

(Cx)   See Box 4.2

Box 4.2 COMPLICATIONS OF TONSILLITIS

- *General*:
  - septicaemia
  - rheumatic fever
  - post-streptococcal acute glomerulonephritis
- *Local*:
  - respiratory obstruction
  - abscess formation

(Px)   Consider tonsillectomy for recurrent attacks over several years

QUINSY (PERITONSILLAR ABSCESS)

(P)   Pus around the fibrous capsule of the tonsil, in the soft tissues
Sequela of tonsillitis

(Sy)   Preceding sore throat, increasing unilateral pain with otalgia, difficulty swallowing

(Si)   'Hot potato speech' (soft palate splinting), spitting out saliva, trismus ('lock-jaw') medialization of a tonsil, deviation of uvula away and soft palate swelling

(Rx)   Aspiration ± incision, i.v. antibiotics

(Px)   Tonsillectomy as above or if recurrent quinsy

EPIGLOTTITIS/SUPRAGLOTTITIS

(P)   Bacterial infection of the supraglottis (area above the vocal cords), which may predominantly affect the epiglottis

(A)   Epiglottitis usually affects children (3–4 years old) and supraglottitis usually adults
Usually *Haemophilus influenzae*, sometimes *Streptococcus*

(Sy)   Odynophagia (painful swallowing), dysphagia

(Si)   Fever, hoarse voice, drooling, stridor or *in extremis* with airway compromise

(Ix)   In adults visualization of the larynx with either a mirror or nasendoscope

(Rx)   Assess and secure airway as required, i.e. intubate or tracheostomy
NB if suspected in children **do not attempt to examine** (may precipitate airway obstruction), call for ENT surgeon, i.v. antibiotics (third generation cephalosporin) and dexamethasone

STRIDOR

(P) High-pitched sound made by turbulent flow through a partially obstructed airway
It is a sign, not a diagnosis

(A) *Congenital*: laryngomalacia, vocal cord palsy, tracheomalacia
Acquired: epiglottitis/supraglottitis, croup, foreign body, vocal cord palsy, trauma, allergy

(Si) Harsh, noisy breathing; cyanosis; collapse

(Ix) Lateral soft tissue neck, fibreoptic nasendoscopy

(Rx) Oxygen, nebulized adrenaline, dexamethasone
Conservative, i.e. observe, or secure airway, e.g. intubate/tracheostomy and treat cause

CHAPTER 5

Urology

Simon Bott and Ben Eddy

THE ACUTE SCROTUM

TESTICULAR TORSION

P *Intravaginal*: rotation within tunica vaginalis, usually peripubertal
Extravaginal: rotation on the spermatic cord, usually neonates

Sy Acute onset pain in the testis ± iliac fossa, nausea and vomiting, often previous similar episodes with spontaneous resolution.

Si Tender swollen testis, overlying scrotal skin may be red
Cremasteric reflex may be absent on affected side

Ix Doppler ultrasound scan may show ↓ arterial flow, but must not delay definitive treatment

Rx Urgent scrotal exploration, untwist testis
Both testes fixed; if the testis is infarcted orchidectomy and fixation of contralateral testis
Differential diagnosis: orchitis, torsion of hydatid of Morgagni, strangulated inguinal hernia, testis tumour

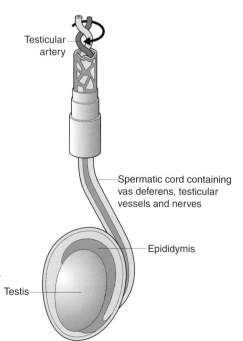

Testicular artery

Spermatic cord containing vas deferens, testicular vessels and nerves

Epididymis

Testis

Figure 5.1 Torsion of the testis results in vascular compromise and subsequent infarction (adapted with kind permission from Abrahams P, Craven J, Lumley J. *Illustrated Clinical Anatomy*, London: Hodder Education, 2005)

EPIDIDYMO-ORCHITIS

(A) Typically *Chlamydia* in sexually active young men and *E. coli* in older men,
May be viral orchitis – mumps, Coxsackie, infective mononucleosis, or bacterial
epididymo-orchitis – *Gonococcus*, TB

(Sy) Unilateral or bilateral testis pain, swelling, fever, frequency, dysuria

(Si) Tender swollen testis, overlying scrotal skin is red

(Ix) Doppler ultrasound scan (USS) may show ↑ arterial flow

(Rx) Once torsion has been excluded treatment is with antibiotics (ofloxacin)

TORSION OF THE HYDATID OF MORGAGNI

(P) Embryological remnant, which can twist and infarct

(A) Usually in pre-pubescent boys

(Sy) Similar to testicular torsion

(Si) May see 'blue-dot' sign through scrotal skin, non-tender testis

(Rx) Usually requires scrotal exploration to exclude torsion

THE PROSTATE

BENIGN PROSTATIC HYPERPLASIA (BPH)

(A) Affects men over 50 years, incidence ↑ with age

(S) *Voiding*: hesitancy, poor stream, incomplete bladder emptying, pis-en-deux (large
second voiding of urine immediately after finishing normal urination)
Storage: frequency, nocturia, urgency
Abdominal examination is usually unremarkable, may palpate an enlarged bladder
and *per rectum* (PR) examination will reveal an enlarged prostate

(Ix) Full blood count (FBC) – anaemia in renal failure, urea and electrolytes (U&E),
mid-stream urine (MSU)
Urinary flow rate and post-void residual urine volume
Consider prostate-specific antigen PSA (? carcinoma), urodynamic investigation

(Rx) See Box 5.1

Box 5.1 TREATMENT OPTIONS IN BENIGN PROSTATIC HYPERPLASIA

- *Conservative*:
  - avoid caffeinated and sugary drinks and evening fluids
- *Medical*:
  - α-blocker, e.g. tamsulosin or alfuzosin
  - 5α-reductase inhibitor, e.g. finasteride or dutasteride (prevents peripheral
    activation of testosterone in prostate)
- *Surgery*:
  - trans-urethral resection of the prostate (TURP), laser vaporization or
    enucleation

(Cx) Acute urinary retention, overflow incontinence, acute renal failure, bladder stones, recurrent UTI and haematuria

Acute retention requires urgent catheterization; record residual urine and whether creatinine is elevated, watch for a diuresis (urine output >200 mL/h), replace with normal saline as necessary

PROSTATE CANCER

(A) 40 per cent of males born in the Western world will develop prostate cancer

10 per cent will be diagnosed with it

3 per cent will die from the disease

Incidence ↓ in Asia, but approaches Western levels in Asian immigrants living in the US. ↑ incidence in African–American men

Risk factors include aging and positive family history (one first-degree relative 2× risk, two first-degree relatives 5× risk)

(Sy) Storage and voiding symptoms (see BPH), haematuria/spermia

Usually diagnosed by PSA screening in asymptomatic men

(Si) Hard nodular prostate on rectal exam

Occasional incidental diagnosis after TURP

Can also present with advanced disease – acute renal failure from ureteric obstruction, bone pain, pathological fracture, spinal cord compression, malaise, weight loss

(Ix) PSA (can monitor course of disease), FBC, U&E, Ca^{2+}, liver function tests (LFT)

Transrectal ultrasound-guided prostatic biopsy – provides Gleason grading

Magnetic resonance imaging (MRI) to assess if cancer is prostate confined or there is lymph node involvement

Nuclear medicine bone scan (? metastases)

INFORMATION BOX: TNM (TUMOUR, NODE, METASTASIS) (2000) STAGING OF PROSTATE CANCER

- *T1*: impalpable and not visible on imaging
- *T2*: tumour confined within the prostate
- *T3*: tumour extends outside the prostate capsule
- *T4*: tumour invades adjacent structures (bladder, pelvic wall, levator ani)

Box 5.2 TREATMENT OPTIONS IN PROSTATE CANCER

- *Localized disease* (prostate confined):
  - active surveillance: monitor PSA and treat if PSA rises or cancer upgraded on repeat biopsy
  - radiotherapy: external beam or brachytherapy (^{125}Iodine seed implantation)
  - surgery: laparoscopic, robotic or open radical prostatectomy
- *Advanced disease*:
  - medical: hormonal manipulation with gonadotrophin-releasing hormone (GnRH) agonist (goserelin, leuprorelin, triptorelin), antagonists (degarelix) or testosterone anatagonists or testosterone antagonist (flutamide, bicalutamide)
  - surgery: castration
  - radiotherapy: treat painful bone metastases

PROSTATITIS

P Complex of symptoms and aetiologies, 50 per cent of men will experience symptoms during lifetime.
– *category 1*: acute infection of the prostate (*E. coli, Pseudomonas, Klebsiella*)
– *category 2*: chronic infection of the prostate (*E. coli, Pseudomonas, Klebsiella*)
– *category 3*: chronic pelvic pain syndrome (without infection but with or without inflammation)
– *category 4*: asymptomatic inflammatory prostatitis (incidental finding) after TURP/prostate biopsy

Sy Pelvic, urethral, perineal or rectal pain, frequency, urgency. If category 1, there may be life-threatening septicaemia and urinary retention

Si PR may reveal exquisitely tender, boggy prostate

Ix Pyuria on MSU. Diagnosis confirmed by prostatic massage and microscopy and culture of prostatic secretions

Rx 3–4 weeks of fluoroquinolone (ciprofloxacin/ofloxacin) treatment, or TURP if abscess. Retention should be treated with suprapubic catheterization
Category 3: notoriously difficult to treat – may get response with α-blocker, non-steroidal anti-inflammatory drugs (NSAIDs), long-term antibiotics, diazepam, prostatic massage, warm baths, avoiding caffeine, alcohol and spicy food, reassurance that it is not life-threatening
Category 4: needs no treatment

HAEMATURIA

BLADDER CANCER

A 12 000 new cases per annum in UK, ♂:♀ 3:1
Risk factors include smoking and exposure to aromatic amines (industries include clothing dyes, printing, petrochemical and aluminium smelting)
Mean age at diagnosis is 65 years

P Latency period after exposure can be up to 20 years
90 per cent are transitional cell carcinoma (TCC)
80 per cent present with superficial disease, 20 per cent have invasive disease
Small proportion are squamous cell carcinoma (risk factors include schistosomiasis, chronic infection, long-term catheterization)

Sy Haematuria most common presenting symptom
Macroscopic haematuria has 25 per cent risk of TCC
Microscopic haematuria has 5 per cent risk of TCC
Can also present with recurrent UTIs and storage symptoms (frequency, urgency)

Ix *Endoscopy*: flexible cystoscopy is gold standard
Imaging: CT urography, USS or IVU are used to look for upper tract disease
Computed tomography is also useful for extravesical spread
Pathology: Urine cytology useful in high-grade disease

INFORMATION BOX: TNM STAGING OF BLADDER CANCER

Superficial disease
- *Ta*: non-invasive papillary
- *Tis*: carcinoma *in situ*
- *T1*: tumour invades lamina propria

Invasive disease
- *T2*: tumour invades muscle
- *T3*: tumour extends outside bladder
- *T4*: tumour invades adjacent organs

(Rx) *Superficial disease*:
  – endoscopic resection, examination under anaesthesia (EUA) and intravesical chemotherapy to reduce recurrence
  – patients need regular surveillance cystoscopies
  Invasive disease:
  – radical cystectomy (50 per cent 5-year survival) or radical radiotherapy (40 per cent 5-year survival)
  – prognosis is related to stage of initial disease

(Px) Overall mortality of 23 per cent for all stages and grades of disease

URINARY STONE DISEASE (UROLITHIASIS)

(A) Increasing incidence over last 50 years
Prevalence of 2 per cent, lifetime risk of 1 in 8 ♂:♀ 3:1
Most common in 4th and 5th decade, 10 per cent bilateral
High incidence in USA, UK and Scandinavia, low incidence in Africa and South America

---

Box 5.3 CAUSES OF RENAL STONES

- Idiopathic
- Infection
- Obstruction
- Prolonged immobilization
- Hot climate
- Hyperparathyroidism
- Oral calcium supplements
- Congenital abnormalities (i.e. horseshoe kidney and duplex systems)
- Genetic (positive family history in 25 per cent)
- Sedentary occupation

(P) *Stone type*:
  – 90 per cent are calcium based therefore are radio-opaque
  – urate stones (5 per cent) are radiolucent, so will not show up on abdominal X-ray

(Sy) Severe loin pain (10/10 intensity). Pain radiating to the iliac fossa, testis, penile tip or labia suggests a mid or distal ureteric stone
  Differential diagnosis: appendicitis, abdominal aortic aneurysm (AAA), biliary colic, diverticulitis, torted ovarian cyst or torted testis

Ⓘⓧ *Urinalysis*: 97 per cent will have microscopic haematuria, if absent then a stone is
    unlikely
    Bloods : FBC, U&E, Ca^{2+}, PO_4^{3-}, urate
    Imaging:
    – CT KUB is the gold standard,
      but many units still use IVU.
      Almost all stones are visible on
      CT, the kidney PC system and
      ureter may be full down to the
      stone, stranding around the
      kidney may be evident. On an
      IVU, look for enhanced
      nephrogram, delayed excretion,
      hydronephrosis, hydroureter
      and standing column
    – common sites of obstruction
      include the pelvic–ureteric
      junction (PUJ), pelvic brim
      and vesico–ureteric junction
      (VUJ)

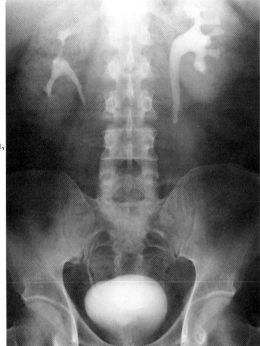

Figure 5.2 IVU showing obstruction of
the left kidney from a ureteric calculus

Ⓡⓧ Analgesia, NSAIDs/opiates
    Small stones <6 mm will usually pass spontaneously (80 per cent),
    Larger stones or complete obstruction – ureteric stent
    Emergency percutaneous nephrostomy if septic and obstructed
    Ureteric stones can be treated with ureteroscopy and stone fragmentation (laser)
    Small (<2 cm) renal stones managed with extracorporeal shockwave lithotripsy
    (ESWL)
    Large (>2 cm) renal stones managed by percutaneous nephrolithotomy
Ⓟⓧ 50 per cent will recur within 10 years

THE KIDNEY

RENAL TUMOURS

Ⓐ 3 per cent of all adult cancers worldwide
    ♂:♀ 2:1
    Average age at diagnosis 70 years
    High incidence in the West, low incidence in Asian countries, cause unknown
    Risk factors include smoking, obesity and chronic renal disease needing dialysis

P Majority are adenocarcinomas, known as renal cell carcinoma (RCC)

Familial variant of RCC known as von Hippel–Lindau disease

S Haematuria seen in 40 per cent

Classic triad of loin pain, haematuria, palpable mass rarely occurs (<10 per cent), and usually indicates advanced disease

Anaemia, polycythaemia, hypercalcaemia, hypertension, malaise, fever or unexplained weight loss

60 per cent detected incidentally as a result of increased use of imaging techniques

Cx Local disease can spread to renal vein, inferior vena cava (IVC) or surrounding structures (e.g. adrenal)

Metastatic disease commonly to bones, lung (cannon ball lesions) and lymph nodes

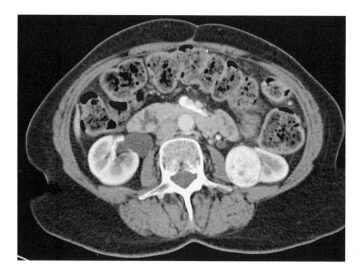

Figure 5.3 Multiple lung metastases secondary to renal carcinoma

Ix USS more sensitive than IVU for renal lesions

CT is the gold standard for imaging and staging local and metastatic disease

Bone scan if symptomatic or raised alkaline phosphatase (ALP)

INFORMATION BOX: TNM STAGING OF RENAL TUMOURS

- *T1*: tumour <7 cm confined to the kidney
- *T2*: tumour >7 cm confined to the kidney
- *T3*: extends beyond the kidney, i.e. renal vein, IVC or adrenal gland
- *T4*: extends beyond Gerota's fascia (connective tissue capsule of the kidney)

Rx Laparoscopic or open radical nephrectomy is the treatment of choice

Surgery for metastatic disease in selected cases

Tumours are chemo- and radio-insensitive so these therapies have limited role, immunotherapy (interferon/interleukins) or tyrosine kinase inhibitors for selected metastatic cases

Px 90 per cent 5-year survival for T1 disease

0–13 per cent 5-year survival for metastatic disease

COMMON PRESENTATIONS

HAEMATURIA

A Very common problem, may be a sign of serious underlying disease

10 per cent of urology referrals

Overall prevalence 5 per cent, up to 20 per cent in those aged over 60 years

P See Fig. 5.4

S Microscopic or macroscopic haematuria

Painful haematuria suggests infection

Pain at start of stream suggests prostatic or urethral origin

Loin pain suggests renal origin

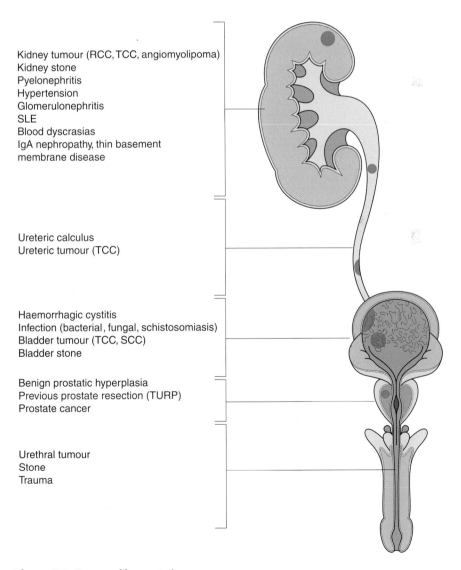

Kidney tumour (RCC, TCC, angiomyolipoma)
Kidney stone
Pyelonephritis
Hypertension
Glomerulonephritis
SLE
Blood dyscrasias
IgA nephropathy, thin basement
membrane disease

Ureteric calculus
Ureteric tumour (TCC)

Haemorrhagic cystitis
Infection (bacterial, fungal, schistosomiasis)
Bladder tumour (TCC, SCC)
Bladder stone

Benign prostatic hyperplasia
Previous prostate resection (TURP)
Prostate cancer

Urethral tumour
Stone
Trauma

Figure 5.4 Causes of haematuria

Ix *Microscopic* (confirmed on two freshly voided urines without infection):
- if aged over 40 years, will need MSU/urine cytology/U&E/PSA (prostate-specific antigen)/IVU (or kidneys, ureters and bladder (KUB) X-ray and USS) and flexible cystoscopy
- investigate if under 40 years if there are risk factors in history, i.e. smoking
- consider renal referral if there is evidence of casts, dysmorphic cells, proteinuria, hypertension or an elevated creatinine

Macroscopic (visible to the naked eye):
- all patients should be investigated
- MSU/urine cytology/U&E/PSA/CT urogram and flexible cystoscopy
- if all normal, probably prostatic in origin, however if persistent, consider magnetic resonance imaging (MRI) or renal angiogram as vascular malformations are rare causes
- novel markers for bladder cancer like NMP-22
- patients may need admission for bladder washouts/transfusion or general anaesthetic cystoscopy and washout in severe cases

URINARY TRACT INFECTION

A Very common health problem
Usually as a result of bacterial ascent along urethra
More common in women, due to shorter urethra, moist environment and proximity to anus

Box 5.4 PREDISPOSING FACTORS TO URINARY TRACT INFECTION
• Sexual activity
• Stones
• Foreign bodies (e.g. catheters)
• Congenital abnormalities (e.g. duplex system, horseshoe kidney, PUJ obstruction)
• Bladder outflow obstruction from BPH or strictures
• Other diseases including TCC or fistulae from adjacent organs

P Common organisms include *E. coli*, *Proteus* spp, *Pseudomonas* spp, *Klebsiella* and *Enterococcus*

S Can be asymptomatic
Cystitis: frequency, urgency, dysuria and suprapubic pain, fever is unusual
Pyelonephritis: loin pain, nausea, fever (temp >38°C), rigors and a leucocytosis

Ix Investigate all men, recurrent infections, children and infections in pregnancy
Urinalysis: leucocytes and nitrites indicate infection
MSU:
- microscopy and culture should be used to confirm infection prior to starting antibiotics
- $>10^3$ colony-forming units (CFUs) in uncomplicated and $>10^5$ CFUs in complicated UTI is diagnostic

Imaging:
- KUB X-ray to rule out stone disease
- renal USS to identify reflux and renal scarring

– consider DMSA (nuclear medicine scan) if scarring seen

Endoscopy: cystoscopy rarely useful in young patients unless there are other risk factors, e.g. haematuria

Rx Conservative measures first, increase fluid intake, hygiene advice, double voiding, emptying bladder after intercourse, cranberry juice

Asymptomatic UTI: needs no treatment (except in pregnancy)

Uncomplicated UTI: 3-day course of antibiotics usually adequate

Recurrent infections: consider prophylactic antibiotics, rotated 3 monthly

Pyelonephritis: needs 2 week course (exclude other causes first)

Antibiotics:
– first-line trimethoprim or amoxicillin (high resistance rates in hospitals)
– second-line consider a quinolone (ciprofloxacin) or cephalosporin (cefalexin)
  – obtain sensitivities before starting treatment if possible

IMPOTENCE

A Common problem, increasing incidence with age

Wide variety of causes (see Box 5.5)

Box 5.5 CAUSES OF IMPOTENCE

- *Neurological*: autonomic neuropathy (usually secondary to diabetes), multiple sclerosis and spinal injuries
- *Vascular*: pelvic/aorto-iliac disease
- *Iatrogenic*: commonly α- and β-blockers, psychotropic agents
- *Alcohol abuse*
- *Psychological*: depression
- *Endocrine*: hyperprolactinaemia, hypo/hyperthyroidism, Cushing's syndrome, androgen deficiency

---

Si Loss of libido is a sign of androgen deficiency and hyperprolactinaemia

Spontaneous morning erections with impotence are suggestive of psychogenic disease

Rx Treat underlying disease if possible

Phosphodiesterase inhibitors (sildenafil, vardenafil and tadalafil) improve penile blood flow via nitric oxide

Testosterone treatment if there is proven hypogonadism

Ophthalmology

Jagdeep Singh Gandhi

In finals in ophthalmology, examiners are fond of only a few subjects such as diabetic and hypertensive retinopathy, the appearances of the optic disc, and III, IV and VI nerve palsies.

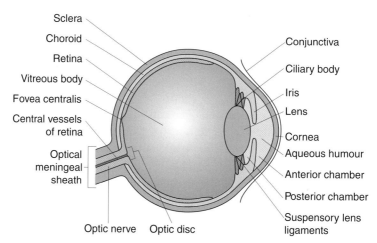

Figure 6.1 Side view of the eye (adapted with kind permission from Abrahams P, Craven J, Lumley J, *Illustrated Clinical Anatomy*, London: Hodder Education, 2005)

THE RED EYE

CONJUNCTIVITIS

P Inflammation of the conjunctiva

A *Infections*:
  - viral (most cases, e.g. adenovirus, herpes simplex),
  - bacterial (e.g. *Staphylococcus, Streptococcus*), *Chlamydia* (in young sexually active patients)

  Allergic: commonly seasonal

  Toxins: chemical splash, chlorine

  Radiation: direct irritation of conjunctival tissue

  Trauma: blinking of very dry eyes

Sy Uncomfortable (typically **not** painful) eye, vision typically normal

Si Redness, sticky discharge, swollen eyelids: follicles (typically in infection) or papillae (typically in allergy), seen as lumps when lid is everted

Ix Usually a self-limiting condition. Conjunctival swabs and viral cultures if persistent, or very severe

Rx Chloramphenicol gives broad-spectrum, bacteriostatic cover. Frequently, ocular lubricants ('artificial tears') alone are adequate and provide symptomatic relief

CORNEAL ULCER

A *Infections*: viral (herpes simplex: 'dendritic' ulcer), bacterial (*Staphylococcus, Streptococcus*), rarely fungal

  Cold sores (herpes simplex virus [HSV]), contact lens wear, lid margin disease (blepharitis)

Sy Pain, photophobia, blurred vision, sensation of foreign body

Si Red eye, corneal opacity, corneal stain with fluorescein, hypopyon (sediment of white cells in the anterior chamber)

Ix If the ulcer is severe or persistent then scrape samples are taken from the cornea for microscopy, culture and sensitivities (MC&S) analysis

Rx *Herpes simplex infections*: aciclovir ointment

  Bacterial keratitis: topical antibiotics

  Topical steroids added only when microbiology is known or there is clinical improvement

IRITIS

P Inflammation of the iris is a common ophthalmic presentation

A Most cases are idiopathic (>95 per cent)

  Remainder are associated with systemic conditions (human leucocyte antigen [HLA]-B27, ankylosing spondylitis, sarcoid, TB, etc.), or an intrinsic eye problem (e.g. corneal ulcer, retinal detachment, etc.)

Sy Pain, photophobia, blurred vision

Si Redness often around the cornea, cells in the anterior chamber, pupil stuck to lens in parts, clumps of cells stuck to inner surface of cornea, ↑ or ↓ intraocular pressure

Ix Screening tests for systemic conditions if iritis is recurrent, severe or bilateral

Rx Topical steroid, cycloplegic/mydriatic (dilating) drops (e.g. cyclopentolate, atropine)

EPISCLERITIS

(P) Usually a self-limiting inflammation of the connective tissue layer overlying the sclera

(A) Most cases idiopathic
Some associated with dry eyes, contact lens wear, rarely rheumatological disease

(Sy) Sore, irritable eye, foreign body sensation

(Si) Localized redness

(Rx) Topical steroid/lubricants given if symptomatic

SCLERITIS

(P) Severe inflammation of the sclera that can potentially result in necrosis and perforation in some cases

(A) Frequently associated with rheumatological disease and vasculitides

(Sy) Deep, boring, severe pain

(Si) Exquisite tenderness

(Ix) Rheumatological and vasculitic screen (e.g. rheumatoid factor [RhF], inflammatory markers, full blood count (FBC), antineutrophil cytoplasmic antibodies [ANCA])

(Rx) Intensive topical/local steroid, systemic non-steroidal anti-inflammatory drugs (NSAIDs) and steroids

ACUTE ANGLE-CLOSURE GLAUCOMA

(A) Important cause of a painful red eye in the older (50+ years) patient

(P) Affected eyes have an anatomical predisposition: shallow anterior chamber

(Sy) Intermittent eye pain, headache, haloes (corneal oedema), blurred vision, severe pain, nausea and vomiting (during acute angle-closure)

(Si) Raised intraocular pressure, red eye, mid-dilated oval pupil, shallow anterior chamber, corneal oedema, other eye also has shallow anterior chamber

(Ix) Gonioscopy (special lens examination) shows an occluded iridocorneal angle in the affected eye and an at-risk configuration in the other eye's angle

(Rx) *Medical*: aimed at lower intraocular pressure with systemic and topical antiglaucoma drugs, e.g. mannitol, pilocarpine
Surgical: peripheral laser iridotomy done to prevent further attack of angle-closure

AGE-RELATED MACULAR DEGENERATION

(A) A common cause of central visual loss in older (50+ years) patients
The central retina (or macula) undergoes degenerative change
'Dry' form of the disease: deposition of particulate debris (drusen) and pigmentary disturbance in the macula
'Wet' form of the disease: abnormal, leaky new vessels grow in the degenerative macula

(Sy) Blurring of central vision or a distortion of straight-edges occurs when abnormal new vessels grow at the macula

(Si) Haemorrhage, lipid exudation and thickened tissue at the macula

(Ix) Fundus angiography and optical coherence tomography to delineate the neovascular complex

(Rx) Injection of growth-inhibitor drugs into the eye (intravitreal therapy) which suppress the neovascular process

DIABETIC RETINOPATHY

(A) Long-standing diabetes, related to poor glycaemic control

(P) Basic problem is damage to the blood–retina barrier

This damage causes occlusion or leakage in the retinal circulation

Diabetic retinopathy consists of a spectrum of lesions

Box 6.1 CLASSIFICATION OF DIABETIC RETINOPATHY

Background retinopathy:
- **H**aemorrhage:
  - leakage of blood into the retina
  - dot, blot, flame-shaped haemorrhages
- **O**edema:
  - leakage of fluid (transudate)
  - diabetic macular oedema can occur even in background disease
- **M**icroaneurysms:
  - outpouchings of venous end of capillaries
  - earliest sign of retinopathy, found in the central macula
- **E**xudates:
  - leakage of lipid
  - yellowish deposits, usually in the macula

Pre-proliferative retinopathy
- *Cotton wool spot*:
  - with blockage of fine retinal capillaries (axoplasmic) flow is slowed, producing a feathery whitish area called a 'cotton wool spot' – this represents a focal infarct
- *Vein abnormalities*:
  - characterize an ischaemic retina
  - venous looping, beading and engorgement can be seen

Proliferative retinopathy
- New vessel growth from the retina
- New vessel growth from the optic disc
- New vessel growth from the iris (rubeosis)

Advanced retinopathy
- Scar tissue is laid down inside the eye
- Tractional retinal detachment (scar tissue associated with neovascular processes pulls on the retina)
- Retinal gliosis (scarring)
- Vitreous haemorrhage

(Sy) Often asymptomatic, in later stages visual field loss

(Ix) Fundoscopy, retinal photography

(Rx) *Medical*: optimize glycaemic control

Laser photocoagulation: can prevent progression from proliferative retinopathy

HYPERTENSIVE RETINOPATHY

(P) In its simplest form, the classical account of hypertensive retinopathy (Keith–Wagener–Barker, see Box 6.2) describes 4 grades

---

Box 6.2 KEITH–WAGENER–BARKER CLASSIFICATION OF HYPERTENSIVE RETINOPATHY

- *Grade I*: arteriolar narrowing
- *Grade II*: arteriovenous nipping
- *Grade III*: flame-shaped haemorrhages
- *Grade IV*: optic disc swelling + macular oedema

(Rx) Blood pressure control

(Cx) Irreversible visual impairment or damage to the optic nerve or macula

CATARACT

(P) Opacification of the crystalline lens

(A) May be congenital (e.g. maternal rubella) or acquired (e.g. trauma)
Risk factors include ↑ age, diabetes mellitus, steroid therapy, trauma, chronic uveitis

(Sy) Blurred vision, haloes, glare

(Si) Loss of red reflex, brownness in the lens under slit lamp examination, a white pupil if the cataract is advanced

(Rx) Commonest operation in ophthalmology
Operation performed when vision affects activities of daily living for a given patient
Two main techniques are phacoemulsification (see Information Box) and occasionally extracapsular extraction

---

INFORMATION BOX: PHACOEMULSIFICATION

In 'phaco', the cataract is divided into portions by an ultrasound cutter and the diseased lens removed. Then an intraocular lens implant is placed within the eye.
A small incision is used so stitches are not routinely necessary. The operation is usually done under local anaesthetic and patients go home the same day.
See Fig. 6.2

With extracapsular surgery, a large corneal incision is made and the lens is removed in one piece

The wound is stitched and a lens implant placed into the eye

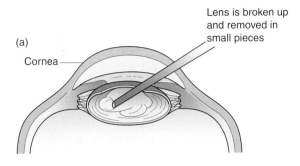

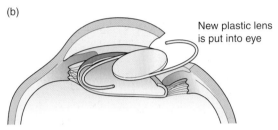

Figure 6.2 (a) Phacoemulsification; (b) posterior chamber lens implantation (copyright © 2001 McKesson Health Solutions LLC. Used with permission of the University of Michigan Health System, April 2006)

NERVE PALSIES

Six muscles are found around the eye.

These are the lateral rectus (*ab*duction), medial rectus (*ad*duction), superior rectus (elevation), inferior rectus (depression), superior oblique (depression combined with adduction, intortion) and inferior oblique (elevation combined with adduction, extortion).

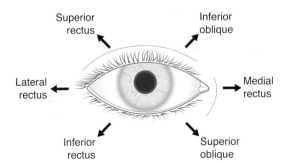

Figure 6.3 The muscles of eye movement (right eye illustrated)

All muscles are innervated by the III nerve, except the lateral rectus (VI nerve) and superior oblique (IV nerve): LR6 SO4 is the time-honoured mnemonic.

THIRD NERVE PALSY

A Cardiovascular risk factors (hypertension, diabetes, dyslipidaemia, smoking), ↑intracranial pressure, vasculitis, demyelination

Si The eye is ptotic and in a 'down and out' (depressed and abducted) position
This orientation follows from suppressed elevation (superior rectus and inferior oblique) and the unopposed pull of the lateral rectus (underactive medial rectus)
The upper lid is ptotic because the III nerve also drives the levator palpebrae superioris (elevates the eyelid)

FOURTH NERVE PALSY

A Head trauma, congenital IV palsy, cardiovascular risk factors

Si The affected eye is elevated relative to the fellow eye in primary position (the depressive effect of the superior oblique is missing)
The eye is unable to look 'down and in', a position which tests the primary direction of pull for the superior oblique

SIXTH NERVE PALSY

A Cardiovascular risk factors, ↑intracranial pressure (false localizing sign), demyelination, vasculitis

Si The eye cannot abduct beyond the midline

THE OPTIC DISC

It is customary to describe the optic disc in terms of cup, colour and contour (the 3 Cs).

CUP

- The cup refers to the bowl-shaped depression in the centre of the disc.
- There is anatomical and pathological variation in the size of the cup.
- In advanced disc swelling, the cup disappears because of the gross swelling of the neuroretinal rim.
- In advanced glaucoma, the cup is enlarged because the neuroretinal rim is destroyed.

COLOUR

- The colour of the disc is usually a pink–red, with the cup being a whitish area in the centre.
- Many conditions can produce pallor of the optic disc.
- These include a space-occupying intracranial lesion, previous optic neuritis, B_{12}/folate deficiency, glaucoma, infarction of the optic disc.

CONTOUR

- The contour refers to the margin of the disc.
- The normal disc has pulsating vessels on the disc (the retinal veins, to which pressure waves in the eye are transmitted).
- Venous pulsation is abolished in the swollen disc (however note that in 20 per cent

of the population there is no detectable physiological venous pulsation).

- The margin can become indistinct in the early stages of disc swelling (especially nasally).
- With advanced disc swelling, the margin of the disc can become blurred.
- With establishment of disc swelling, it is seen that the plane of the optic disc is raised compared to the surrounding retina, an important sign that confirms swelling.

Box 6.3 CAUSES OF OPTIC DISC SWELLING

- *Local*:
  - optic neuritis
  - optic disc vasculitis (e.g. giant cell arteritis)
  - disc infarction
- *Systemic*:
  - intracranial space-occupying lesion
  - severe hypertension
  - leukaemic cell infiltration
  - metastases

OPTIC DISC ATROPHY

P Loss of fibres within the optic nerve

A *Local*: advanced glaucoma, intracranial space-occupying lesion (e.g. pituitary tumour), optic disc infarction (non-arteritic anterior ischaemic optic atrophy)
Systemic: drugs, B_{12}/folate deficiency, tobacco, alcohol

Sy Blurred vision, $\downarrow$ acuity, loss of colour vision

Si Pale optic disc

Rx Treatment of underlying cause if possible

OPTIC NEURITIS

P Inflammation of the optic nerve

A Common first presentation of multiple sclerosis, rarely infections

Si Loss of vision, eye pain, impairment of colour vision, swollen optic disc

Ix Magnetic resonance imaging (MRI)

Rx Treat underlying cause

Oncology

Kirstin Satherley

INTRODUCTION

P Malignancy = ability of a tumour to demonstrate local invasion, lymph node involvement and distant (metastatic) spread, usually via blood or lymphatics

A 300 000 new cases per annum of cancer in UK
  >1 in 3 people will be diagnosed with cancer in their lifetime
  1 in 4 people will die from cancer
  Prevalence ~3.3 per cent of population in UK (2 million people)

Px Survival rates are improving with earlier diagnosis and better treatment

Table 7.1 Incidence of cancers in the UK

Cancer	% Incidence in UK (2007)
Male	
Prostate	24 (36 101)
Lung	15 (22 355)
Colorectal	14 (21 014)
Bladder	5 (7284)
Non-Hodgkins lymphoma	4 (5881)
Female	
Breast	31 (45 695)
Colorectal	12 (17 594)
Lung	12 (17 118)
Uterus	5 (7536)
Ovary	5 (6719)

Adapted from Cancer Research UK. *Cancer in the UK, 2010*. London: Cancer Research UK, 2010

Table 7.2 Deaths from all cancer types in the UK

Cancer type	% of all deaths (male and female, 2008)
Lung	22
Colorectal	10
Breast	8
Prostate	6
Pancreas	5

Adapted from Cancer Research UK. *Cancer in the UK, 2010*. London: Cancer Research UK, 2010

AETIOLOGY AND MECHANISM OF DISEASE

- There is usually no single factor that leads to the development of a tumour in a particular patient – it is a combination of genetic risk factors and environmental influences
- *Environmental risk factors*: e.g. cigarette smoking (accounts for >25 per cent all cancers), UV light, alcohol, obesity, asbestos, hydrocarbons, aflatoxin, viruses (Epstein–Barr virus (EBV), hepatitis B virus (HBV), human papillomavirus (HPV), human T-cell lymphotropic virus type 1 (HTLV-1)
- *Genetic risk factors*: e.g. *BRCA1* and *2* genes for breast cancer. 'Oncogenes' account for an increased risk of certain cancers in 1st degree relatives
- *Hereditary conditions* that predispose to the development of malignancy, e.g. familial polyposis coli
- The combination of genetic/environmental factors leads to structural changes in the DNA molecule, which in turn leads to uncontrolled cell division and tumour growth

TREATMENT OPTIONS

- *Intention of treatment*:
  - curative
  - palliative (i.e. symptom control/prolong life but non-curative)
- *Modes of treatment*:
  - surgery
  - chemotherapy
  - radiotherapy (RT)
  - biological therapy
  - or a combination of above
- Factors affecting choice of treatment: tumour stage (often TNM – tumour, node metastases), performance status, co-morbidity, age, patient preference
- Patients should be discussed at a multidisciplinary team (MDT) meeting (physician, surgeon, oncologist, pathologist, radiologist as minimum) to ensure that the correct and optimum treatment is delivered in each individual case

PRINCIPLES OF SURGERY

CURATIVE

- Surgery is the mainstay for curative treatment: if at operation the tumour can be removed with margins that are clear of microscopic disease
- Can be combined with 'neoadjuvant' or 'adjuvant' chemotherapy or RT:
  - neoadjuvant treatment is given *before* surgery to reduce tumour bulk and limit disease to enable surgery to be curative, or allow less complex surgery to be performed
  - adjuvant treatment is given *after* surgery to decrease the chance of tumour recurrence
- The presence of metastases no longer precludes curative surgery: disease can be firstly downstaged with chemotherapy and then metastasectomy attempted, e.g. limited liver resection

PALLIATIVE

- Surgery can also be a palliative measure, providing significant symptom relief and prolonging life expectancy without removing all the tumour, e.g. to relieve duodenal obstruction from carcinoma of the head of the pancreas or resection of solitary brain metastasis

PREVENTATIVE

- High-risk patients (familial adenomatous polyposis or BRCA1/BRCA2 positive patients) may opt to undergo surgery to remove the organ of interest (large bowel/ both breasts respectively) prior to cancer developing

HISTOLOGY

- Surgery allows sufficient tissue to be obtained for histological diagnosis (further tissue analysis determines further treatment options, e.g. oestrogen receptor status in breast cancer)
- Accurate staging, e.g. Dukes' staging of bowel cancer, lymph node involvement
- Immediate histological examination intra-operatively can inform the surgeon if enough tissue has been resected

NON-SURGICAL INTERVENTION

CHEMOTHERAPY

PRINCIPLES OF CHEMOTHERAPY

- Chemotherapy targets and damages any rapidly dividing cells – hence destroying malignant cells preferentially
- Non-malignant cells that rapidly divide are also affected, which partly accounts for the toxic side-effects of chemotherapy (e.g. hair follicles, gastrointestinal [GI] tract mucosa, bone marrow)
- Normal cell cycle: allows increased number, growth, replacement and repair of cells
- Chromosomes contain DNA and have a regulatory role in cell division
- Chemotherapy affects cell cycle at different points
- Cell regulation is a complex process: if DNA damage is detected then cell cycle is halted and repair of cell damage or apoptosis (cell suicide) occurs
- Drug resistance commonly develops – if tumour recurs after initial treatment then an alternative regime will be needed

CLASSIFICATION OF CHEMOTHERAPY AGENTS

- *Modes of administration*: intravenous (i.v.) bolus, i.v. infusion, oral, intrathecal, intravesical
- *Single versus combination regimes*: combination often has superior effect
- *Side effects*: e.g. nausea and vomiting, change in bowel habit, immunosuppression, skin reactions, alopecia, neuropathy

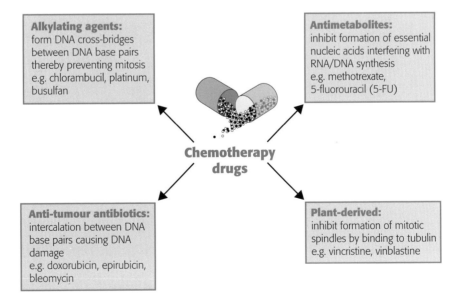

Figure 7.1 Chemotherapy drugs

RADIOTHERAPY

PRINCIPLES OF RADIOTHERAPY

- Radiation (X-rays or radioactivity) causes cell death or damage. RT directs radiation at the tumour, usually by means of an external beam carefully positioned outside the patient
- Alternatively, a radioactive source is placed close to the tumour in the patient (brachytherapy)
- RT can be used for curative and palliative cases. Curative cases tend to receive a course of treatment over weeks; palliative cases receive either a single treatment or a short course
- RT causes irreversible DNA damage directly or indirectly by generating toxic free radicals. Process is oxygen dependent and the most important factor in cell killing – hence need to keep haemoglobin (Hb) >10 g/dL during course of RT treatment
- Effects of RT are dependent on dose, tumour size, tumour growth rate, hypoxia, anaemia and performance status of patient including co-morbidity
- The use of CT and MRI to assist planning of the treatment field has led to dose escalation with less toxicity
- Side-effects are divided into early (<90 days) and late (90+ days)

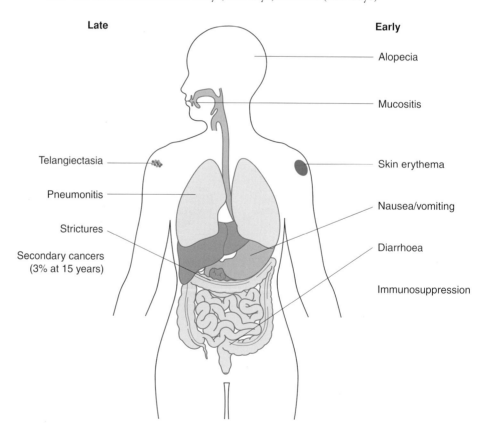

Figure 7.2 Complications of radiotherapy

OTHER TREATMENTS

- *Hormones*: hormone-sensitive or hormone-dependent cancers can be targeted by either reducing the production of the hormone in the body, e.g. goserelin (pituitary down-regulator) or by preventing the hormone reaching the cancer cells, e.g. tamoxifen (partial oestrogen receptor blocker)
- *Biological*: targeted use of the body's natural substances or drugs derived from these substances to either control the growth of cancer cells (e.g. the monoclonal antibody rituximab causing B-cell lysis in NHL, or herceptin which blocks HER2 receptors on breast or gastric cancer cells) or eliminate/reduce the side-effects caused by other cancer therapies (e.g. growth factors, G-CSF/GM-CSF, which stimulate the bone marrow to produce white bloods cells post chemotherapy)
- *Pharmacological*: e.g. bisphosphonates which work in areas of high osteoclastic activity, reducing osteolysis which may allow healing of some osteolytic metastases. This may result in a decrease in the rate of pathological fractures in bone metastases and reduce blood calcium levels

ONCOLOGICAL EMERGENCIES: DIAGNOSIS AND TREATMENT

NEUTROPENIC SEPSIS

(P) Occurs when neutrophil count $<1.0 \times 10^9$/L
Typically occurs 10–14 days after chemotherapy

(A) Common organisms: Gram +ve/−ve bacilli, fungal, atypical (e.g. *Pneumocystis carinii* pneumonia [PCP])

(S) Pyrexia >38°C, rigors, rash, inflammation, infective symptoms, hypotension

(Ix) Blood cultures (peripheral and central from *in situ* line)
Urine/sputum/stool/swab from i.v. line for microscopy, culture and sensitivity (MC&S)
Chest X-ray (CXR)

(Rx) Many patients with curative disease die as a result of delayed diagnosis of neutropenia – do not wait for full blood count (FBC) before giving antibiotics! Prompt detection and treatment are essential to prevent complications. Can be fatal
Start empirical broad-spectrum antibiotics early (according to hospital protocol)
Consider use of granulocyte cell-stimulating factors (G-CSF) to ↑ white cell count (WCC)
Close liaison with microbiologist essential
Barrier nursing

HYPERCALCAEMIA OF MALIGNANCY

(P) Calcium level often >3.5 mmol/L
Due to bone metastases or ectopic parathyroid hormone (PTH) secretion

(Sy) Malaise, nausea and vomiting, drowsiness, constipation

(Si) Polydipsia, polyuria, dehydration, fits, psychosis, confusion, coma

(Rx) *Hydration*: 3–4 L 0.9 per cent normal saline per 24 h
Bisphosphonates: pamidronate, zolendronic acid

Stop thiazide diuretics (cause hypercalcaemia), consider loop diuretics

Treat malignancy

Response expected within 3–5 days

SPINAL CORD COMPRESSION

(P)   70 per cent thoracic; 20 per cent lumbosacral; 10 per cent cervical

(S)   Back pain, weakness, upper motor neurone and sensory signs (sensory level may be identifiable), urinary retention, faecal incontinence

(Ix)   Plain X-rays of spine

Urgent magnetic resonance imaging (MRI) scan (definitive diagnosis)

(Rx)   Consider suitability for neurosurgical decompression

Dexamethasone 4–8mg qds

RT to involved area on urgent basis

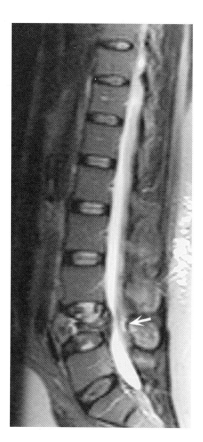

Figure 7.3 MRI (T$_2$W): vertebral deposit at L4 causing thecal compression

SUPERIOR VENA CAVA OBSTRUCTION

(P) 80 per cent lung cancer; 17 per cent lymphoma

(S) Distended thoracic/neck veins, dyspnoea, oedema, feeling of fullness in head, headache, ↑ jugular venous pressure (JVP), plethoric face, tachypnoea

(Ix) Sputum cytology
CXR
Computed tomography (CT) of the thorax

(Rx) Dexamethasone 4 mg qds
Chemotherapy (small cell carcinoma and lymphoma)
RT (squamous cell carcinoma)
Superior vena cava stent insertion (palliative measure only)

SYMPTOM CONTROL

● Common symptoms include pain, nausea and vomiting, constipation, diarrhoea, symptomatic ascites ± pleural effusions, anxiety and depression

PAIN

(A) Multifaceted: physical, psychological, social

(Rx) Assess pain carefully and treat underlying cause
Regular analgesia instead of prn is more effective
Analgesics are more powerful when given prophylactically
Various routes: oral, intramuscular, i.v., subcutaneous (s.c.), *per rectum*, epidural, i.v./s.c. infusion
Methods of providing pain relief (see World Health Organization pain ladder, Fig. 7.4):

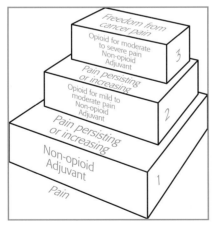

Figure 7.4 World Health Organization analgesic pain ladder:
● Step 1: non-opioid, e.g. aspirin, paracetamol, non-steroidal anti-inflammatory drugs
● Step 2: weak opioid, e.g. codeine, dihydrocodeine ± non-opioid
● Step 3: strong opioid, e.g. morphine ± non-opioid
● Adjuvants: antidepressants, steroids, anti-epileptic drugs
(Reproduced with kind permission from WHO)

– starting dose of strong opioids is dependent on previous analgesia used and hepatic and renal function
– remember there is no upper limit in opiate dose when treating neoplastic pain
Bone pain can be reduced by RT, orthopaedic fixation of pathological fractures, bisphosphonates
Role of pain team – can advise if patient is intolerant to opioid of choice, drug interactions, adjuvant treatment

NAUSEA AND VOMITING

- Often treatment of the underlying cause is sufficient, e.g. hypercalcaemia
- Anti-emetics include antihistamines, e.g. cyclizine, hyoscine, or dopamine antagonists, e.g. haloperidol
- Gastric stasis is best treated with peripheral dopamine antagonists, e.g. metoclopramide, domperidone
- Early chemotherapy-related nausea can be controlled with serotonin ($5\text{-}HT_3$) antagonists, e.g. ondansetron

CONSTIPATION

- Prevention in high-risk patients is the key
- Regular use of laxatives, e.g. bisacodyl, sodium docusate
- If patient is on regular opioids, then co-danthramer is the most effective and the dose is titrated against soft stools
- If the rectum is full, start with glycerin suppositories and consider enemas

DIARRHOEA

- Mainstay of management is rehydration and loperamide
- If infection is the cause, antibiotics may be commenced
- RT-related diarrhoea responds to loperamide and codeine phosphate

CARE OF THE TERMINALLY ILL PATIENT

- The dying phase is an important stage in a patient's illness and is often the stage which most affects the family and carers
- A holistic approach is essential – physical, psychological, social and spiritual needs must be addressed
- Symptom control is a priority of palliative care. Many of the common symptoms are described above, but they also include terminal agitation which is best treated with midazolam or haloperidol
- Medications are often administered to a terminally ill patient by means of a syringe driver which:
  - allows a continuous infusion of medication to be given subcutaneously over a 24 hour period
  - avoids the need for venous access and is suitable for the unconscious patient
  - often contains a 'cocktail' of medication, such as diamorphine, metoclopramide, hyoscine and midazolam
- Multidisciplinary team approach is essential – early involvement of specialist nurses and doctors
- Consider continuing care in the hospice or at home with Macmillan support

CARDIOPULMONARY RESUSCITATION STATUS

- Often a difficult subject for the patient, family and medical team. If a patient shows signs of deterioration and further medical treatment is likely to be unsuccessful then early discussion with the patient can help establish their wishes regarding resuscitation

- Some patients with metastatic disease still have a good prognosis in that they will have a life expectancy of many years (e.g. hormone/chemotherapy-responsive breast cancer or prostate cancer), and these patients may wish to be considered for resuscitation
- If there is an identifiable cause, e.g. septic shock secondary to neutropenic sepsis or cardiac arrhythmia secondary to chemotherapy, then resuscitation can be justified as these are often reversible conditions
- There is no right or wrong answer and each individual case is different
- Ultimately, the final decision regarding resuscitation status is made at consultant level, but this should obviously take into account the patient's wishes
- Any decision not to resuscitate should be clearly documented in the medical notes and conveyed to the nursing staff

Public health

Kinesh Patel

STATISTICS

BASIC DEFINITIONS

- *Prevalence*: the proportion of a population with a disease at any particular time, e.g. 13 in 100 children suffer from asthma
- *Incidence*: the number of new cases of a disease in a particular time period, e.g. 33 in 100 000 people are diagnosed with stomach cancer every year
- *Mortality*: the proportion of people who die from a disease, e.g. 40 per cent of people who are diagnosed with meningococcal septicaemia die
- *Standardized mortality ratio*: the rate of deaths in one population compared with national averages corrected for age, sex, social class, etc.
- *Relative risk*: the risk of developing disease for one population with an exposure compared with a population without the exposure, e.g. smokers are 20 times more likely to contract lung cancer than non-smokers
- *Number needed to treat (NNT)*: the number of people receiving a treatment for one person to derive a benefit, e.g. after myocardial infarction, 18 people need to take an angiotensin-converting enzyme (ACE) inhibitor to prevent one heart attack (NNT = 18)

TESTING

- No diagnostic test is 100 per cent perfect
- To gauge the accuracy of a test, there are several measures used to assess how reliable it is
- These are often expressed as mathematical formulae (see Table 8.1):

Table 8.1 Accuracy of tests

	Test positive	Test negative
Have disease	a (true positive)	b (false negative)
Do not have disease	c (false positive)	d (true negative)

- It is often easier to understand what each of the terms mean if the question they seek to answer is remembered (see Table 8.2)

Table 8.2 Definitions used in testing

Term	Question	Formula
Sensitivity	'If a group of people have a disease, what percentage of them will test positive?'	$\dfrac{a}{a+b}$
Specificity	'If a group of people do not have a disease, what percentage of them will test negative?'	$\dfrac{d}{c+d}$
Positive predictive value (PPV)	'If a person has a positive test result, what chance do they have of actually having the disease?'	$\dfrac{a}{a+c}$
Negative predictive value (NPV)	'If a person has a negative test result, what chance do they have of not having the disease?'	$\dfrac{d}{b+d}$

- Knowing the sensitivity and specificity of a test will influence the decision whether or not to perform it – a test with low sensitivity will not help confirm a diagnosis
- The best tests have sensitivities and specificities near 100 per cent
- The predictive values indicate the likelihood of a positive or negative screening test result meaning the presence or absence of the disease
- Knowing the predictive value will influence the view that an individual does or does not have the disease, once the test result is known

BIAS

- Bias is a systematic flaw with data collection, leading to results from the analysis of the data being incorrect
- Statistical analysis cannot be used to compensate for the effects of bias
- Whereas increasing the size of the study will decrease random error, this will not affect the level of bias
- The best way to avoid bias is effective study design, e.g. double-blind placebo-controlled randomized trial
- There are several types of bias:
  - *selection bias:* those included in a trial do not reflect a typical population, e.g. excluding those aged over 65 years from a study into ischaemic heart disease
  - *information bias:* wrongly assigning trial participants incorrect diagnoses/exposures

- *reporting bias:* cases with disease remember exposures better than those who are disease free
- *interviewer bias:* an interviewer may ask patients with disease more questions about exposures than those who are disease free
- *loss to follow-up:* if a significant proportion of trial participants drop out as time progresses, then the final data cannot be reliably interpreted
- *lead time bias:* earlier diagnosis of a condition results in an apparently longer survival time (see Fig. 8.1)
- *publication bias:* trials with positive results are much more likely to be published

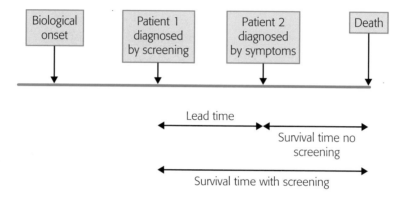

Figure 8.1 Lead time bias

SCREENING

The purpose of screening is to discover latent disease in apparently healthy individuals so that treatment can be offered to improve prognosis

---

Box 8.1 CRITERIA FOR SCREENING

- The condition screened for should be an important health problem
- The natural history of the disease should be well understood
- There should be a detectable pre-clinical stage with a long latent phase
- The pre-clinical stage must have a high prevalence in the target population
- There should be a test for the condition that is:
  - cheap
  - acceptable
  - reliable
  - easy to administer
- There should be a treatment for the disease at the preclinical stage that:
  - is effective
  - is sustainable
  - reduces morbidity and mortality

STUDIES

- There are many different ways of studying populations
- Generally prospective trials are more powerful than retrospective studies
- Randomization is a strategy to decrease the effect of bias on data
- Double-blinding (neither the doctor nor the patient know the treatment given) is another effective way to increase the validity of data
- The two major types of clinical study are case–control and cohort studies
- Case–control studies take a known case of the disease and then match one or more controls to that person to see what differences exist between the affected and unaffected groups
- Cohort studies take two separate groups and follow them

Table 8.3 Advantages and disadvantages of cohort and case–control studies

Type	Case–control study	Cohort study
Advantages	Quick/inexpensive	Valuable for rare exposures
	Easy to study diseases with long latent periods	Can reveal temporal relationship between exposure and disease
	Good for evaluation of rare diseases	Minimizes bias in exposure ascertainment
	Can examine multiple aetiological factors for a single disease	Allows direct incidence calculation
Disadvantages	Inefficient for evaluation of rare exposures	Inefficient for evaluation of rare diseases
	Cannot compute incidence rates in exposed and unexposed individuals	Prospective: expensive and time-consuming
	The temporal relationship between exposure and disease may be difficult to establish	Retrospective: availability of adequate records
	Problems with recall and selection bias	Losses to follow-up can affect results

EVIDENCE-BASED MEDICINE

- Modern medicine is now increasingly based on the principle that patient care should be based on evidence from high-quality trials
- There are difference qualities of evidence, in order of decreasing reliability:
  - meta-analysis (data from several high-quality trials analysed together)
  - multiple randomized control trials
  - single randomized control trial
  - non-randomized control trial
  - uncontrolled trial
  - retrospective studies (case–control, cross-sectional)
  - case series
  - case report
- For rarer conditions, generally there is less high-quality evidence available for clinical use

INFECTIOUS DISEASES

NOTIFIABLE DISEASES

- Some diseases have to be notified to the authorities when diagnosed so that outbreaks of disease can be contained and contacts traced
- It is the responsibility of the doctor to ensure that the local consultant in communicable disease control is notified of any of the diseases shown in Box 8.2

Box 8.2 NOTIFIABLE DISEASES

- Acute encephalitis
- Acute poliomyelitis
- Anthrax
- Cholera
- Diphtheria
- Dysentery
- Food poisoning
- Leptospirosis
- Malaria
- Measles
- Meningitis (meningococcal, pneumococcal, *Haemophilus influenzae*, viral, other)
- Meningococcal septicaemia (without meningitis)
- Mumps
- Ophthalmia neonatorum

- Paratyphoid fever
- Plague
- Rabies
- Relapsing fever
- Rubella
- Scarlet fever
- Smallpox
- Tetanus
- Tuberculosis
- Typhoid fever
- Typhus fever
- Viral haemorrhagic fever
- Viral hepatitis (hepatitis A, hepatitis B, hepatitis C, other)
- Whooping cough
- Yellow fever

Source: Health Protection Agency. Diseases notifiable (to Local Authority Proper Officers) under the Public Health (Infectious Diseases) Regulations 1988. www.phls. co.uk/infections/topics_az/noids/noidlist.htm

---

- The Public Health Laboratory Service aims to identify outbreaks of disease with these data and prevent further spread

VACCINATION

- Vaccination aims to protect individuals from disease by exposing them to an attenuated version of the pathogen

---

Box 8.3 DISEASES FOR WHICH VACCINES ARE CURRENTLY AVAILABLE

Anthrax	Pertussis
Diphtheria	Pneumococcus
Haemophilus influenzae type B	Rabies
Hepatitis A	Rubella
Hepatitis B	Smallpox
Influenza	TB (BCG)
Japanese B encephalitis	Tetanus
Measles	Tick-borne encephalitis
Meningococcus (A and C)	Typhoid
Mumps	Yellow fever

- High levels of population vaccination prevent the spread of disease by reducing the number of cases – so-called herd immunity
- For effective herd immunity, over 95 per cent of the population needs to be vaccinated
- Recent public concerns over the safety of vaccines has led to a general decrease in the level of herd immunity, with consequent increases in cases of diseases such as measles

Table 8.4 Routine childhood immunization schedule

	DTaP/Hib/ polio	Men C	MMR	dTaP/ polio	BCG	Td/polio
Birth					✓*	
2 months	✓	✓				
3 months	✓	✓				
4 months	✓	✓				
13 months			✓			
3–5 years			✓	✓		
13–18 years						✓

DTaP: diphtheria, tetanus, pertussis; Hib: *Haemophilus influenzae* type B; Men C: Meningococcus type C; MMR: mumps, measles, rubella; BCG: Bacille Calmette–Guérin (tuberculosis); *at-risk groups only

CHAPTER 9

Paediatrics

Sarita Depani

NORMAL PAEDIATRIC VALUES

Table 9.1 Normal ranges for heart rate and respiratory rate according to age

Age	Heart rate	Respiratory rate
<1 year	120–160	30–60
1–2 years	90–150	24–40
2–5 years	80–140	22–34
6–12 years	70–120	18–30
>12 years	60–100	12–16

FLUIDS

MAINTENANCE FLUIDS

Usually isotonic fluids, e.g. 0.9 per cent saline/5 per cent dextrose used with 1–2 mmol/kg K^+ (approx. 10 mmol KCl per 500 mL bag)

Table 9.2 Calculating paediatric maintenance fluids

Body weight	Fluid requirement per 24 hours
First 10 kg	100 mL/kg
Second 10 kg	50 mL/kg
Further kg	20 mL/kg

RESUSCITATION FLUIDS

0.9 per cent saline bolus:
- – 20 mL/kg, repeat as required
- – 10 mL/kg in trauma/diabetic ketoacidosis (DKA)

4.5 per cent human albumin: 20 mL/kg in severe sepsis (e.g. meningococcal disease)

Packed red blood cells (RBCs): 10–15 mL/kg in suspected blood loss

NEONATAL MEDICINE

HYPOXIC–ISCHAEMIC ENCEPHALOPATHY

(P) Neonatal brain injury secondary to prenatal, perinatal or postnatal asphyxia. 1–2/1000 deliveries

(A) Abnormal cardiotocograph (CTG), poor Apgar scores (see Table 9.3), metabolic acidosis (pH < 7.0)

Table 9.3 Apgar score: score out of 10 taken at 1, 5 and 10 mins

	Score 0	Score 1	Score 2
Appearance	Blue or pale all over	Blue extremities	Pink all over
Pulse rate	0	< 100/min	≥ 100/min
Grimace	No response to stimulation	Grimace/weak cry when stimulated	Cries/pulls away when stimulated
Activity	None	Some flexion of limbs	Flexed limbs that resist extension
Respiration	Absent breathing	Irregular breathing/ gasping	Regular breathing, strong cry

Score ≤3 at 10 mins indicator of poor outcome.

(S) *Mild*: irritable, increased tone and reflexes, staring eyes, poor feeding
Moderate: lethargy, reduced tone and reflexes, seizures
Severe: coma, reduced tone, absent reflexes, prolonged seizures, multi-organ failure

(Ix) Cerebral function monitor (CFM), electroencephalogram (EEG), magnetic resonance imaging (MRI) brain

(Rx) Respiratory and circulatory support, anticonvulsants, cooling

(Cx) Cerebral palsy, learning difficulties, epilepsy, hearing and visual impairment

(Px) *Mild*: majority have no sequelae

Moderate: 40 per cent serious long term complications, 15 per cent minor disability
Severe: 30 per cent mortality, 50 per cent severe disability, 10 per cent moderate disability

RESPIRATORY DISTRESS IN TERM INFANTS

(A) See Table 9.4

(S) Tachypnoea (respiration rate [RR] 60/min), grunting, intercostal/subcostal recession, tracheal tug, nasal flare, cyanosis

(Ix) Chest X-ray (CXR) (see Table 9.4); Echo if cardiac cause/persistent pulmonary hypertension of the newborn (PPHN) suspected

(Rx) Respiratory support: oxygen, continuous positive airway pressure (CPAP), invasive ventilation
Specific treatment, see Table 9.4

(Cx) Chronic lung disease

Table 9.4 Causes of respiratory distress in term neonates

Diagnosis	Pathology	Chest X-ray findings	Specific treatment
Meconium aspiration syndrome	Aspiration of meconium during delivery causing pneumonitis	Patchy infiltrates	Surfactant
Congenital pneumonia	Congenital infection of lungs	Focal consolidation	Antibiotics
Persistent pulmonary hypertension of the newborn (PPHN)	High pulmonary vascular pressure causing left–right shunting and poor oxygenation	Normal heart size and pulmonary oligaemia	Nitric oxide (pulmonary vasodilator)
Heart failure	Secondary to congenital heart disease (e.g. persistent ductus arteriosus [PDA])	Cardiomegaly and pulmonary oedema	Diuretics
Pneumothorax	May be spontaneous. Often iatrogenic – high-pressure ventilation/ continuous positive airway pressure (CPAP)	Hyperlucency with absent lung markings	Often resolve if small; chest drain if large/ symptomatic

continued ▶

Diagnosis	Pathology	Chest X-ray findings	Specific treatment
Diaphragmatic hernia	Herniation of abdominal contents into chest cavity through diaphragm leading to pulmonary hypoplasia	Bowel loops seen in chest (usually left sided) mediastinal deviation	Surgical repair
Transient tachypnoea of newborn	Delay in resorption of lung fluid, associated with caesarean section, resolves spontaneously	Fluid in horizontal fissure, 'wet lungs'	Resolves in a few days

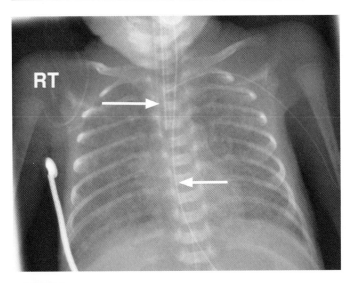

Figure 9.1 Ground glass appearance of lung fields in neonatal RDS. Note: endotracheal tube (bold arrow), and nasogastric tube (thin arrow)

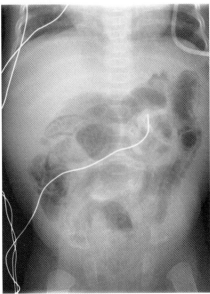

Figure 9.2 Intramural gas in a neonate with necrotizing enterocolitis

PREMATURITY

P Prematurity: 28–36 weeks

Extreme prematurity: 23–27 weeks

Increased morbidity and mortality with decreasing gestation. Care on neonatal unit usually required until expected due date

Cx Susceptible to respiratory distress syndrome (RDS), persistent ductus arteriosus (PDA), necrotizing enterocolitis (NEC), retinopathy of prematurity (ROP), intraventricular haemorrhage (IVH) (see below), hypoglycaemia, hypothermia and sepsis

Rx Require feeding support with high energy nasogastric/orogastric tube (NGT/OGT) feeds ± total parental nutrition (TPN)

Table 9.5 Complications of prematurity

Diagnosis	Pathology	Signs/symptoms	Treatment	Complications
Respiratory distress syndrome (hyaline membrane disease)	Lack of surfactant secreted by Type II pneumocytes	Respiratory distress Tachycardia Hypoxia Chest X-ray (CXR): 'ground glass' appearance, air bronchograms (see Figure 9.1)	Antenatal steroids Exogenous surfactant Respiratory support (invasive ventilation/ continuous positive airway pressure [CPAP]/oxygen)	Chronic lung disease (oxygen requirement at 28 days of life or ≥ corrected age of 36 weeks)
Patent ductus arteriosus	Failure of ductus arterious to close leading to left– right shunting, fluid overload and heart failure	Continuous murmur heard between clavicles Bounding pulses Wide pulse pressure	Medical: fluid restriction, ibuprofen/ indometacin Surgical: ligation of duct	Heart failure Failure to wean off respiratory support
Necrotizing enterocolitis	Ischaemia of gut wall and secondary infection of bowel. Risk factors: prematurity, milk feeding (higher risk with formula), sepsis, ibuprofen/ indometacin	Intolerance of feeds, distended abdomen, vomiting, *per rectum* bleeding Abdominal X-ray (AXR): distended bowel loops, bowel wall thickening, intramural air, perforation (see Figure 9.2)	Nil by mouth, total parental nutrition (TPN) antibiotics, surgery if severe or perforation: bowel resection ± stoma formation	Malabsorption Stricture formation 20 per cent mortality

continued ❯

Diagnosis	Pathology	Signs/symptoms	Treatment	Complications
Retinopathy of prematurity	Proliferation of blood vessels at junction of non-vascularized and vascularized retina. Risk factors: extreme prematurity, excessive oxygen therapy	Asymptomatic. At-risk infants require ophthalmology screening	Laser therapy for severe disease	Retinal detachment. Retinal fibrosis. Severe visual impairment in 1 per cent
Intraventricular haemorrhage	Haemorrhage of fragile blood vessels in germinal matrix secondary to hypoxia/respiratory distress syndrome (RDS)	Cranial ultrasound: bleed graded according to whether periventricular or spread into ventricles/parenchyma	Treatment of ventricular dilatation (cerebrospinal fluid [CSF] taps/shunt insertion)	Hydrocephalus. Cerebral palsy

NEONATAL SEPSIS

(A) Prolonged rupture of membranes (≥24 h), chorioamnionitis, maternal pyrexia/sepsis, maternal carriage of Group B *Streptococcus* (GBS), prematurity, nosocomial (e.g. indwelling central lines, poor hand hygiene)

Pathogens:
- GBS (50 per cent transmission rate from mother, 1 per cent of these develop clinical symptoms, two peaks of disease at 1–3 days and at 2–3 weeks, 10 per cent mortality)
- *E. coli*
- Chlamydia (conjunctivitis in first week, pneumonia at 4 weeks)
- Gonorrhoea (purulent conjunctivitis)
- Listeria
- *Herpes simplex virus* (HSV)
- Coagulase negative *Staphylococcus* (line infections)

(S) Respiratory distress, apnoea, temperature instability, poor feeding. Often non-specific

(Ix) Inflammatory markers (*C*-reactive protein [CRP], white blood cell [WBC]), blood culture, lumbar puncture, urine microscopy, culture and sensitivity (MC&S), CXR

(Rx) Maternal antibiotics when risk factors for sepsis present, broad-spectrum antibiotics (to cover GBS and Gram-negatives), strict hand washing and infection control measures on neonatal unit.

JAUNDICE

(P) Rapid haemolysis of RBCs following birth, reduced lifespan of neonatal RBCs, reduced bilirubin metabolism and breast feeding all cause physiological jaundice. Disorders causing jaundice include pathological haemolysis, infection and liver disease.

(A) *First 24 h:* Rhesus incompatibility, ABO incompatibility, glucose 6 phosphate dehydrogenase (G6PD) deficiency, hereditary spherocytosis, sepsis, bruising
Day 2–14: Physiological/breast milk, causes as above
≥2–3 weeks:
  – *Unconjugated:* physiological/breast milk, UTI, hypothyroidism, galactosaemia, causes as above
  – *Conjugated:* biliary atresia, neonatal hepatitis

(S) Yellow pigmentation of skin, sleepy and lethargic, poor feeding/weight gain (dehydration worsens jaundice), pale stool and dark urine in conjugated hyperbilirubinaemia, hepatomegaly in liver disease

(Ix) Split bilirubin, direct antigen (Coombs') test, full blood count (FBC), reticulocytes, blood film, G6PD assay, liver function tests (LFTs), inflammatory markers, urine MC&S, liver ultrasound scan (USS) (as indicated by history)

(Rx) Phototherapy (blue band of light spectrum converts unconjugated bilirubin into water soluble pigment)
Optimize hydration (top-up feeds, nasogastric feeding, i.v. fluids)
Exchange transfusion (if bilirubin rising rapidly despite phototherapy)
Prompt surgery for bilary atresia (within first 4 weeks)

(Cx) Kernicterus – unconjugated bilirubin accumulation in basal ganglia leading to choreoathetoid cerebral palsy and sensorineural hearing loss.

HYPOGLYCAEMIA

(P) Blood glucose level below 2.5 mmol/L

(A) Prematurity, small for gestational age (SGA), macrosomia, infants of diabetic mothers, sepsis, polycythaemia, metabolic, e.g. hyperinsulinism, galactosaemia, congenital adrenal hyperplasia

(S) Jitteriness, poor feeding, irritability, drowsiness, apnoea, seizures

(Ix) Blood glucose level; metabolic screen if persistent or severe hypoglycaemia

(Rx) Early and frequent milk feeds, i.v. 10 per cent dextrose

(Cx) Seizures, neurological impairment

(Px) Good if treated early; neurological disability if persistent

EXOMPHALOS/GASTROSCHISIS

(P) Congenital herniation of abdominal contents

(S) *Exomphalos:* Herniation through umbilicus. Bowel and viscera covered with membranous sac. Associated with other congenital abnormalities
Gastroschisis: Herniation through abdominal wall defect to right of umbilicus. Bowel not covered with membrane

(Rx) Cover abdomen with clingfilm as high risk of heat and fluid loss especially with gastroschisis. NGT, i.v. fluid replacement. Primary surgical closure if small defect; gradual reduction with silo if large.

OESOPHAGEAL ATRESIA

P Often associated with tracheo-oesophageal fistula.

S Polyhydramnios (fetus unable to swallow amniotic fluid), excessive oral secretions, aspiration and regurgitation when fed

Ix CXR: NGT curled up in oesophagus – unable to pass into stomach (see Figure 9.3)

Rx Surgical repair

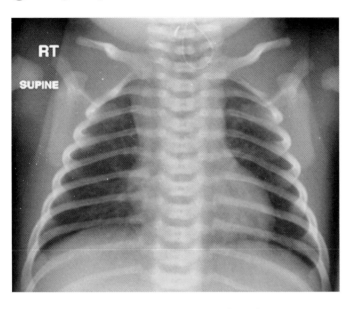

Figure 9.3 Curled nasogastric tube in oesophageal atresia

BIRTH INJURIES

A Large babies, instrumental/difficult delivery

Table 9.6 Common birth injuries

Pathology	Signs	Treatment
Erb's palsy (C5/C6 brachial plexus injury)	Asymmetrical Moro reflex (Limp arm, 'Waiter's tip' position)	Physiotherapy
Klumpe's palsy (C8/T1 brachial plexus injury)	Wrist/hand muscle weakness	Physiotherapy
Cephalhaematoma (Subperiosteal bleed)	Unilateral boggy swelling over skull	Resolve spontaneously
Subaponeurotic bleed	Diffuse boggy swelling over skull – can be significant blood loss	May require blood/platelet support

INFECTION

See the Infectious Diseases section of Chapter 1 (Medicine) for childhood infections: Epstein–Barr virus (EBV), HSV, chickenpox, mumps, measles, tuberculosis (TB)

FEVERISH CHILD

(A) Most common paediatric complaint. Difficulty distinguishing self-limiting viral infection from more serious bacterial infection in early stages.

Mild illnesses: Upper respiratory tract infection (URTI), mild gastroenteritis, non-specific viral infection

Significant illnesses: pneumonia, meningitis, encephalitis, meningococcal sepsis, urinary tract infection (UTI), septic arthritis, Kawasaki's disease

(S) See Table 9.7

(Ix) Clean catch urine dipstick mandatory in all feverish children. ±FBC, CRP, blood culture, CXR, lumbar puncture (LP) as indicated by severity of presentation/age of child

(Rx) *Antipyretics:* safety-netting advice if discharging child

Antibiotics: if clear bacterial focus/child significantly unwell (do not blindly treat with antibiotics if not indicated).

Table 9.7 Identifying risk of serious illness

	Low risk	Intermediate risk	High risk
Colour	Normal	Pallor	Pale/mottled/blue
Activity	Responds normally to social cues Awake/wakens quickly Content/smiling Normal cry	Not responding normally to social cues Wakes only with prolonged stimulation Decreased activity No smile	No response to social cues Appears ill to a healthcare professional Unable to rouse or if roused does not stay awake Weak, high-pitched or continuous cry
Respiratory	No respiratory distress	Nasal flaring Tachypnoea: respiration rate (RR) >50 breaths/min age 6–12 months, >40 breaths/min age >12 months Oxygen saturation ≤95 per cent in air Crackles	Grunting Tachypnoea: RR >60 breaths/minute Moderate or severe chest indrawing
Hydration	Normal Moist mucus membranes	Dry mucous membranes Poor feeding in infants Capillary refill time (CRT) ≥3 s Reduced urine output	Reduced skin turgor

continued ●

	Low risk	Intermediate risk	High risk
Other		Fever for ≥5 days	Age 0–3 months, temperature ≥38°C
			Age 3–6 months, temperature ≥39°C

Adapted from NICE guideline: Feverish illness in children

MENINGITIS

P Inflammation of the meninges

A About 80 per cent of all cases of meningitis (including adults) occur in the first 5 years of life.
Bacterial: *Streptococcus pneumoniae, Haemophilus influenzae, Neisseria meningitidis*
Viral: HSV, enterovirus, adenovirus
Neonatal meningitis: GBS, *E. coli, Listeria*

S Non-specific in young children: fever, irritability, vomiting, poor feeding, bulging fontanelle
Older children: headache, neck stiffness, photophobia, Kernig's sign

Ix LP: if any concerns regarding raised intracranial pressure (ICP), perform computed tomography (CT) on head first
Cerebrospinal fluid (CSF):
  – raised WBC: increased lymphocytes: viral/partially treated bacterial/TB
  – increased neutrophils: bacterial
  – High protein/low glucose in bacterial meningitis

Rx i.v. Antibiotics: benzylpenicillin+gentamicin for neonates, ceftriaxone
Dose of dexamethasone before antibiotics if high index of suspicion (e.g. purulent CSF) reduces rate of hearing impairment

Cx Hearing impairment, hydrocephalus, epilepsy, developmental delay

Px Five per cent mortality; 10 per cent of survivors have neurological sequelae

MENINGOCOCCAL SEPTICAEMIA

P *Neisseria meningitidis* infection

S Mild non-specific, followed by fever, non-blanching petechiae/purpura, rapid onset of septic shock. May be associated meningeal signs (see meningitis)

Ix FBC, CRP, blood cultures, meningococcal polymerase chain reaction (PCR)

Rx Prompt administration of antibiotics (i.v. ceftriaxone/i.m. benzylpenicillin), aggressive fluid resuscitation, cardiorespiratory support (invasive ventilation, inotropes)
Rifampicin (chemoprophylaxis) for close contacts

Cx Necrosis of limbs requiring amputation, hearing loss, neurological sequelae

Px Ten per cent case fatality rate

KAWASAKI'S DISEASE

(P) Immune mediated inflammatory condition leading to coronary aneurysms in up to 30 per cent

(A) More common in Japan. Most common cause of acquired heart disease in childhood in developed countries

(S) Fever for 5 days + four out of five features:
- rash – often blanching, maculopapular
- non-purulent conjunctivitis
- mucosal changes of mouth and lips (strawberry tongue, cracked lips, red pharynx)
- cervical lymphadenopathy
- erythema/oedema of hands and feet followed by desquamation

Inflammation of Bacille Calmette-Guérin (BCG) scar also associated

(Ix) No diagnostic test. Often associated with raised CRP/erythrocyte sedimentation rate (ESR) and thrombophilia

Echo: coronary artery aneurysms (initial echo may be normal, need to be performed serially)

(Rx) Immunoglobin, high-dose aspirin

(Cx) Coronary artery disease

CONGENITAL INFECTIONS

(P) Infection obtained antenatally/perinatally

(A) TORCH infections:
- **T**oxoplasmosis
- **O**ther: HBV, syphilis, varicella zoster, *Human immunodeficiency virus* (HIV), parvovirus B19
- **R**ubella
- **C**MV (cytomegalovirus)
- **H**SV

(S) Microcephaly, chorioretinitis, cerebral calcification, hepatosplenomegaly, jaundice, cataracts

Anaemia (parvovirus B19). Hepatitis B and HIV often asymptomatic at birth; HSV presents with vesicular rash ± meningitis/fulminant sepsis

(Ix) Serological testing of baby and mother

(Rx) High-dose aciclovir

IMMUNODEFICIENCIES

(P) *Acquired:* HIV (most transmission vertical)

Inherited: Immunoglobulin deficiency, e.g. X-linked agammaglobulinaemia

Abnormal phagocytic function (e.g. chronic granulomatous disease)

Thymic aplasia (e.g. DiGeorge syndrome)

Abnormal DNA repair (e.g. ataxia telangiectasia)

Severe combined immunodeficiency (SCID)

(S) Failure to thrive, recurrent infections, chronic diarrhoea

NEUROLOGY

FEBRILE CONVULSIONS

(P) Seizure associated with fever

(A) 6 months–6 years. Incidence 1 in 300

(S) Brief generalized tonic-clonic seizure with associated fever

(Ix) As for febrile child (urine dipstick, inflammatory markers, CXR, LP as indicated)
Consider EEG and brain imaging if atypical seizure (prolonged, focal, neurological signs, poor recovery)

(Rx) Parental reassurance and advice. Antibiotics if indicated. Benzodiazepines if seizure >5 min. Treat status epilepticus with anti-convulsant drugs

(Px) One in three have further febrile convulsion (often in same illness). Background risk of developing epilepsy is 1 per cent (0.5 per cent in general population)

EPILEPSY

(P) Idiopathic, cerebral palsy, brain insult (head injury/meningitis), metabolic, genetic

(A) Overall incidence 0.5 per cent, 10 per cent affected severely

(S) *Generalized*: absence, tonic–clonic, myoclonic, tonic, atonic
Focal/Partial:
  - frontal lobe – simple partial seizures (e.g. Jacksonian march/Todd's paresis)
  - temporal lobe – automatisms, sensory phenomena, déjà vu
  - parietal lobe – vertigo, sensory symptoms, distorted body image
  - occipital lobe – visual symptoms

Table 9.8 Epilepsy syndromes

Seizure disorder	Aetiology	Signs/symptoms	Electroencephalo-gram (EEG)	Prognosis
Absence	3–12 years 1–2 per cent of childhood epilepsy	Transient loss of consciousness for few seconds with immediate resumption of activity	3 Hz spikes Precipitated by hyperventilation	95 per cent remission in adolescence
Infantile spasms (West's syndrome)	4–6 months Often preceded by developmental delay	Repetitive violent flexion of limbs, trunk and head followed by extension of arms (salaam attacks) while awake	Hypsarrhythmia (high amplitude spikes + irregular spikes on EEG)	High rate of associated developmental delay and regression
Lennox–Gastaut syndrome	1–5 years	Myoclonic jerks, atypical absence, atonic seizure	1–2.5 Hz spike + wave	Poor. Developmental delay/ regression

continued ❯

Seizure disorder	Aetiology	Signs/symptoms	Electroencephalo-gram (EEG)	Prognosis
Benign Rolandic	3–10 years	Tonic–clonic seizures during sleep Partial seizures affecting face and arm during day	Rolandic spikes centrotemporal region	Very good – usually stop by mid adolescence
Juvenile myoclonic	10–12 years ♀:♂, 2:1	Myoclonic seizures after waking	Multi-spike with fragmentation	Responds well to treatment

CEREBRAL PALSY

P Disorder of movement and posture associated with a fixed insult to the developing brain

A About 0.2 per cent of live births.
Prenatal, perinatal or postnatal event (ischaemia, congenital infection, neonatal meningitis, prematurity, IVH, kernicterus)

S *Spastic*: increased tone and reflexes, reduced power – hemiplegia, diplegia, quadriplegia
Dystonic/dyskinetic: involuntary movements – athetosis, chorea
Ataxic: hypotonia, wide-based gait, nystagmus, intention tremor

Ix MRI brain, exclude neurodegenerative/metabolic condition if aetiology not clear or signs of regression

Rx Multidisciplinary – medical/physiotherapy/occupational therapy (OT)/speech and language therapy (SALT)/special needs teachers)

Cx Epilepsy, learning and behavioural difficulties, speech and language delay, visual/hearing impairment, feeding difficulties, scoliosis, hip dislocation, contractures.

NEURAL TUBE DEFECTS

P Failure of formation of the neural tube during embryogenesis, affects 1 in 1000 live births
Anencephaly: failure of brain to develop. Stillborn/die shortly after birth
Encephalocoele: extrusion of brain through midline skull defect
Myelomeningocoele: abnormal spinal cord and exposed defect
Meningocoele: normal spinal cord, defect covered with skin
Spina bifida occulta: cord covered with bone, and skin with overlying skin lesion, e.g. lipoma/sinus/hair

A Maternal folate deficiency

S Variable according to defect: lower limb paralysis, sensory loss, neuropathic bladder/bowel, scoliosis, hydrocephalus

Ix MRI

Rx Early surgical closure, shunt if hydrocephalus, intermittent catheterization, laxatives, physiotherapy, correction of contractures/scoliosis

Cx Urinary tract infections, renal failure, scoliosis, contractures, skin damage/ulcers secondary to sensory loss

HYDROCEPHALUS

P Increased ventricular fluid leading to raised intracranial pressure

A *Communicating*: failure to reabsorb CSF – post bleed/infection, Arnold–Chiari malformation. Over-production of CSF – choroid plexus tumour
Non-communicating: obstruction to CSF flow – tumour, congenital malformation

Sy Irritability, poor feeding, headaches, vomiting, seizures

Si Enlarging head size, widened sutures, bulging fontanelle, sunsetting eyes (downward deviation), papilloedema

Ix Cranial USS/CT/MRI

Rx Shunt insertion – usually ventriculoperitoneal (see Figure 9.4)

Cx Shunt blockage/infection, over-drainage of CSF

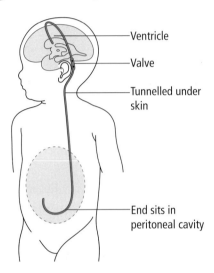

Ventricle

Valve

Tunnelled under skin

End sits in peritoneal cavity

Figure 9.4 Ventriculoperitoneal shunt

SPINAL MUSCULAR ATROPHY

P Degeneration of anterior horn cells

A Type I is most severe; incidence 1 in 20 000. Autosomal recessive

S Progressive proximal weakness. Reduced fetal movements, limb contractures, frog leg posture, muscle wasting, absent reflexes, respiratory distress, bell-shaped chest

Ix Electromyogram (EMG), genetic testing

Px Death by 18 months of age in Type 1

NEUROFIBROMATOSIS

See Chapter 1, Medicine

TUBEROUS SCLEROSIS

P Autosomal dominant but 80 per cent spontaneous mutations

A 1 in 10 000

Sy Developmental delay, seizures (infantile spasms), learning and behavioural difficulties

Ix 'railroad track calcification' on skull X-ray, CT, MRI, gene studies

Px Poor: 30 per cent die before 10 years, 75 per cent before 25 years. Death usually caused by epilepsy

ATAXIA TELANGIECTASIA

(P) Neurodegenerative autosomal recessive disorder of DNA repair affecting cerebellum and thymus causing immunodeficiency

(S) Poor coordination, telangiectasia

(Ix) Elevated alpha-feto protein, white blood cell chromosome fragility

(Cx) Recurrent infections, malignancy – usually acute lymphoblastic leukaemia (ALL; 10 per cent)

(Px) Many wheelchair bound by adolescence, death in 20s secondary to immunodeficiency

FRIEDREICH'S ATAXIA

(P) Progressive ataxia. Autosomal recessive; GAA triplet repeat expansion mutation on Frataxin gene

(A) One in 8000

(S) Sensory and cerebellar ataxia, intention tremor, absent ankle and brisk knee reflexes, extensor plantars, pes cavus, cardiomyopathy, scoliosis, optic atrophy, deafness

(Ix) ECG, echo, nerve conduction studies, gene studies

(Rx) multidisciplinary, treatment of cardiomyopathy

(Px) Death in early/middle adult life

DUCHENNE/BECKER MUSCULAR DYSTROPHY

(P) Inherited disorder of progressive muscle weakness. X-linked recessive. Mutation of Xp21 gene, which produces dystrophin

(A) Duchenne 1 in 3500, Becker 1 in 30 000 of ♂ births

(Sy) Speech and motor delay, waddling gait, cardiomyopathy (Becker)

(Si) Proximal weakness: Gowers' sign positive (when asked to stand from sitting on floor, turns over onto all fours and 'climbs up legs'; Figure 9.5), muscle wasting, calf hypertrophy, absent reflexes

(Ix) Grossly elevated creatine kinase (CK), abnormal EMG and nerve conduction studies, muscle biopsy, DNA testing, MRI of muscles

(Px) *Duchenne*: wheelchair bound by 8–12 years, death by early 20s

Becker: slower progression, often normal lifespan

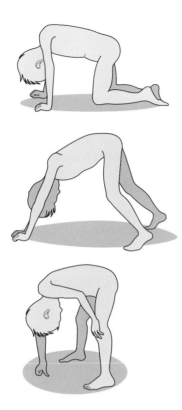

Figure 9.5 Gowers' sign

RESPIRATORY

BRONCHIOLITIS

P Infection and inflammation of bronchioles. Commonest pathogen *Respiratory syncytial virus* (RSV)

A <12 months of age, peak incidence during autumn and spring months

Sy Cough and coryza followed by difficulty in breathing and poor feeding

Si Increased work of breathing (tachypnoea, tracheal tug, subcostal/intercostal recession, head bobbing, grunting), hypoxia, coarse crepitations, wheeze, downwardly displaced liver

Ix CXR: hyperinflation/patchy infiltrative change. Nasopharyngeal aspirate for respiratory viruses

Rx Supportive: oxygen, NG feeds, CPAP/ventilation if severe. Ipratropium nebulizers may help

Palivizumab (RSV monoclonal antibody) given monthly as primary prophylaxis during RSV season to at-risk infants (e.g. chronic lung disease, congenital heart disease)

Cx Chronic wheeze, bronchiolitis obliterans (adenovirus)

Px Most infants make full recovery but half develop recurrent episodes of cough/wheeze

CROUP

(P) Viral laryngotracheal infection

(A) 6 months–6 years. Peak 2 years of age

(Sy) 'Barking' cough, hoarse voice, difficulty in breathing

(Si) Stridor (generally worse when upset/in exertion). Increased work of breathing; hypoxia (in severe cases)

(Rx) Keep calm and avoid upsetting the child (CXR/blood tests not indicated). Dexamethasone p.o. or nebulized budesonide. Nebulized adrenaline in severe cases. Ear, nose and throat (ENT)/senior anaesthetic review if deteriorating

EPIGLOTTITIS

(P) Bacterial infection and inflammation of epiglottis. Now rare with introduction of *Haemophilus influenzae B* (HiB) immunization

(A) 1–6 years of age

(S) Fever, 'toxic' looking child, stridor, drooling, minimal cough (see above, Croup)

(Rx) Keep calm (avoid painful interventions and CXR – may precipitate airway obstruction).
Urgent senior ENT/anaesthetic review to secure airway – may require emergency tracheostomy; i.v. antibiotics

(Px) With correct treatment, most children make a full recovery

WHOOPING COUGH

(P) Bronchitis caused by *Bordetella pertussis* infection

(S) Coryza for 2–3 days followed by episodes of spasmodic coughing ending with an inspiratory 'whoop'. Young babies may present with apnoeas. Symptoms may persist for 10–12 weeks.

(Ix) Per-nasal swab. Lymphocytosis on FBC

(Cx) Pneumonia, bronchiectasis

(Rx) Supportive: admit if history of cyanosis/apnoea. Erythromycin may help reduce spread.

Table 9.9 Wheeze

Pathology	Aetiology	Signs/symptoms	Investigations	Treatment
Viral induced wheeze	Preschool children About 60 per cent grow out of it Those with history/family history of atopy more likely to develop asthma	Wheeze and DIB following cough/coryza	Chest X-ray (CXR): hyperinflation, often not helpful	Bronchodilators: β-agonists; ipratropium bromide useful in infants Limited role for steroids Montelukast (leukotriene antagonist) prophylaxis may help

continued ▶

Pathology	Aetiology	Signs/symptoms	Investigations	Treatment
Asthma	Peak in school aged children (seen in 15 per cent) 'hyperactive' airways, chronic bronchial inflammation Hx of atopy Hx of 'interval' sx (e.g. nocturnal cough/exercise induced wheeze)	Wheeze and difficulty in breathing (DIB) Triggers: viral upper respiratory tract infection (URTI), cold, exercise, allergens (e.g. pets/pollen)	CXR: hyperinflation May show mucus plugging/ collapse/ pneumothorax Peak expiratory flow meter	Bronchodilators Steroids Intravenous aminophylline/ salbutamol if severe Prophylaxis: steroid inhaler, long acting β-agonists, leukotriene antagonists, theophylline
Foreign body (FB) inhalation	Preschool children Preceding history of choking episode	Wheeze Reduced air entry	CXR: visualize FB if radiopaque, collapse of right upper zone (RUZ) (common area of obstruction is right main bronchus)	Bronchoscopy to remove FB
Chronic aspiration/ gastro-oesophageal reflux disease	Usually presents in infancy May be underlying neurological impairment	Choking/ spluttering/ uncomfortable during feeds Failure to thrive Recurrent lower respiratory tract infection (LRTI)	Contrast study Video-fluoroscopy pH/impedance studies	Thickened feeds, H_2 antagonists (ranitidine)/ proton pump inhibitors (omeprazole), domperidone
Mediastinal mass	Rare Monophonic wheeze caused by external compression of bronchi Most common cause is lymphoma	DIB and wheeze which responds to steroid treatment (beware misdiagnosing as asthma), worse on lying down, signs of superior vena cava (SVC) obstruction	CXR: mediastinal mass	Expert oncological input Avoid lying child flat (may precipitate airway obstruction)

PNEUMONIA

(P) Viral or bacterial infection of the lungs. Common pathogens: *Streptococcus pneumoniae, Haemophilus influenzaa, Mycoplasma pneumoniae*

(Sy) Fever, productive cough, tachypnoea, difficulty in breathing (DIB). May present with abdominal pain if lower lobes affected

(Si) Increased work of breathing, inspiratory crepitations, reduced air entry, bronchial breathing

(Ix) CXR – shows areas of consolidation, sputum MC&S (more difficult to obtain in children)

(Rx) Antibiotics, physiotherapy

(Cx) Pleural effusion, syndrome of inappropriate anti-diuretic hormone secretion (SIADH)

(Px) Good with appropriate treatment. With recurrent/unresolving pneumonia consider TB, foreign body aspiration, cystic fibrosis, immunodeficiency, primary ciliary dyskinesia.

CYSTIC FIBROSIS

(P) Autosomal recessive disorder affecting cystic fibrosis transmembrane regulating gene (CFTR) on chromosome 7. Na–Cl channel dysfunction causing thick secretions in lungs and pancreas. Most common mutation is ΔF508

(A) Incidence 1 in 2500 and carrier rate 1 in 25 in White Caucasian population Neonatal screening of immunoreactive trypsin (IRT) now carried out on Guthrie card

(S) Failure to thrive, recurrent chest infections (common pathogens: *Staphylococcus aureus, Haemophilus influenzae, Pseudomonas*), steatorrhoea and malabsorption

(Ix) Sweat test (elevated Na and Cl), gene studies, CXR: bronchiectasis

(Rx) Regular physiotherapy, bronchodilators/inhaled steroids, DNAase, antibiotics, pancreatic enzyme supplementation, high-calorie diet/overnight gastrostomy feeds. Heart/lung transplant for end-stage disease

(Cx) Meconium ileus (neonatal bowel obstruction), distal intestinal obstruction syndrome (DIOS), rectal prolapse, *Pseudomonas/Burkholderia* colonization, diabetes, liver cirrhosis, pancreatitis, infertility in males (absence of vas deferens)

(Px) Improving survival. Life expectancy of newborn is now 40 years

GASTROINTESTINAL/LIVER

COLIC

(P) Persistent crying/discomfort in a healthy thriving infant. Often cause not found. May be secondary to cow's milk intolerance

(A) Present at 3 weeks, resolves by 3 months

(S) Inconsolable crying for 3 h/day, usually evening

(Rx) Parental reassurance. Exclude other pathology. Winding after feeds, and slower rate of feeds may help. Consider trial of cow's milk exclusion/hydrolysed milk.

GASTRO-OESOPHAGEAL REFLUX

(P) Refluxing of milk/acid from stomach back into oesophagus. Gastro-oesophageal *disease* (GORD) when significant sx/failure to thrive

(A) Common. Increased in preterms, neurological disability, post oesophageal atresia/diaphragmatic hernia

(S) Posseting/regurgitation, vomiting, uncomfortable during feeds, failure to thrive, apnoea, dystonic movements if severe (Sandifer's syndrome)

(Ix) pH/impedance study to demonstrate acid/milk reflux; upper gastrointestinal (GI) contrast study

(Rx) *Parental reassurance:* Ensure baby not overfed
Medical: Feed thickeners, Gaviscon, H_2 antagonists (ranitidine), proton pump inhibitors (omeprazole), domperidone increases gastric emptying
Surgical: Nissen fundoplication

(Cx) Pulmonary aspiration, oesophageal stricture

(Px) Most resolve by 12 months

PYLORIC STENOSIS

(P) Hypertrophy of the gastric pylorus causing upper GI obstruction

(A) 2–8 weeks of age. ♂ > ♀ 4:1. +ve family history

(Sy) Projectile milky vomits after every feed, constantly hungry baby, acute weight loss

(Si) Dehydration, palpable olive mass in right upper abdomen, peristaltic wave when feeding

(Ix) Hyperchloraemic, hypokalaemic metabolic alkalosis. Abdominal USS

(Rx) Nil by mouth (NBM). Correct electrolyte abnormalities with i.v. rehydration, NG tube and replace NG losses. Surgical pyloromyotomy

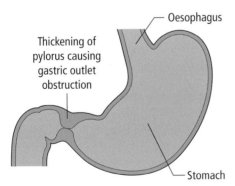

Thickening of pylorus causing gastric outlet obstruction

Oesophagus

Stomach

Figure 9.6 Pyloric stenosis

ALLERGIC COLITIS

(A) Commonest cause of non-infectious diarrhoea in infants

(S) Diarrhoea with blood and mucus, failure to thrive. Most common allergen is cow's milk protein (can be passed through breast milk)

(Ix) Eosinophilia, raised IgE, positive radioallergosorbent test (RAST)/skin prick to specific foods

Rx   Exclude offending food and offer substitute, e.g hydrolysed milk

GASTROENTERITIS

P   Viral/bacterial infection of intestine. Up to 60 per cent rotavirus. Other viruses: adenovirus, norovirus. Bacterial: *Campylobacter*, *Salmonella*, *Shigella*. Highly contagious

A   One of the most common childhood diseases

Sy   Acute onset of vomiting followed by diarrhoea. Fever. Blood in stools indicative of bacterial infection

Si   Signs of dehydration. Abdominal discomfort

Table 9.10 Assessing dehydration in children

Dehydration	Signs/symptoms
Mild (<5 per cent weight loss)	Thirsty, dry mucous membranes
Moderate (5–10 per cent weight loss)	Lethargic, reduced skin turgor, sunken eyes, sunken anterior fontanelle, tachycardia, reduced urine output, reduced tears
Severe (>10 per cent weight loss)	Drowsy, absent urine output, prolonged capillary refill time, weak pulse, low blood pressure (signs of hypovolaemic shock)

Ix   Stool MC&S, urea and electrolytes

Rx   Oral rehydration therapy (ORT) given frequently in small amounts; i.v fluids if not tolerating oral/nasogastric fluids. Good handwashing to prevent spread. Notify public health if bacterial

Cx   Cow's milk protein intolerance

Px   Recovery of acute symptoms within 24–48 h, but diarrhoea may persist for up to 2 weeks.

TODDLER'S DIARRHOEA

P   Benign condition causing frequent loose stool

A   Common. ♂ > ♀. Preschool children. FH of irritable bowel

S   Loose offensive stool with undigested food 'peas and carrots' stool ± mucus.

Ix   Nil indicated

Rx   Parental reassurance. Dietitian review

Px   Majority resolve by 5 years

COELIAC DISEASE

P   Autoimmune small intestinal enteropathy caused by allergy to gluten (wheat, rye, barley, oats). Associated human leucocyte antigen (HLA) DQ2 or DQ8

A   White Caucasian (1 in 2000), particularly Irish populations (1 in 300)

Sy   Failure to thrive, non-specific abdominal pain, vomiting, constipation

Si   Buttock wasting, abdominal distension, short stature, anaemia

Ix   Tissue transglutaminase antibody, endomysial antibodies; upper GI endoscopy and duodenal biopsy (shows villus atrophy)

Rx   Gluten-free diet

Cx   Associated autoimmune conditions, e.g. diabetes, hypothyroidism. Intestinal lymphoma in later life.

INFLAMMATORY BOWEL DISEASE

See Chapter 1, Medicine, p. 31

RECURRENT ABDOMINAL PAIN

P   Recurrent pain for at least 3 months; <10 per cent have organic cause

A   10 per cent of school age children

S   *Irritable bowel*: mucous stools, bloating, tenesmus, alternate diarrhoea/constipation
Abdominal migraine: associated headache and pallor
Dyspepsia: epigastric pain, belching, bloating, heartburn

Rx   Rule out organic cause, e.g. inflammatory bowel disease (IBD), UTI. Ensure child is thriving. Reassurance

CONSTIPATION

P   Difficulty/delay in passing faeces

A   Common. Most caused by low-fibre/high-milk diet.
Other causes: anal stricture, hypothyroidism, hypercalcaemia, allergic colitis.
If delayed passage of meconium, consider Hirschsprung's disease

Sy   Straining, infrequent bowel opening, hard stool, abdominal pain/distension, soiling, encopresis (passage of stool in abnormal places). Painful defaecation leads to anxiety and 'holding on' creating vicious cycle

Si   Distended abdomen, palpable faecal masses. Examine spine and lower limbs to exclude neurological cause

Ix   AXR (faecal loading), serial AXR with radio-opaque marker to demonstrate transit time, rectal biopsy (if Hirschsprung's suspected), thyroid functions tests, serum calcium, allergy testing

Rx   Increase fluid intake, high-fibre diet, reward system, stool softeners, stimulant laxatives

Cx   Megarectum, overflow faecal incontinence, anal fissures

HIRSCHSPRUNG'S DISEASE

P   Absent ganglion cells in anorectum; 75 per cent also involving sigmoid and 10 per cent affect entire colon

A   One in 5000. ♂:♀ 4:1. Familial inheritance

S   Delayed passage of meconium (>24 h after birth), acute bowel obstruction, chronic constipation

Ix   AXR: dilated bowel loops, absent rectal air. Rectal biopsy

Rx   Excision or bypass of aganglionic intestine, which may involve interval colostomy

Cx   Enterocolitis: profuse diarrhoea and hypovolaemic shock

INTUSSUSCEPTION

See Chapter 2, Surgery, p. 124

MALROTATION

(P) Failure of midgut to rotate during embryogenesis. Mobile midgut with short mesentery and propensity to twist

(S) *Infant*: Bile-stained vomiting (may be only sign)
Older child: GORD, vomiting, abdominal pain

(Ix) Contrast study

(Rx) Surgical

(Cx) Volvulus and acute bowel obstruction

BILIARY ATRESIA

(P) Atresia of extrahepatic biliary system leading to disrupted flow and excretion of bilirubin

(A) One in 12 000

(Sy) Prolonged jaundice (beyond 2 weeks), pale stools, dark urine

(Si) Jaundice, hepatomegaly, splenomegaly (portal hypertension)

(Ix) *Blood tests*: conjugated hyperbilirubinaemia, raised alkaline phosphatase (ALP) and liver enzymes
USS: may show absent/contracted gallbladder
Radioisotope scan: uptake by liver but no excretion. Liver biopsy

(Rx) Kasai procedure (hepatoportoenterostomy) most effective if performed before 8 weeks of life

(Cx) Liver cirrhosis. Liver transplant

NEONATAL HEPATITIS

(P) Alpha-1-antitrysin deficiency: AR, 1 in 3000 (see p. 18)
Galactosaemia: 1 in 40 000. Jaundice, vomiting, lethargy when fed milk. Associated *E. coli* sepsis and cataracts. Positive urine reducing substances. Galactose 1 phosphate uridyl transferase (GAL-1-PUT) testing.

WILSON'S DISEASE

See Chapter 1, Medicine, p. 42

NEPHROLOGY

NEPHROTIC SYNDROME

See Nephrology in Chapter 1, Medicine, p. 59

GLOMERULONEPHRITIS

See Nephrology in Chapter 1, Medicine, p. 58

RENAL FAILURE

See Nephrology in Chapter 1, Medicine, p. 61

HAEMOLYTIC URAEMIC SYNDROME (HUS)

(A) Most common cause of acute renal failure (ARF) in children. See Nephrology in Chapter 1, Medicine, p. 60

HENOCH–SCHÖNLEIN PURPURA (HSP)

(P) Small vessel vasculitis

(A) Peak 4–6 years. Often preceded by viral infection

(S) Purpuric rash with predominant thigh and buttock distribution, abdominal pain, transient large joint arthritis

(Ix) Haematuria on urine dipstick, blood pressure (BP; hypertension)

(Cx) IgA nephritis

(Rx) Supportive: analgesia. Steroids if significant abdominal pain/renal involvement

(Px) Self-limited. Completes resolution in most within 1 month. About 1 per cent have long-term renal involvement.

URINARY TRACT INFECTION (UTI)

(A) ♂ > ♀ in infancy ♀ > ♂ after 1 year of age. Overall, 3 per cent of girls and 1 per cent of boys

Increased incidence with vesicoureteric reflux and structural abnormalities

(Sy) *Infants*: often non-specific – fever, poor feeding, vomiting

Older children: dysuria, haematuria, suprapubic/loin tenderness

(Ix) Urine dipstick may be positive for leucocytes ± nitrites/blood. Positive urine culture (important to obtain clean catch urine to avoid contamination)

Recurrent/atypical UTI or in infant <6 months requires imaging:
  – renal USS (structural abnormalities)
  – micturating cystourethrogram/MAG3 (identify vesico-ureteric reflux)
  – radionucleotide DMSA scan (renal scarring).

(Rx) Appropriate antibiotics. Consider prophylactic antibiotics for high-risk children

(Cx) Calyceal dilatation, renal scarring, chronic renal failure

(Px) Fifty per cent have recurrence of UTI within 1 year

STRUCTURAL RENAL ABNORMALITIES

(P) *Renal agenesis* (bilateral incompatible with life)

Horseshoe kidney: kidneys connected along the midline

Pelvic kidney

Duplex system: ranges from bifid renal pelvis to complete duplication of kidneys and ureters

(S) Often asymptomatic. Increased risk of UTI, vesicoureteric reflux, renal stones and pelviureteric obstruction

(Ix) USS, IVU

POSTERIOR URETHRAL VALVES

(P) Mucosal folds causing distal urethral outflow obstruction

(A) 1 in 5000 males

(S) Antenatal oligohydramnios – if severe, leads to pulmonary hypoplasia. Oligo/anuria. Poor urinary stream in older boys

Ix *USS:* bilateral hydronephrosis, dysplastic kidneys, dilated thick-walled bladder. *Micturating cystourethrogram (MCUG):* dilated posterior urethra and vesicoureteric reflux (Figure 9.7)

Rx Suprapubic catheter. Endoscopic transurethral valve ablation

Cx UTI, renal failure

Px Urodynamic abnormalities in 75 per cent. Some require renal transplant.

HYPOSPADIAS

P Abnormal position of urethral opening – see Figure 9.7
May be associated with 'dorsal hood' foreskin (i.e. no foreskin on underside of penis and chordee – bent penis)

S Abnormal appearance. Abnormal urinary stream

Rx Surgical reconstruction if opening on/below shaft of penis. Do not circumcise (foreskin used in reconstruction)

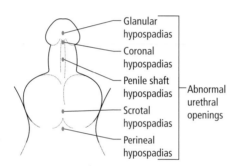

Figure 9.7 Hypospadias

UNDESCENDED TESTES

P Impalpable testes in scrotum. Usually in inguinal region, most descend spontaneously
If undescended bilaterally, consider inter-sex condition

Rx Watch and wait: if not descended by 9 months refer to urologist for surgical exploration

Cx Increased risk of testicular cancer, if left undescended

CARDIOLOGY

NORMAL FETAL BLOOD FLOW

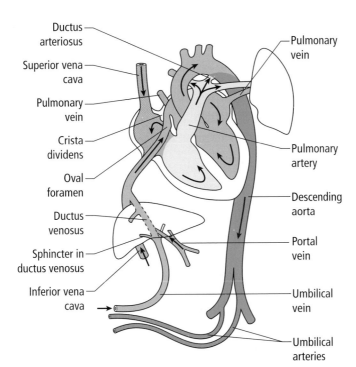

Figure 9.8 Diagram of fetal circulation

Box 9.1 FETAL CIRCULATION

- Only 15 per cent blood enters pulmonary circulation, the rest bypasses via foramen ovale and ductus arteriosus
- After birth, pulmonary vascular resistance falls, pulmonary blood flow increases and the ductus and foramen ovale close

---

INNOCENT MURMURS

P Murmur with no associated structural abnormality

A Heard in up to a third of children at some time

S Murmur:
  - systolic
  - soft (grade 1 or 2)
  - does not radiate
  - typically continuous in left clavicular region (venous hum) or ejection systolic in LSE
  - changes with posture
  - often heard in febrile child (hyperdynamic circulation)

Ix Re-examine when well. Consider ECG, CXR, echo if thought to be significant

---

Box 9.2 CONGENITAL HEART DISEASE

Acyanotic heart disease:
- Ventricular septal defect
- Patent ductus arteriosus
- Pulmonary stenosis
- Atrial septal defect
- Coarctation of the aorta
- Aortic stenosis

Cyanotic heart disease:
- Tetralogy of Fallot
- Transposition of the great arteries

ATRIAL SEPTAL DEFECT (ASD), VENTRICULAR SEPTAL DEFECT (VSD), AORTIC STENOSIS, PULMONARY STENOSIS

See Cardiology in Chapter 1, Medicine p. 10

PATENT DUCTUS ARTERIOSUS (PDA)

See Neonatal medicine above (p. 222)

COARCTATION OF THE AORTA

(A) Associated with Turner's syndrome. Often coexists with VSD

(S) Absent/weak femoral pulses, hypertension in arms but not legs.
Critical stenosis: neonatal shock when ductus closes.
Less critical stenosis: heart failure, murmur from collaterals (heard on back), hypertension

(Ix) *CXR*: 'Rib notching' from collaterals (older child)
ECG: right ventricular (RV) hypertrophy in neonate, left ventricular (LV) hypertrophy in older child. Echo

(Rx) Surgical resection and anastomosis. Balloon dilatation/stenting. Prostaglandin E in critical coarctation to keep ductus open

TETRALOGY OF FALLOT

(P) 1. VSD
2. Right ventricular hypertrophy
3. Overriding aorta
4. Right ventricular outflow tract obstruction (pulmonary stenosis)

(A) Most common cyanotic congenital heart disease. Associated with DiGeorge (22q11 deletion)

(S) May present with cyanosis on closure of the duct. Ejection systolic murmur LSE. Single second heart sound. Cyanotic 'spells' when crying/upset. Child may squat to increase venous return. Clubbing

(Ix) *ECG*: R axis deviation, RV hypertrophy/strain
CXR: small 'boot-shaped' heart. Echo

(Rx) For acute spells – oxygen, morphine, propranolol
Surgical repair at 6 months. Symptomatic infants may require shunt to increase pulmonary blood flow

(Cx) Ventricular arrhythmia

TRANSPOSITION OF THE GREAT ARTERIES

P Aorta arises from right ventricle and pulmonary artery arises from left ventricle creating two parallel circulations. Mixing of blood maintained via PDA/foramen ovale/VSD

S Cyanosis at birth or presentation when duct closes

Ix CXR: 'egg on side' appearance of heart. Echo

Rx Balloon atrial septostomy as emergency procedure. Surgical arterial switch repair

Cx Pulmonary/aortic stenosis, coronary artery disease

ENDOCARDITIS, CARDIOMYOPATHY, PERICARDITIS, MYOCARDITIS, SUPRA-VENTRICULAR TACHYCARDIA

See Cardiology in Chapter 1, Medicine p. 1

RHEUMATIC FEVER

P Immune response following Group A strep infection leading to valvular disease

A Uncommon in developed countries. Age 5–15 years

Box 9.3 JONES CRITERIA FOR THE DIAGNOSIS OF RHEUMATIC FEVER

Diagnosis requires two major criteria or one major and two minor criteria

Major criteria:
- Carditis
- Fever
- Polyarthritis
- Erythema marginatum
- Syndenham's chorea
- Subcutaneous nodules

Minor criteria:
- Polyarthralgia
- Raised acute phase reactants (ESR/CRP)
- Prolonged PR interval
- Previous history of rheumatic fever
- Elevated or rising antistreptolysin O titre

Rx Anti-inflammatory drugs, high-dose aspirin, prophylactic antibiotics

Px Risk of recurrence – repeated episodes increase severity of valvular disease

Cx Commonly mitral stenosis, but may affect the other valves

KAWASAKI'S DISEASE

A Most common cause of acquired heart disease in childhood in developed countries (see Infection, p. 230)

HYPERTENSION

P In children usually secondary to:
Renal: CRF, glomerulonephritis, renal artery stenosis, tumour (e.g. Wilms')
Cardiac: coarctation of aorta
Endocrine: Cushing's syndrome, congenital adrenal hyperplasia, catecholamine release neuroblastoma, phaeochromocytoma

S Incidentally picked up, headaches, lethargy, failure to thrive, facial palsy, convulsions

Rx Antihypertensives, treat underlying cause

MALIGNANCIES

There are 1500 new cases of childhood cancer in the UK each year

---

Box 9.4 CHILDHOOD MALIGNANCIES IN DECREASING ORDER OF INCIDENCE
● Acute leukaemia
● CNS tumour
● Lymphoma
● Neuroblastoma
● Soft tissue sarcoma
● Wilms' tumour
● Bone tumour
● Retinoblastoma

ACUTE LYMPHOBLASTIC LEUKAEMIA

See Chapter 7, Oncology, p. 204

LYMPHOMA

See Chapter 7, Oncology, p. 204

CNS TUMOURS

(A) Second most common childhood malignancy. Usually infratentorial. Most common are astrocytoma and medulloblastoma

(S) Early-morning headache/vomiting, focal neurological signs usually cerebellar, papilloedema

(Ix) MRI brain

(Rx) Surgical resection, chemotherapy, radiotherapy

(Cx) Developmental delay and neuroendocrine effects from treatment

NEUROBLASTOMA

(P) Neuroendocrine tumour arising from sympathetic nervous system. Usually adrenal in origin but can arise anywhere along sympathetic chain

(S) Lethargy, weight loss, abdominal mass, spinal cord compression, bruising/swelling of eye, hypertension; 50 per cent present with metastases

(Ix) Elevated urine catecholamines. MIBG (meta-iodobenzylguanidine) radioisotope scan

(Rx) Chemotherapy, radiotherapy, surgery

(Px) Good if localized tumour, poor if widespread disease

WILMS' TUMOUR

(P) Nephroblastoma

(S) Painless abdominal swelling, haematuria, weight loss, hypertension

(Ix) CT staging, biopsy

(Rx) Surgical resection and chemotherapy

(Px) Ninety per cent 5-year survival

RHABDOMYOSARCOMA

(P) Tumour of skeletal tissue. Can occur at almost any site
(A) About 5–8 per cent of all childhood cancers. Ages 2–6 years, 15–19 years
(S) Lump or pressure symptoms according to site of tumour
(Rx) Surgery ± chemotherapy/radiotherapy
(Px) Fifty per cent 5-year survival

BONE TUMOURS

(P) Osteosarcoma
Ewing's sarcoma
(A) Adolescent boys
(S) Pain, swelling, pathological fractures of long bones
(Rx) Surgical excision, endoprosthetic replacement, chemotherapy, radiotherapy (in Ewing's)

RETINOBLASTOMA

(P) Malignancy of retinal cells; 45 per cent hereditary (Rb gene)
(S) Absent red reflex, squint, visual symptoms; 30 per cent have bilateral disease
(Rx) Chemotherapy, surgery
(Px) About 95–98 per cent cure rate

GENETICS

Table 9.11 Classification of inherited disorders

Disorder	Description	Examples
Chromosomal	Extra or missing chromosome usually caused by failure to separate (non-dysjunction). Also translocation and mosaicism	Down's syndrome (trisomy 21), Edwards' syndrome (trisomy 18), Patau's syndrome (trisomy 13), Klinefelter's syndrome (XXY), Turner's syndrome (XO)
Mendelian inheritance	Single gene disorder	
Autosomal dominant	Affected individual heterozygous (i.e. one normal and one abnormal gene)	Neurofibromatosis, Marfan's
Autosomal recessive	Affected individual homozygous (i.e. two abnormal genes)	Cystic fibrosis, sickle cell disease
X-linked recessive	Carried on X chromosomes – affects males only	Duchenne, Fragile X

continued ●

Disorder	Description	Examples
Trinucleotide repeat	Mendelian inheritance but phenotype depends on size of number of repeat sequences. Increased severity in successive generations	Fragile X, Friedreich's ataxia, Huntingdon's chorea
Imprinting	Only one parental copy of a gene expressed. Abnormal phenotype results if active gene not inherited (i.e both chromosomes from same parent – uniparental disomy)	Prader-Willi (*paternal* 15q11–13 not inherited) Angleman (*maternal* 15q11–13 not inherited)
Polygenic inheritance	Multiple genes involved	Spina bifida, congenital dislocation of the hip, cleft lip/palate, autism

DOWN'S SYNDROME (see Figure 9.9)

(P) Trisomy 21. Usually meiotic non-dysjunction

(A) 1 in 1000. Increased risk with increasing maternal age

(S) Learning difficulties. Dysmorphic features: Round face, flat occiput, protruding tongue, epicanthic folds, upslanting palpebral fissures, brushfield spots in iris, single palmar crease, reduced tone, sandal gap

(Ix) Chromosomes, echo, thyroid function tests (TFTs), tissue transglutaminase

(Rx) Developmental/learning support

(Cx) Hypothyroidism, congenital heart disease (atrioventricular septal defect [AVSD]), leukaemia, duodenal atresia, coeliac disease, hearing/visual impairment, Alzheimer's disease. Life expectancy around 50.

TURNER'S SYNDROME

(P) 45 X0 (only one X chromosome)

(A) Females

(S) Oedematous hands and feet as neonate, short stature, webbed neck, widely spaced nipples, wide carrying angle, horseshoe kidney, normal IQ

(Ix) Chromosomes, echo

(Cx) Coarctation of the aorta, infertility

KLEINFELTER'S SYNDROME

(P) 47 XXY

(A) Undervirilized males, 1–2 in 1000

(S) Tall stature, hypogonadism and small testes, gynaecomastia, behavioural problems

(Ix) Chromosomes

(Cx) Infertility

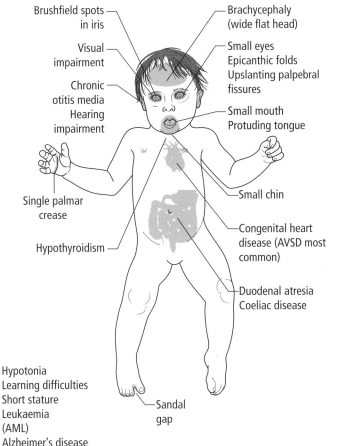

Figure 9.9 Features of Trisomy 21 (Down's syndrome)

Brushfield spots in iris

Visual impairment

Chronic otitis media Hearing impairment

Single palmar crease

Hypothyroidism

Brachycephaly (wide flat head)

Small eyes Epicanthic folds Upslanting palpebral fissures

Small mouth Protuding tongue

Small chin

Congenital heart disease (AVSD most common)

Duodenal atresia Coeliac disease

Hypotonia
Learning difficulties
Short stature
Leukaemia (AML)
Alzheimer's disease

Sandal gap

FRAGILE X

- **P** Trinucleotide repeat expansion disorder. X-linked recessive
- **A** Second most common cause of congenital learning difficulties after trisomy 21
- **S** Low IQ, prominent ears, enlarged testicles

ENDOCRINE/METABOLIC

DIABETES, CUSHING'S SYNDROME, THYROTOXICOSIS, DIABETES INSIPIDUS, SIADH, HYPERPARATHYROIDISM

See Endocrinology in Chapter 1, Medicine p. 63

RICKETS

- **P** Deficiency/abnormal metabolism of vitamin D leading to undermineralized bones
- **A** Deficiency: Afro-Caribbean/Asian populations (diet + reduced exposure to sunlight)
  Chronic renal disease (decreased activity 1α-hydroxylase)
  Hereditary

(S) Swollen wrists, swollen costochondral joints, bow legs
(Ix) Raised ALP, low/normal Ca, low phosphate, low vitamin D levels
Wrist X-ray: cupping and fraying of metaphyses, widened epiphyseal plate
(Figure 9.10)
(Rx) Vitamin D supplements

CONGENITAL HYPOTHYROIDISM

(P) Defective thyroid function from birth. Usually secondary to maldescent of thyroid
(A) One in 4000
(S) Lethargy, prolonged jaundice, enlarged tongue, failure to thrive, coarse facies
(Ix) Universal neonatal screening on Guthrie card, TFTs
(Rx) Levothyroxine (lifelong)
(Cx) Severe learning if levothyroxine not started in first few weeks of life

CONGENITAL ADRENAL HYPERPLASIA

(P) Autosomal recessive disorder leading to abnormal steroidogenesis pathway. Usually 21-hydroxylase deficiency
(A) One in 5000
(S) Failure to thrive
Girls: ambiguous genitalia
Boys: salt-wasting crisis
(Ix) Hyponatraemia, hyperkalaemia, metabolic acidosis, elevated 17α-hydroxprogesterone levels
(Rx) Glucocorticoid $\pm$ mineralocorticoid replacement, corrective surgery for female genitals
(Cx) Short stature, steroid side-effects, infertility

INBORN ERRORS OF METABOLISM

(P) Rare genetic disorders (usually AR) causing abnormal metabolism owing to enzyme defect (e.g. phenylketonuria, galactosaemia, maple syrup urine disease, glycogen storage diseases)
(S) Failure to thrive, vomiting, jaundice, seizures, lethargy, odd smell, developmental delay, learning difficulties, seizures, organomegaly, coarse facies
(Ix) Blood gas (acidosis), blood glucose (hypoglycaemia), lactate, ammonia, urine/serum amino and organic acids. Phenylketonuria screened for on blood spot testing (Guthrie card)

DEVELOPMENT

Table 9.12 Developmental milestones (mean age)

Age	Gross motor	Fine motor/vision	Speech/language and hearing	Social
Newborn	Flexed limbs	Fixes on face	Startles to noise	
2 months	Raises head from prone	Fixes and follows		Smiles
3 months	Rolling	Reaches for objects	Coos, laughs	Shows pleasure to stimuli
6 months	Sitting	Palmar grasp Transfers	Babbles, localizes sounds	Alert, interested
9 months	Crawling	Pincer grip	Understands 'no'	Stranger anxiety
1 year	Cruising/walking	Object permanence	First word	Waves 'bye bye'
2 years	Running	Scribbles Builds tower of six bricks	>20 words Joins two words	Uses spoon
3 years	Climbs stairs	Draws circle Builds bridge from three bricks	Joins three words Gives full name	Can undress
4 years	Rides tricycle	Draws cross Builds three steps from six cubes	Knows nursery rhymes	Dress and undress
5 years	Skips, hops	Draws square	Fluent speech	Washes face

DEVELOPMENTAL DELAY

Global developmental delay

↓

Delay in >2 aspects of development
  Prematurity/HIE
  Genetic disorder
  Neglect
  Inborn errors of metabolism
  Congenital infection

Specific developmental delay

↙ ↘

Motor delay
Cerebral palsy
Muscular dystrophy

Speech and Language delay
Hearing loss
Learning difficulties
Lack of stimulus
Dysarthria (e.g. cleft palate)
Austism

GROWTH

Growth in children assessed according to weight, height and head circumference and plotted on standardized growth centile charts

Table 9.13 Phases of growth

Age	Primary responsible factor for growth
Infantile (0–18 months)	Nutrition
Childhood (1–12 years)	Growth hormone, thyroid hormone
Puberty	Growth hormone, testosterone/oestrogen

FAILURE TO THRIVE

P Failure to maintain normal rate of growth (fall across growth centiles)

A Gastro-oesophageal reflux, coeliac disease, Crohn's disease, chronic renal failure, cystic fibrosis, hypothyroidism, inborn errors of metabolism, neglect

ABNORMAL SEX DEVELOPMENT

P Ambiguous genitalia leading to difficulties in assigning gender

A Excessive androgens causing virilized female (e.g. congenital adrenal hyperplasia)
Androgen insensitivity leading to feminized male
Gonadotrophin insufficiency (e.g. congenital hypopituitarism)
True hermaphroditism with both ovarian and testicular tissue

Ix Adrenal/sex hormone levels, karyotype, USS pelvis

Rx Do not assign gender until Ix complete. Specialist team input required.

DELAYED PUBERTY

P Failure of onset of puberty by 16 years in boys and 14 years in girls

A *Constitutional*: more common in boys, +ve FH
Malnutrition/chronic illness: cystic fibrosis, coeliac disease, chronic renal failure, anorexia nervosa
Endocrine: Cushing's syndrome, growth hormone deficiency (hypopituitarism, craniopharyngioma), hypothyroidism
Chromosomal: Turner's, Klinefelter's

Ix Wrist X-ray for bone age, urea and electrolytes (U&E), TFTs, coeliac screen, chromosome analysis, growth hormone (GH) provocation tests, MRI

Rx Treat underlying cause. Growth hormone for select cases

PRECOCIOUS PUBERTY

P Onset of signs of puberty < 8 years in girls and < 9 years in boys

A *Constitutional in girls*: particularly isolated thelarche (breast development) and adrenarche (pubic hair development)
Central: intracranial tumour, infection, irradiation, hydrocephalus
Peripheral: Congenital adrenal hyperplasia, gonadal/germ cell tumour

Ix Bone age, follicle-stimulating hormone (FSH), luteinizing hormone (LH), pelvic USS in girls, brain MRI

CHILD ABUSE

Table 9.14 Categories and definition of child abuse

Types of abuse	Symptoms/signs
Physical	Bruises, burns, lacerations, deliberate poisoning, torn frenulum, 'shaken' baby (retinal haemorrhage, intracranial haemorrhage) Inconsistent history
Emotional	Withdrawn, low self-esteem
Neglect	Unkempt, ill-fitting clothes, malnourished, poor hygiene/dentition, developmental delay
Sexual	Promiscuous behaviour, withdrawn, signs of sexual assault, sexually transmitted infections (STIs), pregnancy
Fabricated illness	Multiple presentations to health care, symptoms not consistent with signs

(Rx) Child protection involves high level of suspicion, immediate reporting of any concerns regarding welfare of a child, good communication and multi-professional working between doctors, nurses, social workers, health visitors, schools and parents

BEHAVIOUR

AUTISM SPECTRUM DISORDER

(P) Pervasive disorder with difficulty in social interaction, social communication and imaginative play. Spectrum of difficulties
Asperger's: social interaction and communication difficulties but with normal speech and language development

(A) Unknown aetiology. No evidence to associate with MMR (measles, mump, rubella). Often positive FH

(S) Delay in speech and language/social skills, repetitive/obsessive behaviour, poor eye contact, rigidity of thought, lack of imagination

(Rx) Multidisciplinary approach between paediatricians, education, OT, SALT

ATTENTION DEFICIT HYPERACTIVITY DISORDER

(P) Hyperactivity, impulsive tendencies, poor attention span

(Rx) Methylphenidate (Ritalin), cognitive behavioural therapy

BREATH-HOLDING ATTACKS

(A) 1–2 per cent of all children up to 3 years

(S) Precipitated by pain/frustration. Child holds breath and goes red and then blue. May be short loss of consciousness (LOC). Starts breathing again and goes back to normal.

(Rx)   Parental reassurance

(Px)   Benign, self-limiting

ENURESIS

(P)   Bedtime wetting. Usually secondary to reduced sleep arousal and/or failure to produce night-time vasopressin (nocturnal polyuria)
Consider bladder dysfunction (e.g. neuropathic bladder/overactive bladder if daytime symptoms/enuresis every night in a schoolage child)

(A)   ♂ > ♀; 10 per cent of 5 year olds; 1 per cent of 15 year olds

(Rx)   Alarms, desmopressin (vasopressin analogue). Exclude UTI. Treat constipation

CHAPTER 10

Obstetrics and Gynaecology

Jane Borley

MATERNAL CONDITIONS SPECIFIC TO PREGNANCY

PRE-ECLAMPSIA/ECLAMPSIA (OBSTETRIC EMERGENCY)

A Multi-system disorder occurring only during pregnancy

Pre-eclampsia defined as hypertension (>140/90) with proteinuria >0.3 g/L

Eclampsia is characterized by tonic–clonic seizures

Approximately 5–10 per cent of pregnant population (eclampsia 0.05 per cent)

Box 10.1 POSSIBLE SEQUELAE OF PRE-ECLAMPSIA

Mother
- Renal failure
- Liver failure
- Cerebral haemorrhage
- HELLP syndrome (**H**aemolysis, **E**levated **L**iver enzymes, **L**ow **P**latelets)
- Papilloedema
- Pulmonary oedema
- Placental abruption
- Disseminated intravascular coagulation (DIC)
- Eclampsia
- Death

Fetus
- Intrauterine growth restriction
- Intrauterine death
- Iatrogenic preterm delivery

P Disorder of placentation. Failure of trophoblast invasion within the spiral arteries, which leads to uteroplacental ischaemia and widespread endothelial dysfunction

S May be asymptomatic

Headache, malaise, vomiting, epigastric and right upper quadrant (RUQ) pain, visual disturbance and flashing lights

Leg swelling

Sy Hypertension and proteinuria. Peripheral oedema

Hyperreflexia – indicates high risk of seizures

HELLP syndrome: **H**aemolysis (low haemoglobin), **E**levated **L**iver enzymes, **L**ow **P**latelets

Papilloedema

Ix Serial blood pressure (BP)

Urinalysis, urine protein/creatinine ratio

Full blood count (FBC), urea and electrolytes (U&E), liver function tests (LFTs), coagulation, group and save (if delivery thought to be likely)

Cardiotocography (CTG)/ultrasound scan (USS) – to assess fetal well-being

Rx Aim of treatment is to prevent deterioration of disease/complications. Delivery is curative

Medical: magnesium sulphate to prevent seizures, antihypertensives (e.g. methyldopa, labetalol), steroids for fetal lung maturity, induction of labour; avoid ergometrine (precipitates hypertension)

Surgical: caesarean section

OBSTETRIC CHOLESTASIS

A Affects 0.7 per cent of pregnancies, higher in Asians

S Pruritus, jaundice

Ix Weekly monitoring – LFTs, serum bile acids, liver screen, liver USS (normal)

Rx Topical emollients, antihistamines, ursodeoxycholic acid, vitamin K

Fetal monitoring

Popular practice to offer induction of labour (IOL) at 37 weeks but evidence that this prevents intrauterine death (IUD) is limited

Cx *Fetal risks:* increased risk of preterm labour, IUD, iatrogenic prematurity, meconium stained liquor

Maternal risks: vitamin K deficiency (from malabsorption), increased risk of postpartum haemorrhage (PPH)

Increased risk in future pregnancies

MATERNAL DISEASE IN PREGNANCY

Table 10.1 The effect and treatment of maternal disease in pregnancy

Disease	Effects on fetus	Effects on mother	Management
Diabetes	Increased risk of congenital anomalies, perinatal mortality, macrosomia, shoulder dystocia, polyhydraminos	Diabetic nephropathy and retinopathy may deteriorate. Increased risk of miscarriage, pre-eclampsia and operative delivery	Increased insulin requirements. Oral hypoglycaemics are usually avoided. Emphasis on strict glycaemic control Induction of labour at 38–39 weeks is the norm
Epilepsy	Anti-epileptics are teratogenic Increased risk of neural tube defects, orofacial clefts and heart defects	For most women, pregnancy does not affect the frequency of seizures. But seizure frequency may increase due to poor compliance, hyperemesis in early pregnancy, or changes in drug bioavailability	Folic acid 5 mg once daily –reduces neural tube defects (NTDs) Medication should be continued in the majority to prevent mortality and morbidity associated with seizures Vitamin K from 36 weeks (risk of haemorrhagic disease of the newborn)
Anaemia	Associated with low birth weight and preterm delivery	Increased risk through pregnancy owing to iron deficiency Increased risk of postpartum haemorrhage (PPH) and need for blood transfusion postnatally	Full blood count (FBC) at booking and around 28 weeks to identify anaemia Treat the cause of the anaemia. Majority are iron deficient and thus need iron supplements

continued ❯

Disease	Effects on fetus	Effects on mother	Management
Hypothyroidism	Severe untreated hypothyroidism associated with developmental delay If secondary to treated Graves' disease, thyroid-stimulating hormone (TSH) receptor antibodies may cross placenta and cause fetal thyrotoxicosis	May require increased dose of levothyroxine	Continue on pre-pregnancy dose of levothyroxine Thyroid function tests (TFTs) in each trimester and adjust dose accordingly
Asthma	Depends on severity of condition but if well controlled no adverse effects Severe uncontrolled disease related to increased perinatal morbidity, preterm birth, intrauterine growth restriction (IUGR)	Acute exacerbation is uncommon	Important to continue treatment of disease as in non-pregnant population Reassurance to mother that treatment is safe and outweighs risks of stopping treatment
Venous thromboem-bolism (VTE)	Thrombophilia – antiphospholipid syndrome, is associated with increased pregnancy loss and IUGR	VTE is leading cause of maternal death, treatment and prevention are necessary interventions	Anticoagulation by low-molecular weight heparin is mandatory in those with current deep vein thrombosis (DVT) or pulmonary embolism (PE) Thromboprophylaxis should be considered in those with risk factors or following caesarean delivery

INFECTIONS IN PREGNANCY

Table 10.2 Sequelae of infectious diseases in pregnancy

Infection	Maternal signs and symptoms	Trimester of risk	Effects on fetus/ infant	Treatment
Human immunodeficiency virus (HIV)	Screening offered at booking May be asymptomatic	Highest in late third trimester, delivery and breastfeeding	Transmission rate 25–30 per cent, reduced to <2 per cent with highly active anti-retroviral therapy (HAART)/ caesarean delivery and no breastfeeding	HAART to all women No breastfeeding If high viral load i.v. Zidovudine prior to delivery and given to the infant Caesarean section Vaginal delivery may be possible if low viral load
Rubella	Symptomatic in 50–70 per cent Maculopapular rash, lymphadenopathy and arthritis	First trimester Very small risk in second and third trimester	Sensorineural deafness, cataracts, congenital heart defects, developmental delay	No treatment available if infected Management concentrates on prevention with rubella vaccination in teenage girls and identification of at risk mothers (vaccine offered postpartum)
Varicella zoster virus (VZV)	Fever, lethargy, pruritic rash with characteristic vesicles. Increased morbidity and mortality in pregnancy – pneumonia, hepatitis and encephalitis	All trimesters. <20/40; highest risk of fetal varicella syndrome >20/40; varicella of the newborn if infant born during infective episode	Fetal varicella syndrome: limb hypoplasia, skin scarring, deafness, developmental delay Varicella of the newborn	Avoid exposure VZV immunoglobulin to prevent infection in susceptible women with significant exposure Aciclovir if infection develops

continued ●

Infection	Maternal signs and symptoms	Trimester of risk	Effects on fetus/ infant	Treatment
Herpes zoster	Most risk associated with primary infection Genital vesicles, pain, dysuria	Infant at risk if delivered vaginally within 6 weeks of primary infection	Neonatal herpes localized to skin/ eye/mouth Central nervous system (CNS) disease (encephalitis) Disseminated infection	Avoid exposure during pregnancy Deliver by caesarean if within 6 weeks of primary exposure (after 6 weeks maternal antibodies have developed which cross placenta and protect fetus) Aciclovir if severe
Cytomegalo- virus (CMV)	Usually asymptomatic May present with fever, lethargy	All trimesters Most infected fetuses not affected	Intrauterine growth restriction (IUGR), microcephaly, intracerebral calcification, developmental delay, cataracts and deafness	Supportive management
Toxoplasmosis	Often asympto- matic. Fever, lethargy, lym- phadenopathy	First and second trimester Average 50 per cent transmission to infant	Hydrocephaly, chorioretinitis, intracerebral calcification	Spiramycin If fetal infection suspected or confirmed needs pyrimethamine
Listeriosis	Flu-like illness, fever, backache, myalgia	All trimesters	Miscarriage, preterm delivery, meconium- stained liquor Cerebral haemorrhage, pneumonitis, developmental delay	Ampicillin or co- trimoxazole

continued ▶

Infection	Maternal signs and symptoms	Trimester of risk	Effects on fetus/ infant	Treatment
Parvovirus B19	Lymphadenopathy, arthropathy	All trimesters	Miscarriage, haemolytic anaemia, non-immune fetal hydrops, intrauterine death (IUD) No congenital syndrome	Supportive management If fetus severely affected preterm delivery or intrauterine transfusion may be needed
Group B *Streptococcus* (GBS)	Approximately 25 per cent of women are carriers in genital tract. May have PV (per vaginam) discharge but most asymptomatic	Risk of infection once membranes have ruptured	Neonatal GBS disease; pneumonia, sepsis, death	i.v. Benzylpenicillin to carriers when in labour

FETAL CONDITIONS

DOWN'S SYNDROME AND SCREENING

A   Commonest cause of severe mental handicap. Incidence increases with advanced maternal age, 1 in 1500 in under 25 year old, and 1 in 100 at 40 years

P   Trisomy 21. Commonly caused by non-dysjunction at meiosis

Ix   See Table 10.3

Table 10.3 Screening tests for Down's syndrome

Trimester	Test	
First trimester	Combined test	Nuchal translucency and human chorionic gonadotrophin (hCG) and pregnancy-associated plasma protein-A (PAPP-A)
First and second trimester	Integrated test	Combined test (first trimester) and α-fetoprotein (AFP), oestriol and inhibin A (second trimester)
Second trimester	Quadruple test	hCG, estriol, AFP and inhibin A
Second trimester	Anomaly ultrasound scan (USS)	Nuchal translucency ≥ 6 mm or ≥ 2 soft markers on USS

(Rx) If risk following screening is <1 in 250, definitive diagnosis by karyotyping is offered
Chorionic villus sampling
Amniocentesis

RHESUS DISEASE

(A) Since the introduction of anti-D immunoglobulin (anti-D Ig) incidence has dramatically reduced. Infant deaths fell from 46/100 000 to 1.6/100 000

(P) Occurs in rhesus (Rh) −ve mothers who have a Rh +ve fetus. If there is mixing of fetal and maternal blood (delivery, placental abruption, invasive procedures, e.g. amniocentesis, evacuation of retained products of conception [ERPC], miscarriage), maternal IgM antibodies are produced to Rh antigen (do not cross the placenta). In future pregnancies IgG is produced (crosses placenta) and causes haemolytic disease in the fetus

(Cx) Fetus: haemolytic disease, intrauterine growth restriction (IUGR), hydrops fetalis (fetal ascites, pleural and pericardial effusions), death

(Rx) Prevention is the key. All Rh −ve mothers are given prophylactic anti-D IgG antenatally and at sensitizing events and after delivery
If anti-D antibodies are detected at booking the fetus is at risk if Rh +ve
Fetal surveillance: USS, fetal blood sampling
Fetus affected may require early delivery or *in-utero* blood transfusion

MULTIPLE PREGNANCY

(A) Increasing incidence because of assisted fertility treatment
Twins: 1 in 80 pregnancies, dizygotic > monozygotic
Triplets: 1 in 4000 pregnancies

(P) Dizygotic (two eggs) twins will each have their own placenta and membrane (dichorionic, diamniotic). This differs from monozygotic (one egg) twins where chorionicity depends on when splitting of the embryo occurred

---

Box 10.2 RISKS OF MULTIPLE PREGNANCY

Maternal	**Fetal**
• Miscarriage	• Preterm labour
• Hyperemesis	• IUGR
• Anaemia	• IUD
• Pre-eclampsia	• Twin–twin transfusion syndrome
• Gestational diabetes	• Congenital anomalies
• Operative delivery	• Malpresentation
• Post-natal depression	

(Mx) Hospital-led care
Serial USS for growth and presentation
Mode of delivery will depend on presentation of twin 1, maternal wishes and chorionicity

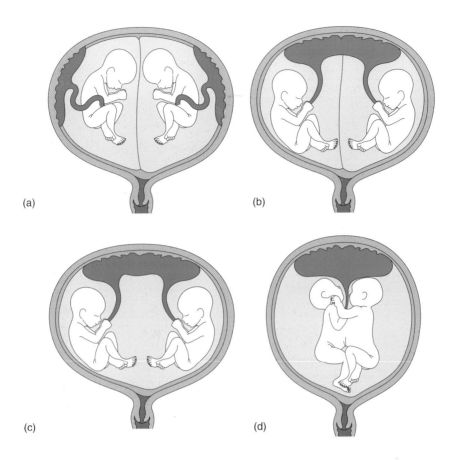

(a)

(b)

(c)

(d)

Figure 10.1 Monozygotic twinning varieties dependent on time of splitting after fertilization. (a) <3 days, dichorionic diamniotic; (b) 4–7 days, monochorionic diamniotic; (c) >8 days, monochorionic monoamniotic; (d) late, conjoined

INTRAUTERINE GROWTH RESTRICTION (IUGR)

P Low-birthweight infants (below 10th centile) may be 'constitutionally small', having reached their growth potential or 'growth restricted' as a result of a pathological process

Up to 40 per cent of stillbirths are small for gestational age

A *Maternal:* poor nutrition, smoking, alcohol and drug abuse, maternal disease

Fetal: abnormality and infection

Placental: failure of trophoblast invasion leading to reduced oxygen transfer to the fetus

S Small symphyseal–fundal height, may be difficult to detect on examination alone

Ix Ultrasound assessment: fetal size, oligohydramnios, Doppler for blood supply

Mx Observe for pre-eclampsia (potential risk of abnormal placentation)

Delivery depends on gestation, fetal blood supply and other risk factors.

INTRAUTERINE DEATH

A   Approximately 1/200 births

P   Birth of an infant over 24 weeks with no signs of life

Box 10.3 POTENTIAL CAUSES OF FETAL DEATH

Fetal
- Chromosomal abnormalities
- Infection
- Umbilical cord accidents
- Twin–twin transfusion syndrome

Maternal
- Chronic disease
- Obstetric cholestasis
- Rhesus disease
- Thrombophilia

Placental
- Abruption
- Pre-eclampsia
- Smoking

Ix   Suspected IUD should be confirmed by USS
Identify possible causes – infection, thrombophilia screen, offer post-mortem examination of the infant

Mx   Aim for vaginal delivery by induction of labour
Counselling, psychological support

OBSTETRIC COMPLICATIONS

ANTEPARTUM HAEMORRHAGE (OBSTETRIC EMERGENCY)

Box 10.4 Causes of vaginal bleeding during pregnancy

- Placental abruption
- Placenta praevia
- Vasa praevia
- Miscarriage
- Ectopic pregnancy
- Cervical/vaginal mass

PLACENTA PRAEVIA

A   A placenta that is partially or wholly covering the lower uterine segment
0.5 per cent pregnancies

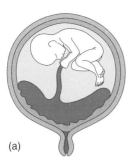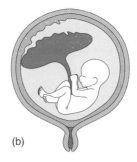

(a)   (b)

Figure 10.2 (a) Placenta praevia; (b) placental abruption

(S) May be asymptomatic or present with painless PV bleeding, which can range from light to torrential

(Ix) Low-lying placenta identified at 20-week anomaly USS. Needs confirmation in third trimester as many will migrate away from lower segment

(Rx) Delivery by caesarean section. Timing depends on whether bleeding has occurred

(Cx) High risk of postpartum haemorrhage

PLACENTAL ABRUPTION

(A) Premature separation of the placenta from the uterine wall

(P) Usually unknown. Can be related to trauma or following rupture of membranes
Higher risk in multiple pregnancy, polyhydramnios, pre-eclampsia, smokers

(S) Painful PV bleeding. May be concealed and present as abdominal pain with or without fetal/maternal compromise
Classical finding is a 'woody' hard uterus

(Rx) Management depends on amount of bleeding and fetal/maternal compromise and gestational age
Vaginal delivery may be achieved

AMNIOTIC FLUID EMBOLISM (OBSTETRIC EMERGENCY)

(A) Rare, 1 in 80 000 pregnancies; 80 per cent mortality

(P) Anaphylactic reaction to the presence of amniotic fluid and fetal matter into the maternal lungs. Leads to pulmonary hypertension and hypoxia

(S) Maternal collapse, respiratory distress, central cyanosis, DIC

(Rx) Resuscitation and correction of coagulopathy, immediate delivery
Supportive management thereafter

ANTENATAL CARE

The aim of antenatal care is to allow appropriate education and support to the pregnant woman and her family, assess and identify those deemed as high risk where more support is necessary, screen for fetal and maternal complications and determine timing and mode of delivery.

Table 10.4 An example of antenatal care for a low-risk woman

Gestation (weeks)	Recommended action
10–13	Booking – identify risk factors. Lifestyle advice, smoking, alcohol, folic acid
	Blood pressure (BP), urinalysis
	Full blood count (FBC), haemoglobin (Hb) electrophoresis
	Blood group, autoantibodies and rhesus status
	Human immunodeficiency virus (HIV), syphilis and hepatitis screen, rubella susceptibility
	Dating ultrasound scan (USS)
	Down's syndrome screening
16	To discuss results of above
	BP, urinalysis
18–20	Anomaly USS
24	BP, urinalysis
	Measure symphysis–fundal height (SFH)
28	BP, urinalysis, SFH
	FBC
	Anti-D for rhesus –ve mothers
	Glucose tolerance test for those at high risk of developing gestational diabetes
31	For nulliparous: BP, urinalysis, SFH
34	BP, urinalysis, SFH
	Discuss mode of delivery, preparation for labour and birth
	Discuss blood results taken at 28 weeks
36	BP, urinalysis, SFH
	Identify presentation
	Discuss breastfeeding and care of newborn
38	As for 36 weeks
40	As for 36 weeks
41	BP, urinalysis, SFH
	Discuss induction of labour (IOL) and membrane sweep

INTRAPARTUM

BOX 10.5 LABOUR

- Defined as regular uterine contractions with progressive cervical change
- Most women labour between 37 weeks and 42 weeks gestation (term)
- 1st stage: cervical change from closed os to 10 cm (full) dilatation
- 2nd stage: full dilation of cervix to expulsion of baby
- 3rd stage: following delivery of baby to expulsion of placenta, cord and membranes

PRETERM LABOUR

(A) Defined as labour and delivery before 37 weeks gestation, 6 –15 per cent of deliveries
Most important cause of adverse infant outcome

Box 10.6 RISK FACTORS FOR PRETERM LABOUR

- Acute illness
- Low body mass index (BMI)
- Multiple pregnancy
- Polyhydramnios
- Preterm rupture of membranes
- Previous cervical surgery
- Previous preterm delivery
- Smoking
- Uterine abnormalities

(Rx) The mother should deliver in a unit where adequate facilities to care for the neonate
are available. *Intra utero* transfer may be necessary to achieve this
Medical: corticosteroids – associated with significant reduction in rates of neonatal
death, respiratory distress syndrome, and intraventricular haemorrhage in the
newborn. Tocolytics – atosiban, nifedipine
Surgical: cervical cerclage (suture) for those at risk or identified short cervix

(Px) Most mortality and morbidity occurs in those born before 34 weeks
Approximate overall survival is 20 per cent at 23 weeks, 50 per cent at 25 weeks and
>95 per cent at 30 weeks

FETAL COMPROMISE IN LABOUR

Box 10.7 INDICATIONS FOR CONTINUOUS ELECTRONIC FETAL MONITORING IN LABOUR

- Prematurity
- Meconium-stained liquor
- Decelerations heard on sonocaid
- IUGR
- Oxytocinon use

Box 10.8 CTG INTERPRETATION

A normal CTG (Figure 10.3) should display:
- *Baseline:* between 110 and 160 bpm
- *Variability:* ≥5 bpm
- *Deceleration:* Absence of decelerations. Decelerations are defined as a drop of
  >15 beats below the baseline for >15 s. May be defined in relationship to
  contractions, early, with the contractions or late, after contraction. Most are
  variable in that their shape and timings are variable
- *Acceleration:* presence on accelerations. This is defined as a rise of >15 beats
  above the baseline for >15 s.
- *Contractions:* Comment should be made on presence or absence of contractions
  and frequency
- A deviation away from the normal parameters indicates a suspicious
  (Figure 10.4) or pathological CTG which should prompt investigation and
  treatment

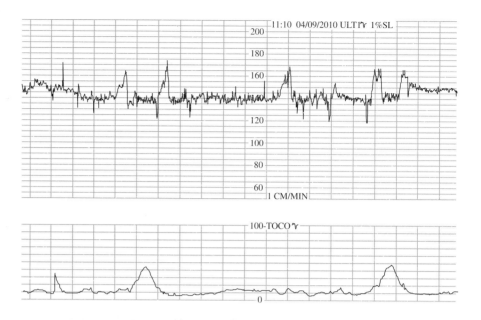

Figure 10.3 CTG trace

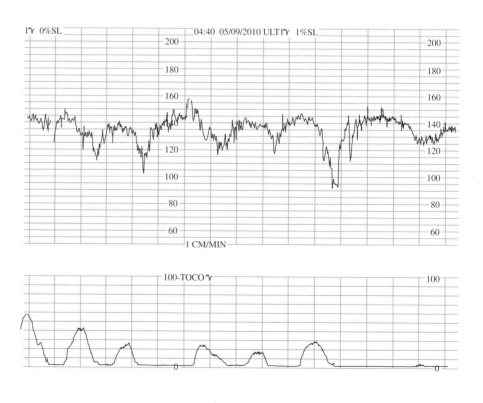

Figure 10.4 CTG trace

INDUCTION OF LABOUR

(A) One in five deliveries is induced

Box 10.9 INDICATIONS FOR IOL	
● Postmaturity	● Gestational diabetes
● Pre-labour rupture of membranes	● Pre-eclamptic toxaemia (PET)
● Suspected IUGR	● IUD
● Obstetric cholestasis	● Maternal request

(Rx) *Medical:* vaginal prostaglandins (prostaglandin E2 [PGE2]), oxytocin infusion
Surgical: membrane sweep, artificial rupture of membranes (amniotomy), cervical balloon

(Cx) Higher risk of instrumental and operative delivery, uterine hyperstimulation, failed induction, cord prolapse, uterine rupture

MALPRESENTATION

(P) Commonest malpresentation is breech presentation (3–4 per cent at term). Other malpresentations include brow, face and shoulder

(A) Often no cause identified. Increased risk in multiple pregnancy, polyhydramnios, uterine abnormalities, placenta praevia, congenital abnormalities

(Rx) *Breech:* external cephalic version. If remains breech, caesarean delivery is recommended because of risk of head entrapment
Face: vaginal delivery is possible in mento-anterior (chin lies behind symphysis pubis). Ventouse delivery is contraindicated
Transverse lie: no presenting part in the pelvis as the lie is transverse
Risk of cord prolapse if there is spontaneous rupture of membranes
Stabilizing induction with external cephalic version followed by artificial rupture of membranes may be possible, otherwise delivery is by caesarean section

CORD PROLAPSE (OBSTETRIC EMERGENCY)

(P) Descent of the umbilical cord through the cervix alongside or past the presenting part. Cord presentation describes the umbilical cord presenting between the cervix and presenting part

(A) Incidence 0.1–0.6 per cent

(S) Cord visible outside of vagina or palpable on vaginal examination

(Rx) Call for help
Immediate delivery:
– forceps vaginal delivery if cephalic presentation, fully dilated and low
– emergency caesarean section
Once delivered neonatal resuscitation as appropriate

(Cx) Infant death, cerebral palsy and hypoxic encephalopathy caused by cord compression and vasospasm

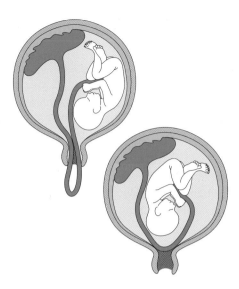

Figure 10.5 Cord prolapse versus cord presentation

SHOULDER DYSTOCIA (OBSTETRIC EMERGENCY)

P   A delivery that requires additional obstetric manoeuvres to release the shoulders after gentle downward traction has failed. Anterior shoulder impacts on maternal symphysis pubis

Box 10.10 RISK FACTORS FOR SHOULDER DYSTOCIA	
• Previous shoulder dystocia • Macrosomia • Diabetes mellitus • Maternal BMI >30	• IOL • Prolonged first and second stage labour • Forceps/ventouse delivery • Oxytocin

Cx   High risk of fetal mortality and morbidity: hypoxic encephalopathy, cerebral palsy and even death. Brachial plexus injury of the newborn, Erb's palsy
Maternal risks include higher rate of PPH and significant perineal trauma

Rx   The HELPERR mnemonic is the defined treatment for shoulder dystocia

Box 10.11 THE HELPERR MNEMONIC	
H	Call for **H**elp
E	**E**valuate for episiotomy
L	**L**egs (McRobert's manoeuvre)
P	Suprapubic **P**ressure
E	**E**nter manoeuvres (internal rotation of anterior shoulder)
R	**R**emove posterior arm
R	**R**oll the patient onto all fours and begin the cycle

POSTPARTUM

POSTPARTUM HAEMORRHAGE (OBSTETRIC EMERGENCY)

A *Primary PPH*: >500 mL blood loss within first 24 hours of delivery
Secondary PPH: >500mL blood loss after 24 hours of delivery
Risk factors: Prolonged delivery, multiparity, previous PPH, assisted delivery

P The four 'Ts':
– Tone – uterine atony
– Trauma – cervical, vagina and perineal tears
– Tissue – retained placenta or membranes
– Thrombin – coagulation disorder

S PV bleeding will be evident. Dependent on amount of blood loss and preceding haemoglobin levels patient may present with tachycardia, tachypnoea and hypotension

Rx An obstetric emergency, management should be aimed at resuscitation of the patient and treating the cause
Fluid resuscitation, uterine massage, drugs to stimulate uterine contractility (e.g. oxytocin, ergometrine)
Examination to exclude retained tissue and perineal trauma

Cx If simple measures fail to stem the bleeding, further surgical options include:
– insertion of intrauterine balloon
– uterine artery embolisation
– uterine artery ligation
– hysterectomy

PERINEAL TRAUMA

A Common, affects up to 90 per cent of nulliparous women
Third and fourth degree tears are much less common and affect 1 per cent of all vaginal deliveries

Table 10.5 Classification of perineal trauma

Degree	Extent of injury
1st	Involves skin only
2nd	Involves skin and perineal muscle
3rd	Involves the anal sphincter
4th	Extends through internal and external anal sphincter and through the anal mucosa

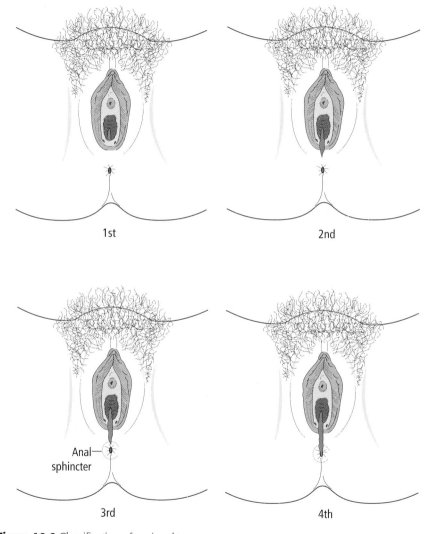

Figure 10.6 Classification of perineal trauma

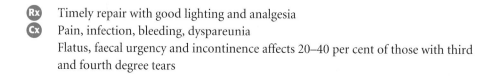

Rx   Timely repair with good lighting and analgesia

Cx   Pain, infection, bleeding, dyspareunia

Flatus, faecal urgency and incontinence affects 20–40 per cent of those with third and fourth degree tears

PUERPERAL PYREXIA

(A) Maternal pyrexia (>38°C) within first 14 days of delivery
Before antibiotics leading cause of maternal death:
  - genital/urinary tract infection
  - mastitis
  - wound infection
  - venous thromboembolism (VTE)

(S) Fever, rigors
Mastitis – painful, engorged, erythematous breast, purulent nipple discharge
Endometritis – abdominal pain, offensive vaginal lochia

(Rx) Empirical antibiotics based on likely cause
Involve microbiology if failure to respond or suspected severe infection

POSTNATAL PSYCHIATRIC DISORDERS

Table 10.6 Signs and symptoms of postnatal psychiatric disorders

Disorder	Signs and symptoms
'Baby blues'	Tearfulness and anxiety
	Common following first delivery (50 per cent)
	Self-limiting
	Normally resolves by day 3
Postnatal depression	Symptoms as per depression but related to pregnancy and childbirth
	Incidence 10–15 per cent
	Suicide is a leading cause of maternal mortality
	Identification and treatment with antidepressants
	Most cases resolve with supportive treatment
Puerperal psychosis	Severe mental health disorder usually presents within first 4 weeks of delivery
	Hallucinations, irrational ideas and negativity towards baby
	Rare
	Needs psychiatric team management
	Admission to mother and baby unit for supervised medical treatment

EARLY PREGNANCY

HYPEREMESIS GRAVIDARUM

(A) 0.1–1 per cent of pregnancies. However, general nausea and vomiting in pregnancy is common and affects >50 per cent

(P) Level of hCG is directly related to severity: higher incidence in multiple pregnancy and molar pregnancy

(S) Nausea, vomiting, dehydration, electrolyte imbalance
Ketonuria

Occasional muscle wasting

Rarely may precipitate thyrotoxic crisis (hCG and TSH similar subunits) or Wernicke's encephalopathy (owing to vitamin B_1 deficiency)

(Ix) FBC, U&E, LFT, TFT. Pelvic USS. Urine microscopy, culture and sensitivity (MC&S)

(Rx) Inpatient or outpatient. Fluids, antiemetics, potassium replacement, thromboprophylaxis, vitamin B_1 replacement

(P) Usually improves by 12 weeks gestation as hCG levels fall

Severe cases may require prolonged hospital stay and in rare cases total parental nutrition (TPN)

MISCARRIAGE

(P) Pregnancy loss less than 24 weeks gestation

Most occur due to chromosomal abnormality of the fetus

Recurrent miscarriage, defined as loss of three or more consecutive pregnancies, can be associated with chromosomal abnormalities (balanced translocation) in the parents, antiphospholipid syndrome and uterine abnormalities

Table 10.7 Classification of miscarriages

Type of miscarriage	Signs and symptoms
Threatened	Pain and bleeding, associated with a closed cervical os and viable intrauterine pregnancy on ultrasound scan (USS)
Inevitable	Pain and bleeding with an open cervical os
Missed	Symptoms and signs often minimal. Diagnosis on USS if no fetal heartbeat/fetal pole identified
Incomplete	Evidence of retained products of conception (RPOC) on USS
Complete	Products of conception passed, cervical os closes, no evidence of RPOC on USS

(A) 10–20 per cent of clinical pregnancies

Majority occur in first trimester

(Rx) Dependent on volume of bleeding and wishes of the patient

Anti-D is needed for Rh −ve mothers with spontaneous miscarriage >12 weeks gestation, or receiving medical/surgical management to prevent Rh sensitization

Expectant management: 'watch and wait' for spontaneous resolution (half of all cases)

Medical management: mifepristone orally followed by misoprostol PV

Surgical management: evacuation of retained products of conception, especially if persistent excessive bleeding, clinical instability, evidence of infected POC, molar pregnancy

ECTOPIC PREGNANCY

(A) One in 100 pregnancies. Commonest site is tubal (98 per cent), other sites include abdominal, ovarian and cervical

Factors associated include previous pelvic inflammatory disease (PID), previous tubal surgery or ectopic pregnancy, intrauterine contraceptive device, assisted reproduction

(P) Implantation into the tube with invasion through the muscularis layer and subsequent rupture and bleeding into the abdominal cavity.

(S) Lower abdominal pain, bleeding (normally light), syncope, cardiovascular collapse USS will confirm absence of intrauterine pregnancy and may demonstrate adenexal mass corresponding to a tubal ectopic

(Ix) Transvaginal ultrasound scan (TVUSS), hCG and progesterone, FBC, group and save and cross-match if intra-abdominal bleeding suspected. Diagnostic laparoscopy

(Rx) *Surgical*: laparoscopic salpingectomy of affected tube. Salpingostomy (surgical incision into fallopian tube and extraction of ectopic pregnancy) if contralateral tube is absent or damaged. Laparotomy if patient is haemodynamically unstable *Medical*: methotrexate i.m. if haemodynamically stable, minimal symptoms, no evidence of bleeding *Expectant*: for clinically stable, asymptomatic patients with a falling serum hCG

(P) 60–70 per cent of women will have intrauterine pregnancy in the future. Repeat ectopic risk increases to 10–15 per cent, therefore early USS in following pregnancies is recommended.

MOLAR PREGNANCY

See Gestational Trophoblastic Disease, p. 281

TERMINATION OF PREGNANCY (TOP)

(A) >150 000 TOP are performed each year in England and Wales The 1967 Abortion Act allows legal terminations dependent on one of five clauses (see Table 10.8). Two doctors have to agree. Most terminations are performed under Clause C.

Table 10.8 Termination of pregnancy legal clauses

Clause	Criteria
A	The continuation of the pregnancy would involve risk to the life of the pregnant women greater than if the pregnancy was terminated
B	The termination is necessary to prevent grave permanent injury to the physical or mental health of the pregnant woman
C	The pregnancy has not exceeded its 24th week and the continuation of the pregnancy would involve risk, greater than if the pregnancy were terminated, of injury to the physical or mental health of the pregnant woman
D	The pregnancy has not exceeded its 24th week and the continuation of the pregnancy would involve risk, greater than if the pregnancy were terminated, of injury to the physical or mental health of any existing child(ren) of the family of the pregnant woman
E	There is substantial risk that if the child were to be born it would suffer from such physical or mental abnormalities as to be seriously handicapped

Rx *Surgical:*
- first trimester – vacuum aspiration
- second trimester – dilatation and evacuation

Medical:
- mifepristone and misoprostol
- If >20 weeks gestation, feticide with intracardiac potassium chloride followed by medical management

GYNAECOLOGICAL MALIGNANCY

CERVICAL INTRA-EPITHELIAL NEOPLASIA (CIN)

P CIN is disordered growth and development of the epithelial lining of the transformation zone of the cervix. Gradual progression of this abnormality continues and 30–80 per cent of CIN 3 will eventually develop into cervical carcinoma

A *Human papilloma virus* (HPV) infection prerequisite for development of CIN/ cancer. HPV types 16 and 18 are high-risk subtypes

S Asymptomatic

Sy NHS cervical screening programme has been designed to identify women at risk of CIN and thus aims to reduce incidence and mortality of cervical carcinoma; 26 per cent reduction in incidence since screening began

Eligibility aged 25–64 years. Smear test every 3 years <50 years, every 5 years when >50 years

---

Box 10.12 CRITERIA FOR REFERRAL TO COLPOSCOPY

- Three consecutive inadequate smear samples
- Three borderline smears (squamous)
- Mild, moderate or severe dyskaryosis
- Suspected invasive disease

Rx Colposcopy involves inspection of the ectocervix under magnification. Acetic acid and Lugol's iodine is applied to identify abnormality. Histological diagnosis is achieved with biopsies of abnormal area

CIN 1 may be managed conservatively

CIN 2 and 3 are commonly treated with large loop excision of the transformation zone (LLETZ)

Px Regular smears required after treatment of CIN to ensure adequate treatment

CERVICAL CANCER

A Twelfth most common female malignancy

Approximately 2800 new cases per year

(P) 80–90 per cent squamous cell, 10–20 per cent adenocarcinoma

(S) May be asymptomatic. Irregular PV bleeding, postcoital bleeding. Pelvic examination or colposcopy may demonstrate a classical hard, craggy, bleeding cervix

Late cases may present with disease progression; renal failure following ureteric obstruction or bowel and bladder involvement

(Ix) *Histology*: cervical biopsy

Imaging: magnetic resonance imaging (MRI) pelvis/computed tomography (CT) chest, abdomen, pelvis to assess spread

(Rx) Depends on stage

Table 10.9 Staging and treatment of cervical cancer

Stage	Features	Treatment	5-year survival (per cent)
1	Carcinoma strictly confined to the cervix	Dependent of size of lesion, local treatment may be enough Radical surgery for bigger lesions	75–99
2	Carcinoma that extends into the parametrium or upper two-thirds of vagina	Radical hysterectomy and pelvic lymphadenectomy±adjuvant radiotherapy/chemotherapy	66
3	Carcinoma that has extended to pelvic side wall, lower one-third of vagina or causes hydronephrosis	Radiotherapy Ureteric stents if obstruction Chemotherapy	40
4	Carcinoma that has extended beyond the pelvis	Radiotherapy±chemotherapy +palliative care	15

ENDOMETRIAL CANCER

(A) Fifth most common female malignancy. Second commonest gynaecological malignancy

Approximately 7000 new cases per year

Incidence is increasing due to obesity

(P) 95 per cent adenocarcinoma

Box 10.13 RISK FACTORS FOR ENDOMETRIAL CANCER

Risk factors are associated with unopposed oestrogens:
- Obesity
- Tamoxifen therapy
- Early menarche/late menopause
- Estrogen secreting tumours
- HRT
- Endometrial hyperplasia with atypia
- Genetic predisposition – Lynch syndrome

(S) Post-menopausal bleeding (PMB) is the most common feature and 8 per cent of women with PMB have endometrial carcinoma. Majority of patients present with early stage disease.

(Ix) TVUSS – to establish endometrial thickness
Endometrial pipelle biopsy
Hysteroscopy and curettage
Staging MRI pelvis/(CT) chest, abdomen, pelvis

(Rx) Depends on stage (see Table 10.10)

Table 10.10 Staging and treatment of endometrial cancer

Stage	Features	Treatment	5-year survival (per cent)
1	Carcinoma strictly confined to the uterus	Total abdominal hysterectomy and bilateral salpingo-oophorectomy	75–95
2	Carcinoma extended to the endocervix (2A) or cervical stroma (2B)	Radical total abdominal hysterectomy (TAH)+bilateral salpingo-oophorectomy (BSO) +radiotherapy ±lymphadenectomy	65
3	Spread to serosa of uterus, pelvic peritoneum or pelvic lymph nodes	Surgery+radiotherapy or radiotherapy alone	30
4	Local metastasis to bladder/bowel (4A) or distant metastasis (4B)	Palliative radiotherapy	10

OVARIAN CANCER

(A) Fourth most common female malignancy. Most common gynaecological malignancy

(P) Majority are epithelial cell adenocarcinoma (e.g. mucinous, serous)
Can also originate from sex-cord stroma (granulosa cell) and germ cells (dysgerminoma, teratoma)

(S) Often have non-specific bowel symptoms, bloating, early satiety, and loss of appetite which makes early diagnosis difficult. Overlap with irritable bowel syndrome (IBS) symptoms.

(Sy:) There may be no clinical signs or findings of an adnexal mass on pelvic examination
Late-stage disease may present as a large pelvic mass, ascites, palpable lymph nodes and pleural effusion

(Ix) Pelvic USS
Carcinoma antigen 125 (Ca125)
Staging MRI pelvis/CT chest, abdomen, pelvis

Colonoscopy/OGD may be indicated if there is a possibility of primary gastrointestinal malignancy

Rx Depends on stage (see Table 10.11)

Table 10.11 Staging and treatment of ovarian cancer

Stage	Features	Treatment	5-year survival (per cent)
1	Tumour limited to the ovaries	Total abdominal hysterectomy and bilateral salpingo-oophorectomy and omentectomy ±chemotherapy	85
2	Tumour involves one or both ovaries with pelvic extension	As per stage 1 ±Lymphadenectomy, with surgical effort to remove all disease	65
3	Tumour with peritoneal implants outside the pelvis or retroperitoneal and or inguinal nodes	As per stage 2 May require neoadjuvant chemotherapy to reduce tumour mass before surgery	30–58
4	Tumour with distant metastasis	As per stage 3 Palliative chemotherapy	18

Px Survival has been shown to be directly related to the success of debulking and absence of residual disease. Lowest overall 5-year survival compared with endometrial and cervical carcinoma owing to typical late presentation

GESTATIONAL TROPHOBLASTIC DISEASE (MOLAR PREGNANCY)

A Abnormal placental development, causing overgrowth of abnormal pregnancy tissue. Rare disease, incidence of 1/714 live births
Benign: complete or partial hydatiform mole
Malignant: choriocarcinoma

P Majority of cases are caused by disorder of fertilization, either duplication of haploid sperm into an empty ovum or dispermic fertilization

S PV bleeding in early pregnancy, hyperemesis, pelvic mass or diagnosed at time of first USS in early pregnancy. Rarely present with disseminated disease

Ix Majority of cases are diagnosed on USS by classical appearance of 'snowstorm' within endometrial cavity. Partial moles may have evidence of fetal parts
hCG will be grossly elevated

Rx Surgical evacuation to obtain histology
Once molar pregnancy confirmed by histology, serial hCG to monitor disease
Persistent ↑ hCG levels indicate active disease and warrant chemotherapy

VULVAL AND VAGINAL CARCINOMA

(A) Rare gynaecological malignancy, disease of older age group

(S) Itching, bleeding, vulval/vaginal lesion

Inguinal lymphadenopathy

(Rx) Depends on extent of tumour

Wide local excision for small tumours, with or without inguinal lymph node dissection

Adjuvant chemoradiotherapy

More radical surgery required for larger tumours

BENIGN GYNAECOLOGY

PELVIC INFLAMMATORY DISEASE

(A) Common condition

(P) Usually the result of ascending infection from the endocervix causing endometritis, salpingitis, tubo-ovarian abscess, peritonitis

Common causative organisms are *Chlamydia trachomatis* and *Neisseria gonorrhoeae* transmitted by unprotected sexual intercourse

(S) Constant lower abdominal pain, purulent vaginal discharge, deep dyspareunia.

Pyrexia, cervical excitation, irregular PV bleeding, adnexal tenderness

---

Box 10.14 DIFFERENTIAL DIAGNOSIS OF LOWER ABDOMINAL PAIN IN A YOUNG WOMAN

- Ectopic pregnancy
- Acute appendicitis
- Endometriosis
- Irritable bowel syndrome
- Ovarian cyst accident – rupture/torsion
- Urinary tract infection

(Ix) FBC, C-reactive protein (CRP), ensure hCG negative, mid-stream urine (MSU), high vaginal swab (HVS) and endocervical swabs, blood cultures if febrile, pelvic USS

(Rx) *Medical management*:

   – mild: oral ofloxacin + metronidazole for 14 days

   – moderate: intramuscular ceftriaxone + oral doxycycline + metronidazole for 14 days

   – severe: inpatient intravenous therapy if clinically unwell and severe disease

Surgical management: may be indicated in severe cases with evidence of pelvic abscess

Contact tracing for sexual partners

(Cx) Long-term sequelae of PID include infertility, ectopic pregnancy and chronic pelvic pain.

ENDOMETRIOSIS

(A) Common. Incidence 6–15 per cent. Increased detection because of increased use of laparoscopic surgery

(P) Presence of endometrial-like tissue outside the uterus, which induces a chronic inflammatory reaction, usually pelvic organs and peritoneum. Very rarely bowel and lung
No correlation between symptoms and severity of disease

(S) Dysmenorrhoea, deep dyspareunia, chronic pelvic pain, and ovulation pain, infertility, dyschezia (pain on defaecation). Tenderness and/or palpable nodules on bimanual examination, frozen pelvis.
21 per cent of women investigated for infertility have endometriosis

---

Box 10.15 CAUSES OF DYSMENORRHOEA

- Endometriosis
- Pelvic adhesions
- Chronic PID
- Ovarian cysts
- Pelvic venous congestion
- Uterine fibroids

(Ix) *Pelvic USS*: large nodules or endometriomas may be visible
MRI pelvis: if severe disease suspected and surgical planning necessary
Diagnostic laparoscopy: gold standard

(Rx) *Medical*: non-steroidal anti-inflammatory drugs (NSAIDs)/combined oral contraceptive pill, danazol, Mirena intrauterine system (IUS), gonadotrophin-releasing hormone (GnRH) agonist
Surgical: aim to diagnose and surgically remove endometriosis, can range from laparoscopic ablation of lesions to hysterectomy and bilateral salpingo-oophorectomy

BARTHOLIN'S ABSCESS

(A) Commonest cause of vulval swelling. Higher incidence in diabetes

(P) Dilatation of the Bartholin's gland caused by blockage to the outflow tract. Abscess formation can then occur

(S) Pain, swelling, dyspareunia. Unilateral fluctuant vulval swelling. Abscess erythematous and exquisitely tender to palpation

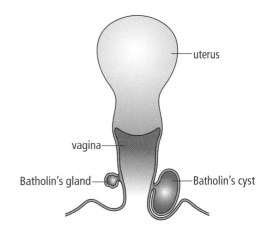

Figure 10.7 Bartholin's cyst

(Rx) Incision and drainage and marsupialization (inner cyst wall is sutured to the skin to create new duct opening)
10 per cent risk of recurrence

MENSTRUAL DISTURBANCES

MENORRHAGIA

(P) Heavy menstrual bleeding (>80 mL per cycle)
(A) See Box 10.16

Box 10.16 CAUSES OF MENORRHAGIA
• Uterine fibroids
• Dysfunctional uterine bleeding
• Coagulopathies
• Pelvic malignancies

(Ix) FBC, TFTs, pelvic USS, hCG
Hysteroscopy and endometrial biopsy if simple treatment fails or suspicious features
(Rx) Dependent on pathology

Box 10.17 TREATMENT OF MENORRHAGIA	
Medical management	**Surgical management**
• Tranexamic acid/mefenamic acid	• Trans-cervical resection of submucous fibroids
• Combined oral contraception	• Endometrial ablation
• Progesterones, medroxyprogestone orally, depot injection, Mirena IUS	• Myomectomy
• GnRH analogues	• Hysterectomy

FIBROIDS (LEIOMYOMAS)

Benign tumours arising from the myometrium. Vary in site and size. Symptoms vary according to this.

(S) May be asymptomatic, or associated with menorrhagia, pressure symptoms on bladder/bowel
Pain secondary to fibroid degeneration
Large fibroids are palpable abdominally. Uterus may be enlarged on pelvic examination

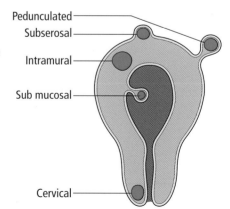

Figure 10.8 Fibroids

(Ix) Pelvic USS to define size and location

(Rx) Treatment as per management of menorrhagia.

Medical: less likely to be effective if fibroids are large and distorting cavity

Surgical:
- for submucous fibroids, if >50 per cent of fibroid is within cavity they may be amenable to trans-cervical resection
- intramural and subserosal fibroids – myomectomy
- hysterectomy

Interventional radiology: uterine artery embolization and MRI-guided ultrasound ablation of fibroids may be possible in specialist centres

AMENORRHOEA/OLIGOMENORRHOEA

(P) *Primary amenorrhoea*: absence of the onset of menses by the age of 14 years with the absence of development of secondary sexual characteristics or absence of the onset of menses by the age of 16 years with development of secondary sexual characteristics

Secondary amenorrhoea: absence of menstruation >6 months in a woman who has previously menstruated

Oligomenorrhoea: interval of more than 35 days between periods

Box 10.18 CAUSES OF AMENORRHOEA
• Pregnancy
• Polycystic ovarian syndrome
• Hypothalamic disorders
• Hyperprolactinaemia
• Ovarian failure/menopause
• Thyroid disease
• Anatomical disorders of outflow

(Ix) hCG, TFTs, luteinizing hormone (LH), follicle-stimulating hormone (FSH), prolactin, chromosomal karyotype

Pelvic USS

Progesterone challenge test: oral progesterone for 5 days, if there is endogenous oestrogen and normal anatomy, withdrawal bleeding will occur

(Rx) Treat the cause

For primary/premature ovarian failure – combined oral contraceptive pill to prevent osteoporosis and sequelae of low oestrogen

Anatomical causes – imperforate hymen/transverse septum are amenable to surgery

PREMENSTRUAL SYNDROME

(P) Distressing physical, behavioural and psychological symptoms in the absence of organic or underlying psychiatric disease, which regularly recurs during the luteal phase of menstruation and which disappears/regresses at the end of menstruation

(A) Five per cent of women experience severe symptoms but up to 92 per cent report one or more symptoms

(S) Depression, anxiety, irritability, mood swings, bloating, mastalgia, increased appetite

(Rx) Behavioural; cognitive behavioural therapy, exercise
Vitamin B$_6$
Combined oral contraception – new generation (e.g. Yasmin/Cilest)
Selective serotonin reuptake inhibitors
GnRH analogue and add back hormone replacement therapy (HRT)
Total abdominal hysterectomy and bilateral salpingo-oophorectomy

POLYCYSTIC OVARIAN SYNDROME

(A) Common disorder

(S) Two of the three following criteria
- polycystic ovaries on USS
- oligo-ovulation or anovulation
- clinical (hirsutism, acne) or biochemical signs of hyperandrogenism

(Sy) Oligomenorrhoea/amenorrhoea, excessive hair growth, obesity, acne, subfertility

(Cx) Long-term risk factors of type 2 diabetes, sleep apnoea, cardiovascular risk, endometrial hyperplasia and carcinoma

(Ix) Pelvic USS, testosterone and sex-hormone binding globulin, glucose tolerance test, BP

(Rx) Weight loss and exercise
Oral contraceptive pill (OCP), progesterone – to induce withdrawal bleeds
Weight reduction medications (e.g. orlistat)
Cosmetic therapies for hirsutism

CONTRACEPTION AND STERILIZATION

Table 10.12 Contraceptive methods

Type	Mode of action	Contraindications	Benefits	Problems	Failure rate*
Barrier methods (condoms, diaphragm, caps)	Prevent sperm transport	Nil	Protect against sexually transmitted disease (STD)	Diaphragms and caps require correct size and fitting	5–15
Combined oral contraception	Inhibits ovulation Thickens cervical mucus Inhibits implantation	Cardiovascular disease (CVD) Migraine Previous or current venous thrombo-embolism (VTE) Smoker >35 yrs Body mass index (BMI) >35 Liver conditions Breastfeeding Hormone dependent tumour	Improved premenstrual syndrome (PMS), lighter periods Reduction ovarian cysts Reduction endometrial/ ovarian cancer	Weight gain, hypertension, headaches, breakthrough bleeding	0.2–3
Progestogen-only contraception	Inhibits implantation Thickens cervical mucus	Severe liver disease Current VTE Hormone dependent tumour	Useful for those contra-indicated to using combined oral contraceptive pill (COCP) Amenorrhoea	Erratic bleeding, nausea Needs timely dosage	0.3–4
Depot-Provera	Inhibits ovulation Thickens cervical mucus Inhibits implantation	As progestogen only pill (POP)	As POP May be more suitable in those who forget to take pills daily	Menstrual irregularities Delayed return to fertility Weight gain	<0.5
Implant (Implanon)	Prevents ovulation	As POP	Oligomenor-rhoea/amen-orrhoea Long term	Delayed return to fertility Irregular bleeding	0.1

continued ▶

Type	Mode of action	Contraindications	Benefits	Problems	Failure rate*
Copper intrauterine device	Prevents implantation	Menorrhagia Copper allergy Uterine abnormalities Acute pelvic inflammatory disease (PID) Pregnancy Cervical/ endometrial cancer	Long term	Increased menstrual flow and dysmenorrhoea possible Ectopic pregnancy Perforation and expulsion PID	0.3–4
Mirena intrauterine system	Prevents implantation	Uterine abnormalities Acute PID Pregnancy Cervical/ endometrial ca	Long term Oligomenorrhoea/amenorrhoea	Ectopic pregnancy Perforation and expulsion PID	0.09
Female sterilization	Prevents tubal transport	Uncertainty High BMI Comorbidities that contraindicate general anaesthetic	Permanent	Risks associated with surgery; pain, bleeding, visceral damage Ectopic pregnancy Regret	0.5
Male sterilization	Blocks sperm transport	Uncertainty	Permanent Can be done under local anaesthetic	Pain Bleeding Additional contraception for 2–3 months Need semen analysis at 3 months to ensure effective	0.05

*Failure rate defined as pregnancy per 100 woman years

EMERGENCY CONTRACEPTION

Box 10.19 EMERGENCY CONTRACEPTION

Progesterone only
- Single dose taken within 72 hours of unprotected sexual intercourse
- Efficacy 95–58 per cent dependent on how soon tablet is taken

Copper intrauterine device
- Can be inserted up to 5 days after unprotected sexual intercourse
- Efficacy 98 per cent
- Need prophylactic antibiotics to prevent PID

MENOPAUSE AND HRT

P Lack of menstruation for >1 year

S See Box 10.20

Box 10.20 SYMPTOMS AND SIGNS OF THE MENOPAUSE

- Hot flushes and night sweats
- Atrophy and thinning of vaginal epithelium
- Dryness of vagina
- Dyspareunia
- Overactive bladder symptoms – frequency, urgency
- Mood changes
- Loss of libido
- Osteoporosis
- Increase in cardiovascular risk
- Increased risk of Alzheimer's

Ix FSH and LH are diagnostically high, oestrogen will be low

Rx Recommended for women with premature menopause, or to treat menopausal symptoms in women who are aware of the risks of treatment

Combined HRT (oestrogen and progestogen) for women with a uterus

Oestrogen alone for those with hysterectomy

Can be given sequentially (monthly withdrawal bleeding), or continuous (period-free)

Cx HRT is associated with increased risk of:
- venous thromboembolism
- breast cancer
- endometrial cancer
- gall bladder disease
- vascular disease

INFERTILITY

 Affects between 9 and 14 per cent of couples; 84 per cent of couples will conceive in 1 year

Primary infertility: unprotected sexual intercourse for over 1 year and no history of pregnancy

Secondary infertility: unprotected sexual intercourse for >1 year with a previous history of pregnancy

Table 10.13 Causes of infertility

Causes	Examples	Frequency (per cent)	Investigations
Ovulatory dysfunction	Polycystic ovarian syndrome (PCOS) Ovarian failure – premature menopause – abnormal karyotype (Turner's) – surgical removal/ radiochemotherapy Hypothalamic pituitary failure – hyperprolactinaemia – weight loss/stress – Sheehan's syndrome	25	Follicle-stimulating hormone (FSH), luteinizing hormone (LH) Oestrogen Day 21 progesterone (confirms ovulation) Prolactin Pelvic ultrasound scan (USS) Karyotype if indicated
Tubal dysfunction	Previous pelvic inflammatory disease (PID) Endometriosis Sterilization Uterine abnormality	25	Hysterosalpingogram Diagnostic laparoscopy and dye test
Male factor	Failure of production – abnormal karyotype (Klinefelter syndrome) – previous orchiditis (mumps, tuberculosis) Failure of transport – sterilization – cystic fibrosis – impotence	35	Semen analysis FSH, LH Karyotype if indicated
Unexplained		15	Exclusion of all of the above with normal results

Ix Aim to find the cause and thus modify treatment

Rx Ovulation induction
- laparoscopic ovarian drilling
- clomifene
- GnRH

Tubal surgery

Sperm donation

Oocyte donation

Intrauterine insemination

In-vitro fertilization (IVF)

Intracytoplasmic sperm injection (ICSI)

Px Success depends on woman's age and cause of infertility. For IVF women < 35 years have a > 20 per cent success rate per cycle, if > 40 years this is reduced to 6 per cent.

OVARIAN HYPERSTIMULATION SYNDROME

A Affects 33 per cent of IVF cycles, 3–8 per cent are moderate or severe

P Systemic disease resulting from hyperstimulated ovaries. Vasoactive products are released causing increased capillary permeability. In severe forms this can cause marked ascites and pleural effusions, renal and respiratory failure and VTE

S Abdominal pain and bloating, increasing abdominal girth, nausea, vomiting, dyspnoea

Ix Pelvic USS to determine ovarian size and presence of ascites

Chest X-ray (CXR) (if symptoms of pleural effusion)

FBC – haematocrit and white blood cell (WBC), U&E, LFT

Fluid balance

Rx Analgesia, antiemetics, inpatient management for moderate and severe cases, fluid restriction

Paracentesis – if abdominal pressure caused by ascites is leading to reduced renal output

UROGYNAECOLOGY

STRESS INCONTINENCE

S Urine leakage on coughing, laughing, sneezing, exercise, sexual intercourse May be demonstrated on examination with a full bladder. Severity ranges from mild to severe

Ix MSU

Urodynamics

Rx *Conservative:* Pelvic floor exercises, lifestyle modifications (e.g. weight loss, reducing intake of caffeine, alcohol)

Medical: duloxetine

Surgical:
- tension-free vaginal tape
- colposuspension
- urethral bulking agents

URGE INCONTINENCE

(P) *Urge incontinence:* involuntary loss of urine when there is involuntary detrusor activity

Overactive bladder syndrome: symptoms of urgency and frequency with or without associated incontinence

(S) Symptoms of urgency – and incontinence if unable to reach toilet, nocturia, frequency

(Ix) MSU, urodynamics

(Rx) *Conservative:*
- physiotherapy
- bladder retraining
- lifestyle modifications

Medical:
- anticholinergics

Surgical:
- Botox injections
- clam cystoplasty
- urinary diversion

UTEROVAGINAL PROLAPSE

(A) Common condition. Caused by weakening of pelvic floor normally secondary to child birth

(S) Complaints of 'mass down below', 'dragging sensation'

May be association with urinary incontinence

May need to digitally reduce to enable bowel motion

Dyspareunia

(Sy) Sims speculum examination should be performed with the patient in left lateral position or standing

1st degree prolapse: prolapse still contained within vagina

2nd degree prolapse: prolapse extending beyond intraoitus

3rd degree prolapse (procidentia): uterus completely prolapsed out of vagina

(Rx) Dependent on severity and patient wishes

Conservative:
- pelvic floor exercises
- ring and shelf pessaries

Surgical:
- vaginal hysterectomy
- anterior and posterior vaginal wall repair

Psychiatry

Sophie Atwood and Scott Cherry

History and examination are as essential in psychiatry as in any other branch of medicine, but there are some important additions in psychiatry. For full details on psychiatric history, see Tatham and Patel *Complete OSCE Skills for Medical and Surgical Finals*, London: Arnold (2010). Generally ICD 10 (WHO) and DSM IV are used to guide diagnoses in psychiatry.

Table 11.1 Mental State Examination

Appearance and behaviour	How was the patient dressed and behaving?
	What was their eye contact like?
	Could you build a rapport with them?
	Paint a 'mental picture' of the patient to the examiner
Speech	Rate, tone, volume, rhythm
	Content: neologisms, grandiosity, perseveration, etc.
Mood	Subjective assessment: the patient's description of their mood, e.g. 'feeling low/high'
	Objective assessment: the range of emotional reactivity observed during the interview = affect e.g. reactive, flat, blunted, labile, elated
	Symptoms and signs of mood disorders, including biological symptoms (see Mood (affective) disorders, p. 295)
	Thoughts/plans/acts of harm to self or others and evidence of neglect
Thoughts	Form: evidence of thought alienation (thought echo, insertion, withdrawal or broadcast), loosening of associations, flight of ideas, content (e.g. delusions, preoccupations)
	Content: delusions, neologisms, grandiosity, perseveration, obsessions, etc.

continued ▶

Perceptions	Hallucinations – auditory, visual, tactile, gustatory, olfactory
	Are they responding to hallucinations during the interview?
Cognition	Orientation in time, place and person.
	Ideally also Mini Mental State Examination (30-point) and appropriate additional tests (frontal lobe, clock face, etc.)
Insight	What does the patient think the problem is?
	Do they believe they are unwell?
	What treatment would they accept?
	If lacking insight, is admission/treatment under the Mental Health Act necessary?

SCHIZOPHRENIA

(A) *Genetic*: twin and family studies show increased risk

Environmental: urban living, migration, stress and traumatic life events, cannabis use, perinatal complications, intrauterine infection (especially viral)

Personality: schizotypal personality can develop into schizophrenia

♂ = ♀, men present at younger age. Lifetime prevalence 1 per cent. Annual incidence 1/10 000 per year

(P) Neurotransmitters (e.g. dopamine hypothesis including hyperactivity of dopaminergic transmission at D2 receptor)

(Sy) Fundamental and characteristic distortions of thinking and perception; inappropriate or blunted affect.

Box 11.1 ICD-10 DIAGNOSIS OF SCHIZOPHRENIA

One month plus one of the following:
- Thought echo/insertion/withdrawal/broadcast
- Delusions of control/influence/passivity or delusional perception
- Third person auditory hallucinations
- Persistent delusions

or two of:
- Persistent hallucinations
- Thought disorder: incoherent or irrelevant speech or neologisms
- Catatonic behaviour
- 'Negative' symptoms (marked apathy, little speech, blunting/incongruous affect, social withdrawal)
- Persistent change in behaviour: loss of interest, aimlessness, self-absorbed attitude, social withdrawal

---

(Rx) Early diagnosis, referral and treatment are important as this affects outcome and prognosis. Always consider risk issues – neglect, harm to self, harm to others

Pharmacological:
- atypical antipsychotic (e.g. olanzapine, quetiapine – 6- to 8-week trial)
- treatment-resistant schizophrenia (failure to respond to 2+ antipsychotics) – clozapine

    – depot antipsychotic (intramuscular injection every 2–4 weeks) if patient prefers/
non-compliant

Psychological:

    – psycho-education and support for patient, family and carers

    – cognitive behavioural therapy

    – family interventions

    – art therapy

(Px) After first psychotic episode: 20 per cent never have recurrence, 50 per cent have relapsing and remitting illness, 30 per cent have ongoing symptoms

Suicide in 10 per cent, especially soon after diagnosis

MOOD (AFFECTIVE) DISORDERS

DEPRESSION (DEPRESSIVE EPISODE)

(A) More common in females, onset commonest in 30s. Lifetime risk: 5–12 per cent ♂, 9–26 per cent ♀

Genetics: family/twin/adoption studies show increased risk

Personality: e.g. cyclothymic, depressive

Psychosocial stressors: life events, expressed emotion in family

Physical illness: endocrine disorder, viruses, chronic pain, etc.

Psychological factors: Beck's cognitive triad/distortions

(P) *Neurotransmitters*: monoamine hypothesis (e.g. 5-hydroxytryptamine [5-HT]/ noradrenaline [NA] underactivity)

Neuroendocrine factors: hypothalamo–pituitary–adrenal (HPA) axis, thyroid axis, melatonin all implicated

(Sy) Duration at least 2 weeks. Not better accounted for by another mental illness (e.g. schizophrenia/bipolar disorder)

Mild: At least two 'core' symptoms plus 'other' symptoms; total ≥4

Moderate: At least two 'core' symptoms plus 'other' symptoms; total ≥6

Severe: All three 'core symptoms' plus other symptoms; total ≥8

For mild/moderate – subclassify as 'with/without somatic syndrome'

For severe – subclassify as 'with/without psychotic symptoms'

More than one episode is 'recurrent depressive disorder'

Box 11.2 SYMPTOMS OF DEPRESSION

- *'Core symptoms'*: ↓ mood, ↓ interest/enjoyment, ↓ energy (fatigability)
- *'Other symptoms'*: ↓ attention/concentration, ↓ confidence/self-esteem, ideas of guilt, pessimism regarding future, ideas of suicide/deliberate self-harm (DSH), ↓ sleep, ↓ appetite
- *'Somatic syndrome'*: ↓ interest/enjoyment, ↓ weight >5 per cent in 1 month, psychomotor changes, early morning wakening >2 hours before normal, ↓ libido, diurnal mood variation: feeling worse in mornings

---

(Rx) See Table 11.2

Table 11.2 Treatment of depression

Classification	Treatment
Mild	Monitoring, self-help, cognitive behavioural therapy (CBT), exercise rather than medication
Moderate	Use antidepressant medication (selective serotonin reuptake inhibitors [SSRI] first-line), CBT
Severe without psychotic features	Antidepressant medication plus CBT
Severe with psychotic features	Antidepressant plus antipsychotic medication
Treatment-refractory	Switch antidepressant or augment with lithium/antipsychotic

Electroconvulsive therapy (ECT) is only used for severe, treatment-resistant depression

Px Chronic and recurrent – 75 per cent have multiple episodes, 15 per cent have chronic course

Better if medication continued for ≥6 months (single episode), ≥2 years (recurrent)

Suicide rate 15 per cent

BIPOLAR DISORDER

A Similar to depression, onset commonest in 20s

Sex ratio equal, lifetime risk both around 1 per cent

P See Table 11.3

Table 11.3 Comparison of hypomania and mania

Hypomania	Mania
Duration of at least 4 days	Duration at least 1 week
≥4 of the following symptoms: ↑ mood, ↑ energy, ↑ sociability, ↑ talkativeness, ↑ libido, overfamiliarity, ↓ sleep	As for hypomania but more symptoms, more exaggerated degree with significant impact on functioning, psychotic symptoms, grandiosity and flight of ideas may be seen
Normal life disrupted but can still function	Subclassify as 'with or without psychotic symptoms'

Sy ≥2 episodes of mood disturbance (includes recurrent mania). Not better accounted for by another mental illness (e.g. schizophrenia)

Rx *Acute phase*:
  – stop any antidepressants
  – start an antipsychotic, lithium or sodium valproate
  – consider adding a short-term benzodiazepine
  – if response inadequate, combine antipsychotic with lithium/valproate
  Maintenance:
  – lithium/olanzapine/valproate/quetiapine for at least 2 years

– antidepressants/cognitive behavioural therapy (CBT) for intercurrent episodes of depression

– combine mood-stabilizers for refractory/rapid cycling (≥4 episodes in 1 year) illness

Px Relapse rate high ≤90 per cent
Suicide risk 15 per cent

ANXIETY DISORDERS

PHOBIAS

A Genetics, psychological factors (conditioning), life events
♀ > ♂ except for social phobia where sex ratio is equal
High rates of comorbid anxiety disorders, depression, substance misuse, OCD
Lifetime prevalence varies widely – around 10 per cent

Sy Avoidance is key
Anxiety symptoms include, autonomic arousal ($\uparrow$ heart rate [HR], $\uparrow$ respiration rate [RR], $\uparrow$ blood pressure [BP], sweating, shaking, palpitations, etc.), feeling faint, chest pain, choking, fear of dying/losing control/going mad
Symptoms not better explained by another condition (e.g. schizophrenia)
Agoraphobia: anxiety in ≥2 of: crowds, public places, travelling away from home/alone
Social phobia: anxiety restricted to/predominates in particular social situations
Specific phobia: anxiety restricted to specific situations (e.g. heights)

Rx CBT/exposure therapy is the treatment of choice
Benzodiazepines useful in short-term crisis only, SSRI antidepressants may help

Px Childhood phobias nearly always improve
Adults: 20 per cent unchanged, 40 per cent better, 40 per cent worse at 5 years

PANIC DISORDER

A As for phobias
Onset rare after age 40 years, ♀ > ♂ 2:1
Lifetime risk and prevalence around 1 per cent

Sy Recurrent unpredictable attacks of severe anxiety, usually lasting a few minutes only
Several attacks within 1 month

Rx CBT. If response to CBT is inadequate, SSRI can be added. If still symptomatic, or if unable to use SSRI, Imipramine or Clomipramine can be tried after 3 months (beware increased toxicity in overdose)

Px Highly variable course, 60 per cent mild impairment, 10 per cent severe disability

GENERALIZED ANXIETY DISORDER (GAD)

A As for phobias
Prevalence 2–6 per cent, earlier, more gradual onset than other anxiety disorders

Sy Generalized, persistent, free-floating anxiety, present on most days for several weeks

(Rx)   CBT, applied relaxation, first line. If patient requests drug treatment, SSRIs can be used (Sertraline as first choice). If those do not work or cannot be tolerated, use SNRI (serotonin and noradrenaline reuptake inhibition), e.g. Venlafaxine, Duloxine, Pregabalin.

(Px)   60 per cent improved at 5 years
High co-morbidity with alcoholism
10 per cent severe impairment

OBSESSIVE–COMPULSIVE DISORDER

(A)   ♂ = ♀. Onset usually childhood or early adulthood. Prevalence 1/50

(Sy)   *Obsessions*: repetitive thoughts, images or impulses, unsuccessfully resisted, recognized as the patient's own
Compulsions: non-enjoyable repeated rituals or stereotyped behaviours that the patient believes may prevent harm to self or others. Patient recognizes as pointless or ineffective and tries to resist
Diagnosis: obsessions and/or compulsions must be present on most days for at least two successive weeks, causing distress or interference with daily activities

(DD)   Depressive disorder, obsessive compulsive (anankastic) personality disorder, part of Tourette's syndrome or schizophrenia

(Rx)   *First line*: cognitive behavioural therapy (including exposure and response prevention)
Second line: anti-depressants (SSRIs)

POST TRAUMATIC STRESS DISORDER

(P)   Delayed and/or protracted response to stressful event or situation of exceptionally threatening or catastrophic nature. Onset within 6 months of the event.

(A)   ♀ > ♂ 2:1. Risk factors: experiencing major trauma, past mental health problems and personality factors, depression after trauma, lack of social support

(Sy)   Re-experiencing: flashbacks and/or nightmares
Avoidance of stimuli that may lead to recollection of the trauma
'*Numbness*': emotional blunting, detachment from other people, anhedonia
Hyperarousal: hypervigilance, exaggerated startle response, difficulty sleeping
Co-morbidities: depression, suicidality/self-harm, substance misuse

(Rx)   *Psychological interventions*:
  – individual debriefing immediately after event no longer advised
  – trauma-focused CBT has the best evidence base
  – EMDR (eye movement desensitization and reprocessing)
  Pharmacological interventions: paroxetine (SSRI) or mirtazapine

(Px)   Symptoms often continue several years after diagnosis

EATING DISORDERS

ANOREXIA NERVOSA

(A) Prevalence 0.2–0.7 per cent. ♀ > ♂ 10–20:1. Social classes 1 and 2. Family history of eating disorder, depression, anxiety or OCD
Temperament: perfectionism, negative self-evaluation, extreme compliance

(P) Body weight at least 15 per cent below that expected, or body mass index (BMI) 17.5 or below because of fear of eating

(Sy) *Weight loss:* self-induced by dieting/vomiting/purging, excessive exercise, use of appetite suppressants/diuretics
Body image distortions: fear of fatness as over-valued idea
Endocrine disorder: females – amenorrhoea; males – reduced libido/potency
If onset is pre-pubertal, puberty is delayed or arrested

(DD) Depressive disorder, obsessive compulsive disorder, personality disorder, somatic causes of weight loss: chronic debilitating diseases, neoplasia, intestinal disorders such as Crohn's disease or a malabsorption syndrome

(Rx) *Psychological interventions:* cognitive analytic therapy, CBT, interpersonal psychotherapy and family interventions – focused specifically on eating disorders
Pharmacological interventions: Little evidence for pharmacological intervention, not recommended
Hospitalization: minority of patients will require hospital admission with a structured symptom-focused weight-restoration programme, with careful monitoring during re-feeding, combined with psychosocial interventions.

(Px) Mortality of 5–20 per cent. Recovery in one-third.

BULIMIA NERVOSA

(A) Often have a history of anorexia nervosa. ♀ > ♂ 10–9:1. Prevalence: 1 per cent, equal social class distribution.

Box 11.3 RISK FACTORS FOR BULIMIA
● Obesity
● Mood disorder
● Sexual or physical abuse
● Parental obesity
● Substance misuse
● Low self-esteem

(Sy) Persistent preoccupation with eating. Irresistible cravings leading to binges
Attempts to counteract 'fattening foods' by self-induced vomiting, purgative abuse, alternating periods of starvation, use of appetite suppressants, thyroid preparations or diuretics, neglect of insulin treatment in diabetics
Morbid dread of fatness, sets self sharply defined weight threshold, well below optimal and pre-morbid weight

(DD) Upper gastrointestinal (GI) disorders, depressive disorder, personality disorder (where the eating disorder may coexist with alcohol dependence and petty offences, e.g. shoplifting)

(Rx) First line: evidence-based self-help programme
Cognitive behavioural therapy for bulimia nervosa (CBT-BN)
Antidepressants (SSRIs, specifically fluoxetine)
Involve family members in treatment – psycho-education/behavioural management/communication

(Px) Around 50 per cent make full recovery, 30 per cent partial recovery, 20 per cent continue to have symptoms

PERSONALITY DISORDER

(A) Environmental (attachment difficulties, family dysfunction)
Neurological – electroencephalogram (EEG) abnormalities in some groups (e.g. antisocial)
Genetic (especially schizotypal and antisocial)
Approximate general prevalence: community 10 per cent, general practice 20 per cent, psychiatric outpatients 30 per cent, psychiatric inpatients 40 per cent

(Sy) ICD-10 General Criteria: severe disturbance in character/behaviour, usually involving several areas of the personality, associated with considerable personal/social distress. Diagnosis usually inappropriate before 16–17 years
Categories in ICD-10 include schizoid, dissocial (antisocial), emotionally unstable (impulsive/borderline), histrionic, anankastic, anxious (avoidant), dependent

(Rx) Most research focused on 'borderline' and 'dissocial' personality disorder. Beware of co-morbidity and increased risk of other psychiatric conditions
Thorough assessment and 'biopsychosocial' approach is needed
Multidisciplinary approach/psychotherapy
Prescribing in the short-term may be indicated for co-morbidity and crises.
National Institute for Health and Clinical Excellence (NICE) discourages prescribing in the medium to long term as evidence is weak.

(Px) High morbidity and mortality. High rates of co-morbidity (e.g. with psychosis/affective disorder). High risk of suicide (6× standard mortality rate [SMR]) in 20- to 39-year age-group. Antisocial/borderline less evident with increasing age; anankastic/schizotypal have a more stable course.

OLD-AGE PSYCHIATRY

DEMENTIA

(A) See Table 11.4

Table 11.4 Causes of dementia

Disease	Pathology
Alzheimer's	Amyloid plaques (extracellular), neurofibrillary tangles (intracellular)
Vascular	Atherosclerosis risk factors (e.g. ↑ blood pressure (BP), ↑ lipids, smoking, diabetes)
Frontal lobe dementia	Genetics more clearly implicated includes Pick's disease (fronto-temporal lobe atrophy)
Parkinson's/Lewy body dementia (DLB)	Unclear, possibly related to Lewy bodies in cortex
Others	Creutzfeldt–Jakob disease (CJD), normal pressure hydrocephalus, *Human immunodeficiency virus* (HIV), neurosyphilis

Approximate overall prevalence of Alzheimer's disease: 5 per cent at 65 years, 15 per cent at 75 years, 25 per cent at 85 years (varies according to type)
Excess of vascular dementia in males

Sy 6 months or more, decline in memory and thinking including impairment of activities of daily living ADLs. Clear consciousness (i.e. not delirium)
Mini-mental state examination (MMSE): ≤10 – severe, 10–20 – moderate, 20–30 – mild
Alzheimer's: early (≤2 years) cognitive impairment, later neuropsychiatric symptoms (e.g. depression/anxiety/personality change, progressive inability to self-care)
Vascular: step-wise deterioration, vascular risk factors (e.g. diabetes mellitus [DM], hypertension [HTN]) – often difficult to distinguish from Alzheimer's)
Frontal lobe dementia: younger onset (e.g. ≤65 years), insidious onset, marked frontal lobe features, language dysfunction, memory loss variable
Parkinson's/DLB: dementia developing in a patient with Parkinson's; if extrapyramidal symptoms (EPS)/dementia develop at the same time then consider a diagnosis of DLB, especially if consciousness is fluctuating and there are visual hallucinations

Rx Multidisciplinary approach essential
Medications may be needed for depression (SSRIs), agitation/psychosis (neuroleptics/benzodazepines [BZDs]) – controversial/use with caution)
Alzheimer's: cholinesterase inhibitors (ChEIs; e.g. donepezil): NICE recommends treatment for moderate dementia only, only specialists should initiate; review every 6 months
Vascular: control risk factors, growing evidence for ChEIs but not licensed
Frontal lobe dementia: no specific treatment
Parkinson's/DLB: optimize Parkinson's treatment, DLB may respond well to ChEIs

Px *Alzheimer's/vascular*: mean survival 7–10 years, earlier onset has poorer prognosis
Frontal lobe: mean duration 8–11 years

CHILD AND ADOLESCENT PSYCHIATRY

ATTENTION DEFICIT HYPERACTIVITY DISORDER/HYPERKINETIC DISORDER (ADHD)

(A) Prevalence 1–5 per cent. ♂ > ♀ 5:1. Genetic predisposition + psychosocial stress: family dysfunction, attachment difficulties

(Sy) Symptoms evident in more than one situation (e.g. home, school and in clinic), before age 6 years, leading to moderate to severe psychological, social and/or educational or occupational impairment
- impaired attention
- overactivity

Associated features:
- recklessness in potentially dangerous situations
- impulsive flouting of social rules – difficulty waiting their turn, interrupting activities
- co-morbidity common (e.g. conduct disorder/depressive disorder/autism)

(Rx) Parenting-training/education programme
Schools to implement behavioural programme
Group treatment (cognitive behavioural therapy/social skills training for child)
Pharmacological interventions: methylphenidate or atomoxetine

(Px) Up to 60 per cent can have residual symptoms in adulthood. Increased risk of conduct disorder, antisocial personality disorder, substance misuse, criminal justice system interventions

AUTISTIC SPECTRUM DISORDER (AUTISM, ASPERGER'S SYNDROME, ATYPICAL AUTISM)

(A) *Prevalence:* autistic spectrum disorder 10/1000; autism 3/1000; ♂ > ♀ 4:1. ↑ prevalence in learning disability population
Genetics: concurrence in monozygotic (MZ) twins > dizygotic (DZ) twins; Fragile X – dysfunction of X chromosome, leads to autism-like symptoms.
Tuberous sclerosis and neurofibromatosis 1 (NF1) also linked to autism.

(Sy) Abnormalities affecting individual's functioning become apparent before age 3 years:
- Impairment in reciprocal social interaction
- Impairment in communication
- Restricted, repetitive and stereotyped patterns of behaviour, interests and activities

Associated features: lack of cognitive of behavioural flexibility, altered sensory sensitivity, sensory processing difficulties, emotional dysregulation

(Rx) Psychoeducation
Specialist education and behavioural programmes in mainstream or specialist school
Treatment of co-morbidities

(Px) Lifelong condition. Many adults with autism require long-term care

Index

Note: page numbers in **bold** refer to diagrams, page numbers in italics refer to information contained in tables and boxes.